The Silver Bullet Real MCATs Explained with Verbal Reasoning Prep

Welcome to the Family.

Go for the Gold!

MCAT-prep.com
DrFlowersMCAT.com

The only prep you need.™

RuveneCo inc

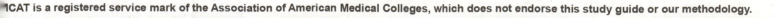

THE SILVER BULLET

Real MCATs Explained
with Verbal Reasoning Prep

Authors

James L. Flowers BSc MD MPH
Brett L. Ferdinand BSc MD-CM

Illustrators

Daphne McCormack
Li Xin

Special Thanks

Ren Yi   Janice Moreland
Noemie Chagnon   Ivory Young
Pamela Simon   Jason Sparks
Nedaa Asbah   Vish Parameswaran

RuveneCo
Inc

Visit MCAT-prep.com's Education Center at www.mcat-prep.com.
Get More Real MCATs Explained at DrFlowersMCAT.com.

Address all inquiries, comments, or suggestions to the publisher.
RuveneCo Publishing
559-334 Cornelia St
Plattsburgh, NY 12901

E-mail: learn@mcat-prep.com

Online resources: www.MCAT-prep.com; www.DrFlowersMCAT.com; www.MCAT-bookstore.com
RuveneCo Inc. and DrFlowersMCAT.com are neither associated nor affiliated with the Association of American Medical Colleges, which produces the Medical College Admission Test (MCAT). Printed in Canada.

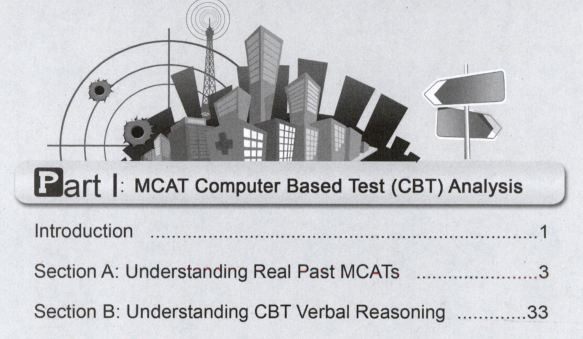

Part I: MCAT Computer Based Test (CBT) Analysis

Part II: Understanding AAMC Practice Test 3

Part III: Understanding AAMC Practice Test 4

∏ntroduction

We have no special relationship with the the Association of American Medical Colleges (AAMC). Simply put, we are both medical doctors who have aced the MCAT and have been writing about the exam and teaching for, combined, 50 years. Dr. Flowers wrote the first comprehensive MCAT text - yes, before Kaplan and Princeton Review - in the 1970s while at Harvard. Dr. Ferdinand wrote *The Gold Standard MCAT* textbook, currently in its 16th edition, as well as produced related teaching videos, MP3s and flashcards. We have taught thousands of students and have reached hundreds of thousands through our publications. We have also developed interactive websites which deliver our teaching experiences to you.

Who do you trust for your MCAT prep?

Us? Your friends? Your premed advisor with a Masters in architecture? A commercial prep company who hires premeds to teach? What about the anonymous guy in the online forum who has taken the test 3 times without success? Your cat? You may want to listen carefully to your experienced premed advisor, but ultimately …

Trust yourself.

It's your car and it's time to drive. Now you need a map and everyone wants to sell you one. There is only one official map for the MCAT: the AAMC. Most commercial MCAT books contain information that is not on the new MCAT CBT. Most contain question types that have not been on the real exam in more than 10 years. Before you waste your time and energy, get a clear idea of where you are going.

The AAMC has published an official guide with a layout of what is covered on the new MCAT. They also have a list online **(aamc.org)**; either way, it is information that you need before you get started. You also must be committed to the idea of taking one of their practice exams very early in your review process. Some call it a "diagnostic test." We call it "Diagnosis with Prescription." Why? Because we believe that once you have a clear idea of your strengths and weaknesses, you need a clear plan to lead you to good academic health. We can help.

We suggest that you start with AAMC Practice Test 3. Currently, this full length test is free at **www.e-mcat.com**. They do provide explanations. In this book, *The Silver Bullet: Real MCATs Explained*, we provide detailed explanations and analysis. We analyze all your options, the topics you must review, the concepts specific to the new MCAT CBT, and an examination of test-taking skills - one question at a time. You will find cross references as well: for example, **SB A.2.2** leads you to Section A, 2.2 in *The Silver Bullet*. There are also references to the complete science review from the most recent edition of *The Gold Standard MCAT* textbook: **ORG 5.3** refers to organic chemistry, Chapter 5, subsection 5.3 for background information.

Before doing more practice tests, use *The Silver Bullet* to get an in depth understanding of Practice Test 3. We will help you avoid memorizing useless data by providing you with a firm grasp of what the real MCAT requires. If you need more support, we have you covered. You will find specific multimedia products at **MCAT-prep.com** ranging from clear teaching on video to simulated practice MCAT CBTs to live online courses. You can also purchase all available AAMC practice tests at **DrFlowersMCAT.com** with detailed explanations and analysis (as you will see in *The Silver Bullet*). There are many other features of **DrFlowersMCAT.com** including cross-referencing, an online dashboard, interactive forum and more.

Of course we closely examine all the sciences but we decided to go the extra mile for verbal prep. So yes, practice practice practice, everyone knows (or should know!) the mantra for Verbal Reasoning (VR). But what about being well prepared before you practice? We'll take you there.

You will also find in this book, a degree of VR MCAT CBT analysis that has never been done before. It is amusing to see prep companies claim that they have the One approach to VR. The irony, of course, is that when you ask students who have aced this section for advice, you will find that there is no One best technique for everyone. So we break down VR into 3 approaches and we use all 3 to provide explanations to Practice Test 3. Then for Practice Test 4, we lay it out like a workbook. This is your opportunity to truly express your understanding of a real past MCAT using techniques that we will teach you. Then, because you own this book, you can go to **DrFlowersMCAT.com** and get free online access to our 3 approaches to respond to Practice Test 4 VR.

So now you understand part of the title: *Real MCATs Explained including Verbal Reasoning Prep.*

But what about *The Silver Bullet*? Isn't that supposed to be fast?

Yes.

Two to three hundred pages to explain 1 test is fast?

Yes.

Why?

Consider the alternative. You have heard the stories; students who have tried so many books, so many courses and rode so many rumors into dead ends. Unlike other standardized exams (LSAT, GMAT, etc) there are not dozens of real past MCATs to use for practice. This means that they should not be treated in the same way you would take some prep company's practice exams to use, get a score and then jump to the next. If you are serious about this exam, then you must seriously examine past tests, one at a time, learn, grow and get ready to attack the next one. We will get you there.

Now let's begin . . .

Section A
MCAT CBT ANALYSIS

UNDERSTANDING REAL MCATs

Section A

UNDERSTANDING REAL PAST
MCAT TESTS

Explanations and Analysis for
the new MCAT CBT

The following skills were detected and developed after analysis of all of the AAMC practice tests which were available. These are not generic test-taking skills touted by other prep programs; the skills below are specific for the new MCAT.

A.1 Stem Option Analysis Skills

A.1.1 Stem Option Analysis General Comments

This analyzes the stem and the options for patterns that may be useful to help solve the problems of the MCAT. The techniques are derived from careful and long term study of the MCAT practice tests. These techniques are not possible using simulated tests, because it is the structure of the tests, real MCATs, that is important and not the content. The only way to get at the structure of the MCAT is to take the real test or use the practice tests. None of these techniques are 100% applicable and must be used with General Subject **(SB A.2.2)** knowledge and careful deliberation to be helpful.

The stem is the question part of the problem; it precedes the options or answers. The options are the possible answers and are lettered as A, B, C, or D. These are not Option Elimination Analysis techniques per se. Each of the AAMC practice test questions, for the science and the verbal questions, are categorized as to the Stem Option Analysis categories.

These Skills are:

1. Best Option **(SB A.1.2)**
2. Camouflage and Distraction **(SB A.1.3)**
3. Three or More Steps Analysis **(SB A.1.4)**

A.1.2 Best Option

This is part of Stem Option Analysis **(SB A.1)** (refer to that discussion for references for CBT questions). A question may have one or more options that are true or false. The critical decision you have to make is which one is the best option to the question (stem) being asked.

For every option, there are always two steps you must perform. First, you have to determine if the option is true or false. This will be based on your knowledge and on the passage, if present. Next, you have to determine if the statement, true or false, answers the questions; either may occur!

This dichotomy of terminology is important to follow the logic used in discussing the solutions to the problem.

True or false is used to determine if the option, as it stands alone, is a true statement or is a false statement.

Correct and incorrect are used to relate the statement to the solution of the question (stem) or problem.

A true statement may be correct (if it answers the question) or incorrect (if it does not answer the question).

A false statement may be correct (if it answers the question) or incorrect (if it does not answer the question).

In Basic Positive Questions and positive Multiple Choice Questions, the correct answer is a true statement. In Negative Questions (which may be a Multiple Choice Question), the correct answer may be a false statement.

If the question is a positive question of some type, then the answer (option) you choose must be a true statement. If only one of the four options is true, then that option must be the correct option (answer). If two or more of the options are true, then you have to determine which one best answers the question.

An example from the AAMC Practice Tests:

Stem: Why is ammonia a Lewis Base?

Option A - Nitrogen is a nonmetal.
Option B - Nitrogen tends to form negative ions.
Option C - Nitrogen is found in Group VA of the periodic table.
Option D - Nitrogen has a free pair of electrons.

Answer: All the options, A, B, C, and D, are true statements. However, only option D addresses and answers the problem. A Lewis Base has to have a free pair of electrons. The other three true options, A, B, or C, do not answer the question being asked.

In some questions, two or more options are true and do appear to answer the question. In these situations, you have to pick the one that is the best option for the question being asked. In the previous example, you might have remembered that bases tend to be negative ions. Then you might have felt that not only is option B true, but it may also explain why nitrogen (found in ammonia) is basic. While it is true that bases generally will form negative ions (and nonmetals for that matter), it is not the best answer. The best answer has to explain not only why ammonia is a base, but why it is a Lewis Base. This requires you to know the definition of a Lewis Base, which is: "A Lewis Base is an electron pair donor." Then between options B and D, option D is very specific as the answer to the question and becomes the "best option." So, to determine between two nearly equal options, you have to look for more specific or detailed characteristics which distinguish them and answer the question being posed.

Similar arguments would hold for a negative question. If the previous question was:

Stem: All of the following characteristics are consistent with the high electronegativity of nitrogen EXCEPT:

Option A - Is found in the upper-right area of the periodic chart.

Option B - Is a nonmetal.

Option C - Tends to withdraw electrons in a chemical bond with carbon.

Option D - Tends to form positive ions.

Answer: It is the "EXCEPT" that makes this a negative question. In this problem, options A, B, and C are all true and are incorrect as answers. Option D is false and is the correct answer.

When you have two or more options that appear to be the correct answer, you must carefully reread the questions and determine which characteristic(s) is being asked for and then compare the options based on this (these) characteristics. Make sure your answer is the best option and best answers the question being asked.

A.1.3 Camouflage and Distractions

This is part of Stem Option Analysis (SB A.1) (CBT questions relating to concept are found from that location). These are pervasive techniques used by test makers when they present questions. There is nothing unethical about this. You will also encounter camouflage and distractions when you start to practice medicine, and it is a critical skill for test takers and physicians to understand and work through them. Part and parcel of the test-taking skill of understanding camouflage and distractions are the following concepts, among others: camouflage, distraction, recognizing the concept, rephrasing of questions, alternative solutions, and lack of trickery.

Distractions represent a variety of data/ information presented in the passage or in the specific question that has nothing to do with the solution of the question. There is no requirement that you be presented only with the information needed to answer the question. One of the skills you will need for this test and will definitely need in the practice of medicine is how to sort through a large amount of data to get to the key information needed to solve the problem at hand. The distracting information may come in any form, such as a statement, a graph, or an equation. The distraction will be greatest when the information appears to be relevant to the question; this is intended by the test makers. In general, you will have to pay attention to the information provided and know what question is being asked. If that information does not fit with the other data in the passage or is not consistent with your prior study, then you will have to ignore it and move on to other data and means to solve the problem. For example,

Stem: A 12-year-old male child is in the rear open cockpit of a plane being flown by his father. The plane is moving at 200 m/s horizontally and is 2000 m above the ocean. The child throws a rock weighing 25 g from the horizontally moving plane at 4 m/s. The rock is thrown perpendicular to the motion of the plane. Approximately how far will the rock fall in 2 s if air resistance is ignored?

Option A - The rock follows a parabolic path and distance cannot be determined.
Option B - 400 m
Option C - 56 m
Option D - 28 m

This entire question is asking is how far the rock will fall in 2 s. The concept being tested is free fall motion. In free fall motion, the only factors involved are the up-down, or vertical, speed or motion, and the equations of uniformly accelerated motion are used. You select an equation from free fall motion,

$$d = v_0 t + at^2/2$$

where

$$v_0 = 4 \text{ m/s}$$
$$a = g = 9.8 \text{ m/s}$$
$$t = 2 \text{ s}$$

The answer is d = 4(2) + (9.8)(2^2) /2
= 8 + (10)(2)(2) /2
= 8 + (10)(2)
= 28 m (see Approximation).

All of the other information and data are irrelevant and are distracters: the father, the speed of the plane, the height of the plane (although this would be important if the rock were to hit the surface of the water first but the distance is very large compared to the time for the rock to fall), and the weight of the rock. If you did not focus and fully understand the question and concept being asked, i.e. free fall motion, you could have wasted valuable time trying to figure out how to use the other data and information presented. Note that option A is out in left field; even though it is partially true, it is not correct (see Complex Sounding Options; **SB A.2.2**).

A camouflaged type of question can be very difficult to tackle if you cannot recognize the concept (see the following) or fact that is being tested. There are a number of questions on the MCAT of this type. A question is posed that on the surface has nothing directly to do with the concept or fact being tested. An example:

Stem: A chemist ran the following exothermic reaction, catalyzed by iron, until it was at equilibrium:

$$N_2(g) + 3 H_2(g) \leftrightarrows 2 NH_3(g)$$

Pressure = 320 atm
T = 450 °C.

The chemist then made a number of changes. Which change will cause the concentration of ammonia to increase?

Option A - Increase the concentration of iron catalyst.

Option B - Decrease the temperature of the reaction.

Option C - Decrease the concentration of hydrogen.

Option D - Increase the pressure of the reaction.

This question is only mildly camouflaged; camouflaging may be less obvious in other questions, but this question is typical of how camouflaging is implemented over and over again. You are given a set of conditions or descriptions or data. The concept being tested is not stated or broadcast (there are other questions in which the concept is stated, though). You have to infer from the conditions or descriptions what concept is being tested (see Rephrasing of Question; **SB B.7.7**). The concept being tested here is Le Chatelier's principle. This is presented as an example because this concept arises so frequently on these tests. The key to your seeing through the camouflage are the key words, phrases or description. In this stem, the key words are "equilibrium" (or just the double arrows) and "change." In this context, you have to ask, is this question on Le Chatelier's principle? Once you recognize that all that is being tested is Le Chatelier's principle, you can then proceed to answer the question by applying it. If you have adequately studied and comprehended the concept of Le Chatelier's principle, this question becomes relatively simple and you get the correct option, which is D.

So, camouflaged questions present data/ situations/information, but do not declare the concept. You have to recognize the cues being presented to get to the concept as quickly as possible to solve the problem (inference). In more difficult camouflaged questions, the cues may not be as obvious or distractions may be added, making them even more difficult to recognize. If the problem begins to appear very difficult to solve by the obvious method, you should start to think that there is some concept, usually rather simple, being camouflaged, that can be applied to solve the problem. Also, when the obvious method to solve the problem does not work, you should abandon the question and return at a later time. Remember, each question counts the same and there are probably easier questions down the road. It is so important to remember that you are only going to be tested on Basic Knowledge **(SB A.2.2)**, which you can learn by studying this Web site, or by careful reading of the passage.

Alternative solutions should be considered for solving problems that appear to be very complex. These solutions represent a type of camouflage, as just discussed. In these questions, the stem presents information or data that appears to direct you to the solution of the problem when, in reality, there is a camouflaged concept that may be used to solve the problem much more easily or quickly. Remember that you only have a little more than a minute, on average, to solve each question. Initially, if you "see" a way of solving the problem that is very complex and time consuming, you may want to quickly consider alternative camouflaged approaches. Of course, you will only have alternative approaches to consider if you have done a comprehensive study. An example (you don't need the diagram to appreciate the problem):

Stem: A 5 kg block, at the bottom of an incline (with a vertical height of 5 m and a horizontal length of 20 m) is lifted by the force vector shown but maintains contact with the surface of the incline:

How much work is required to move the object from the bottom to the top of the incline? (arctan 0.25 = 14°, sine 14° = 0.24, cosine 14° = 0.97)

Option A - need more information
Option B - 200 J
Option C - 50 (2)$^{1/2}$ J
Option D - 245 J

This problem is an excellent example of this principle. In solving mechanics problems, either a "force" approach or an "energy" approach could be used. The problem may be solved by either approach, but one may be easier for a given problem. If you try to solve it by the force approach, you know W = Fd, where F is the force in the direction of motion or the motion in the direction of the force. This will lead you down a dead-end path to an incorrect answer. The camouflaged approach is related to energy concepts.

In this problem, the energy approach is much simpler and easier than trying to use the previous obvious force approach. The work is equal to the potential energy that results when the object is moved from the bottom to the top; the potential energy is independent

of the path and only depends on the initial and final heights. The gravitational potential energy (U_g) will equal the work done. This is an application of the Law of Conservation of Mechanical Energy.

$$U_g = mgh$$
$$= (5 \text{ kg}) (9.8 \text{ m/s}^2) (5 \text{ m})$$
$$= 245 \text{ J}$$
$$= \text{work done.}$$

This question also has significant distractions that could lead you down the wrong path: the trig functions and the force vector. Lack of Trickery is another component of camouflage and distractions that you must understand. To illustrate, the following is an example taken partially from one of the AAMC practice tests:

Information in the passage: oxides of sulfur and nitrogen are acidic in water and acid rain is formed.

Stem: The pH of acid rain found in industrialized areas would increase if the release to the atmosphere of which of the following were decreased?

I. SO_2
II. CaO
III. N_2
IV. NO

Option A - I and IV only
Option B - II and III only
Option C - I, II, and IV only
Option D - I, II, III, and IV

This question is asking you to determine the acid-base properties of substances to answer the question of pH change in acid rain. There is no requirement for you to have studied acid rain in your preparation. You were required to have studied acid-base properties in general and pH. You are not required to know all the acid and base substances.

The essence of this question is for you to decide which of the listed substances are acids or bases. If you did not have to prepare for these specific substances as acids or bases, the only way for you to determine if they are is to ask:

(1) is there some reasonable way from your study to determine if they are acid or base?
(2) is there something in the passage that helps you determine if they are acid or base?

There is no specific requirement (from the descriptions in the AAMC Student Manual) that you know that SO_2, NO, or CaO are acids or bases. You should know that N_2 is not acidic or basic, being a neutral gas. Since you did not have to know that these compounds are acids or bases from your study, the only way to know this is from the passage. The passage does tell you that oxides of sulfur and nitrogen form acids in water. So, you know the status of SO_2 and NO. Now, what is the status of CaO? If you remembered the oxides of metals are basic, then you can eliminate CaO. However, this is not a general knowledge requirement. This is where you have to believe in the quality

of your study, assuming you have done a quality review for the test, and remind yourself that the test is not out to trick you. If you had to be given a passage clue about the oxides of sulfur and nitrogen for you to know if they were acids or bases, the same would have to be done for the oxides of metals, because you were not required to know this.

Since there is no information about the acid-base nature of CaO, you can at least be sure it is not an acid; take time to try to understand what is being stated here. You have to believe that the test makers are not out trying to trick you. The MCAT is a difficult but fair test, without trickery. Again do a good solid study, review and be confident enough to realize what you should know from study and what should be in the passage. Then be confident enough to eliminate options that are not assessable as for the CaO.

What is true of several of the previous examples is that you are required to recognize the concept being tested. This is typical about this test, because of camouflage and distractions, and other tests in the future. A description of a situation or problem will be presented. From that picture, you have to assess what knowledge, principles, and concepts you can apply to it to solve the problem. How do you learn to do this? I am convinced this is not done by trickery or any other method other than good solid study and understanding of the basics.

In medicine, this will be the mode of presentation of every new patient you see. You will be given a collection of symptoms and signs from which you must induce the condition. Patients do not walk into your office with a big sign on their forehead declaring their condition. Study the questions and solutions given and then try to apply them over and over; this is the best way to learn these techniques. Review the previous examples and note that there were concepts being tested that were not declared but could be deciphered by carefully assessing the question and information given.

One of the methods of recognizing the concept is by Rephrasing of Questions (SB B.7.7). You can get around the camouflage and distraction by restating the question in terms of what it is really asked for. Sometimes this will be helpful; but it will only be helpful and feasible if you have done a thorough study. It takes time to rephrase and rethink the question; time is valuable on this test. However, if you can quickly rephrase the question to a more direct and easier one, then you will actually save time. An example from a question on the AAMC Practice Tests:

Information in the passage: HIV is caused by a RNA virus.

Stem: Which of the following vaccines would pose the highest risk to a person NOT infected with HIV?

Option A - A vaccine containing short peptides identical to those of the HIV protein coat

Option B - A vaccine containing small amounts of untreated HIV
Option C - A vaccine containing protein coats removed from active viruses
Option D - A vaccine containing certain enzymes from denatured HIV

This is a classic type camouflage and distraction question requiring rephrasing to get to the answer quickly; 90% of students got this question correct so the camouflage and distractions were not great, but they do illustrate the point. The apparent question is about HIV or vaccines, neither of which is required for the MCAT per se. Both of these are part of the camouflage and distraction. The real question being asked, the rephrased question, is simply, what substances are responsible for replication of organisms? The answer is the nucleic acids, primarily DNA but also RNA. Or the question could have been what part of the virus is responsible for its replication? The answer still returns to the first question. So, to find the correct option, find the option that contains the nucleic acid: option B.

If you rephrase the question, it should also be to cut through the distractions and camouflage in the question and give you a more direct and easily answered question. You must often use the options themselves as clues to how to rephrase the question.

A.1.4 Three or More Steps Options

This is part of Stem Options Analysis (SB A.1) (also contains questions from CBT). All questions have two steps by default that are different from this question type. In every question, you must first decide if each option is true or false, and then you must decide which is the correct option.

In a three or more step analysis type of question; one question/problem must be answered/solved first, then the true/false decision of the options is made, and finally the correct option is determined. Sometimes there is an additional step involved. These problems tend to be more difficult and time consuming. Remember, the correct option will have to be correct for both questions. Because these types of questions are time consuming, it is advisable to omit them in your first pass through the test. This type of question is a kind of Guess Question (SB A.2.4). It is advisable to practice this kind of question to be able to quickly recognize it and then learn how to most efficiently solve it.

In some of these, you will have some idea of the key concept (the first step) and then will have to apply it (the second step) to reach a conclusion not directly evident from the concept to determine whether the options are true or false. Another type of three or more step analysis is when you have to make one calculation or Inference (SB B.5) to get some information necessary in the second step to correctly solve the problem.

The reason these problems are important is that the time constraint is so significant. This means if you have a problem that appears to require three or more steps, you first of all skip it and return later if it will actually take three or more steps to solve. Also, you should seriously question if you are using the best approach and think of Alternative Ways (SB A.1.3) to solve the problem.

An example of a three or more step analysis problem from the AAMC practice tests:

Stem: A 0.5 kg ball accelerates from rest at 10 m/s^2 for 2 s. It then collides with and sticks to a 1.0 kg ball that is initially at rest. After the collision, approximately how fast are the balls going?

Option A - 3.3 m/s
Option B - 6.7 m/s
Option C - 10.0 m/s
Option D - 15.0 m/s

The steps are:

1. To determine the speed of the 0.5 kg ball when it impacts the 1.0 kg ball: must use uniformly accelerated motion equations;
2. To decide to use the conservation of momentum equations and solve for the combined speed to determine which of the options are true or false;
3. To determine which option is correct (the one that is true in step 2).

Steps 2 and 3 are done for all problems; step 1 is an additional step.

A common situation of this concept is when you are given a result and then must explain it. An example from the AAMC practice tests is:

Stem: As the atomic number increases in a horizontal row of the periodic table, ionization energy generally:

Option A - Increases, because of increasing effective nuclear charge.

Option B - Increases, because of increasing atomic radius.

Option C - Decreases, because of

decreasing effective nuclear charge.

Option D - Decreases, because of increasing atomic radius.

The steps are:

1. For each "increase" or "decrease," determine if the reason given matches it.
2. If both parts match, are they true or false (if #1 was false, this step is done).
3. Then determine if the option is correct (answers the question).

Steps 2 and 3 are done for all problems; step 1 is an additional step.

A.1.5 Analyses of AAMC Tests for the Stem Option Analysis Skills

Stem Option Analysis is the analysis of how the question (the stem) and options (the answers) are presented. This breakdown is found only for the science subtests. This is not a means to guess more effectively. However, it identifies categories of questions that may be positively or negatively affecting your scores on the MCAT. For example, there are questions in which you need to exhibit the skill of selecting the Best Option **(SB A.1.2)**; are you having problems with questions of this type? There are many questions in which "camouflage" and/or "distractions" are presented in the stem; are you able to pick these types apart and answer them correctly?

The Stem Option Analysis **(SB A.1)** is of utmost importance for the science questions. So, in the analysis of the AAMC CBT practice tests (click "Test Report" on the bottom menu, click "CBT", click either "Physical Sciences" or "Biological Sciences" and scroll down the leftmost panel to find the "Stem Option Analysis" breakdown), there will be a breakdown of each of the categories of Stem Option Analysis for you to use. You will then be able to direct your studies and focus on any areas of weaknesses using the CBT Solutions provided in the Study Center. We cannot emphasize it enough; first, you have to study the concept of each type of analysis, then you have to study multiple applications

Analysis for the new MCAT CBT

of the concept as found in the CBT Solutions of the real AAMC MCATs.

Best Option (SB A.1.2)
Best Option teaches you when and how to determine which option is the best choice when two or more options appear to be correct.

Camouflage and Distractions (SB A.1.3)
Camouflage and Distractions is a frequently used method in the construction of questions for the MCAT. It is most frequently used in the science subtests. You will be given multiple modes of camouflage and distraction, and you will be instructed on how to recognize and deconstruct these types of questions to your advantage.

Three or More Step Options (SB A.1.4)
Three or More Step Options are important for you to recognize as they are usually more difficult questions. These types of questions take more time and may be better left for the second pass through the test.

Lessons from the analysis of Stem Option Analysis:

- Does not apply to Verbal Reasoning.
- Camouflage and Distractions is the most common method, especially for Physical Sciences.
- This analysis shows that Camouflage/ Distractions are found most often in the Physical Sciences. So, when you are studying Physics and General Chemistry, you must really learn the concepts inside out. You must be able to infer the concepts from the information given in the stem of the question. Then you must apply that concept to determine the correct option.
- About 10% of science questions require multiple steps to solve.

Detailed Analysis of AAMC Practice Tests: Results for Stem Option Analysis

Description	Verbal Reasoning		Physical Sciences		Biological Sciences		Total	
	#	%	#	%	#	%	#	%
Best Option	0	0	9	1.9	20	4.2	29	2.2
Camouflage/Distractions	0	0	120	25.2	44	9.3	164	12.5
Three or More Step Analysis	0	0	47	9.9	51	10.8	98	7.5
None	360	100.0	301	63.1	357	75.6	1018	77.8
Total	360	100.0	477	100.0	472	100.0	1309	100.0

A.2 Option Elimination Analysis Skills

A.2.1 Option Elimination Analysis (OEA) General Discussion

This is the single most important technique to master of all of the test taking skills because it can most directly help you increase your probability of answering questions correctly. This is one of the categories you can use to assess your performance and to learn how to enhance your performance using the CBTs and the Test Report. With Option Elimination Analysis, you are able to intelligently eliminate options to increase your chance of guessing correctly, if the need arises. The skill takes advantage of any basic knowledge you may possess and then develops skills that are independent of it. This means some of the techniques can be used with Study knowledge or Passage knowledge to enhance the skill. You can apply your knowledge to any skill. In general, when you apply knowledge to a skill, this makes success more likely and it should take precedence over pure guessing skills/ applications.

The elimination of incorrect, or probably incorrect, answers will greatly increase your odds if you should have to guess; all of us will have to guess at some time. The odds of getting the correct answer if guessing: Some options may be eliminated directly by your basic knowledge or from the passage information. Additional options can be eliminated by mastering the following techniques:

• Complex Sounding Options **(SB A.2.2)**,
• Dichotomy of Options **(SB A.2.3)**,
• Guess Questions **(SB A.2.4)**,
• Internal Inconsistency of Options **(SB A.2.5)**,
• Mutually Excluding Options **(SB A.2.6)**,
• Similar Pair Options **(SB A.2.7)**, and
• Three Out of Four Options **(SB A.2.8)**.

Number of Options Eliminated	Percentage Correct by Guessing
None	25%
One	33%
Two	50%
Three	100%.

A.2.2 Complex Sounding Options

These are very important to recognize and not be fooled by. These are part of the general test skill of Option Elimination Analysis **(SB A.2)** (also contains links to CBT questions for Complex Sounding Options). This technique is mainly applicable to the science questions.

The critical component of Complex Sounding Options is the concept of Basic Knowledge. It is through Basic Knowledge that you will be able to recognize Complex Sounding Options and make proper option eliminations. Basic Knowledge has two parts: Study Knowledge and Passage Knowledge.

Study Knowledge is knowledge that you should have brought to the MCAT through proper reading of the AAMC Student Manual or by studying this Web site. Passage Knowledge is knowledge you get from the passage itself, either directly or by proper interpretations. Then, any option that is not Study Knowledge or Passage Knowledge cannot be correct and should be eliminated, except that coming under General Knowledge. On the MCAT, there appear to be a limited number of questions that fall into this category of General Knowledge. These questions/options are not answerable based on the proper and reasonable study suggested by the MCAT (Study Knowledge). They are not answerable based on the direct or indirect information found in the passage or question (Passage Knowledge). It appears

you have to apply your General Knowledge, or "common sense," to answer them.

This type of question/option is probably best left to the end of the test unless the answer is obvious; remember all questions count the same. When you do tackle the question, try to eliminate any option that you can. Then try to logically deal with the other options. Fortunately, there are not many General Knowledge based questions on the test. Complex Sounding Options are more frequent in persuasive type questions and questions that may have a greater passage reading component.

Complex Sounding Options will take several different forms. Some will sound very plausible scientifically or simply sound "scientific." Others will be complex in the manner in which they are stated. Still others will be a rather long drawn-out explanation. All of these will only sound as though they could be the answer when you are not sure of the topic or concepts being discussed (not sure of your Study Knowledge or Passage Knowledge). If you are on target for the concept, then the Complex Sounding Option will appear to be out in left field. As an example from the AAMC practice tests:

Information in the passage: a discussion of experiments of BAT (brown adipose tissue) using hamsters; there is a discussion of pineal glands in hamsters; it is stated that

BAT produces thermogenesis effects; there is no mention of fish in the passage.

Stem: Would fish be expected to have BAT?

Option A - No, because fish cannot significantly regulate their body temperatures metabolically

Option B - No, because fish use mechanisms such as vasoconstriction of skin capillaries for metabolic thermoregulation

Option C - Yes, because it is the most effective means of generating heat in the water

Option D - Yes, because, as in hamsters, temperature regulation in fish is controlled by the pineal gland

Two out of four of these options could be considered to be Complex Sounding Options. Options C and D are the most outrageous. Both C and D are very "scientific-sounding options." A general way to assess whether or not the option is too complex or too scientific is to have done a solid study (your Study Knowledge) and be aware of what your limits are. The amount of information and knowledge required for the MCAT is very basic. If the option goes beyond a very basic understanding or application of the concept, then it will only be correct if the answer is found in the passage (your Passage Knowledge).

If the answer is not found in the passage (Passage Knowledge) and it is beyond study knowledge (Study Knowledge), it is probably incorrect. Your Basic Knowledge is found by applying the principle that only information found in the basic first and second year college texts will be on the test (for your Study Knowledge). Anything beyond this level of information must be presented in the passage (for your Passage Knowledge).

Option C requires that you know about the effect of different heat generating mechanisms and their relative effects in water! Where in your Study Knowledge were you required to know this? Nowhere! If the means to answer this question is not from your Study Knowledge, then to be correct it must be Passage Knowledge. There was no discussion of this concept in the passage. So, is it General Knowledge? No! The average college student isn't going to know the relative means of generating heat in water by organisms. Because option C cannot be determined from Study, Passage or General Knowledge, it cannot be correct and you can eliminate it.

Option D is similar. You cannot know this from Study Knowledge because this type of detail is not required for the MCAT. Likewise, it is not General Knowledge. The only possible way for this to be correct is if it is directly or indirectly in the passage; as there is nothing in the passage even close to this, it cannot be answered by Passage Knowledge. Therefore, option D cannot be correct. Option B uses a valid concept pertinent to the issue of temperature regulation (vasoconstriction) that is from your Study Knowledge. This is something you are supposed to know through Study Knowledge, and so it is a possible answer. Option A is also a statement you should know based on your Study Knowledge of energy metabolism. So, options A and B are legitimate scientific statements. You will have to use other means to distinguish between A and B, but you have eliminated C and D and have increased your guess rate by 100% from 25% to 50%.

Generally, you should give simple and basic sounding options more weight unless you have compelling reasons based on the passage or on clearly remembered study to go for a more complex option. When you have a good control of your Basic Knowledge component of Study Knowledge combined with Passage Knowledge, good results happen. Two very important results of having a solid control of Basic Knowledge are to recognize bogus options and to conserve time.

To recognize bogus options; you must understand that any information or concept or skill that is beyond the Study Knowledge must be presented in the passage (Passage Knowledge) if it is a viable correct option for the question. The only way you can know if something presented is beyond the Study Knowledge is if you have studied the information present in the AAMC Student Manual, you have adequately prepared based on that information, and you have confidence in your knowledge. If the knowledge required is not from your Study Knowledge, the only way you can answer the question is from information presented in the passage.

Passage information, Passage Knowledge, can come in several forms. The simplest is just as data or facts that you assess by reading the passage (data type). The next level is information contained in the text that requires reading and minimal interpretation (direct type). The last level is information that must be used with prior knowledge or analyzed to get the correct answer (indirect type). The information becomes more time consuming and difficult as you progress from the first to the last type. If there is no information presented in the passage, then the option cannot be a correct one (if it is not from Basic Knowledge).

Please be careful in applying this principle. If you have not done a thorough study and are not confident in your study (your Study Knowledge), then you will not be able to apply this principle. The second benefit of Basic Knowledge is in time conservation. Making a rapid and accurate and confident determination that you can answer a question with your Study Knowledge will allow you to solve that problem without having to refer back to the passage. Time is very important on this test regardless what the test makers are telling you. As you go through this Web site, questions that can be answered with your Study Knowledge will be pointed out to you (see CBT Solutions).

A.2.3 Dichotomy of Options

This is one of the test skills of Option Elimination Analysis **(SB A.2)** (has links to CBT questions on Dichotomy of Options). A dichotomy question is one that has two sets of options that are mutually exclusive. The two sets may be distinguished from each by two means. One means of separating the sets is by some knowledge you have from your study (Study Knowledge) or from the passage (Passage Knowledge). The other means is simply by some feature that is unrelated to Study Knowledge or Passage Knowledge. If you can identify the dichotomy and then determine in what direction the answer must lie, you can immediately eliminate 50% of the options. This is the key to dichotomy questions. If you can eliminate half the options, it will save you valuable time and increase your successful guessing. An example from the AAMC practice tests:

Stem: As atomic number increases in a horizontal row of the periodic table, ionization energy generally:

Option A - increases, because of increasing effective nuclear charge.
Option B - increases, because of increasing atomic radius.
Option C - decreases, because of decreasing effective nuclear charge.
Option D - decreases, because of increasing atomic radius.

The most obvious dichotomy is the "increases" or "decreases" division; you have two sets: a dichotomy. The "increases" set is options A and B, and the "decreases" set is options C and D. Based on your study (Study Knowledge), you would know that ionization energy does increase as one goes from left to right in a horizontal row of the periodic table. Therefore, the correct half of the dichotomy will be the "increases," or options A or B. So, you eliminate options C and D and concentrate on A or B for your answer or your guess.

In a double dichotomy type question, two dichotomies are present, and if you can successfully eliminate the incorrect half of both dichotomies, you will be left with the correct answer! The previous example is actually a double dichotomy. You have already picked one of the dichotomies, A and B. The other dichotomy is between "effective nuclear charge" in options A and C and "increasing atomic radius" in options B and D. Again, based on your basic study (Study Knowledge) of periodic trends and ionization energy, it was stated that it is effective nuclear charge that was important for the trend of ionization energy. This means the dichotomy of A and C must be correct. Therefore, since A is the only option in both dichotomies (the double dichotomy), it must be the correct answer!

The distinction between the two dichotomies does not always depend on your Study Knowledge. As stated, it may depend on the passage (Passage Knowledge) or simply on some characteristic that you notice. But the best separation is when you can use Study Knowledge or Passage Knowledge.

When you see a dichotomy type question, try to determine what the dichotomy is and what part of the dichotomy is correct (or which part is incorrect). Then you can focus on the difference between the two remaining options. This can greatly cut down the time you have to spend and, of course, greatly increase your chance of guessing correctly if it becomes necessary.

An observation found for Similar Pairs Options may be of value in certain dichotomy of options questions. This is the mirror image/opposites finding. When one half of the dichotomy is of this type, the correct answer probably comes from that half. As an example from an actual AAMC practice test:

Stem: An acetylcholinesterase inhibitor increases nasal secretions because it:

Option A - blocks acetylcholine release from parasympathetic nerve endings.
Option B - blocks acetylcholine response at acetylcholine receptors.
Option C - increases parasympathetic activity at acetylcholine receptors.
Option D - decreases parasympathetic activity at acetylcholine receptors.

Options C and D are of the mirror image/opposite type because of the "increases" and "decreases." Note that options A and B are not of this type. Your guess would be better from options C or D (and in this question, the answer is C or D).

A.2.4 Guess Questions

They are very important to recognize. They are a type of test skill under Option Elimination Analysis (OEA) **(SB A.2)** (has links to CBT Questions for Guess Questions). They are under Option Elimination Analysis even if you may not be able to eliminate any of the options.

These are questions that appear to be very difficult and may be outside of your area of Study Knowledge. They are also questions that may require time consuming analysis of the passage, or graph, or experiment.

Additionally, they may mix difficult concepts and require some Passage Knowledge.

Remember, you have a little more than a minute per question; time is important. This approximate time includes reading of passages; there are some very long passages in Verbal Reasoning, so you have even less time on the questions themselves (this why Skimming **(SB B.4.1, B.4.3)** and Highlighting **(SB B.6, B.7)** is so important).

If most of the questions appear too difficult,

then you have not properly prepared yourself. I would suggest that 10% or fewer of the questions should be in this category with good preparation on your part.

When you encounter one of your Guess Questions, guess what you should do? That's right; just stop and guess with your lucky letter of the day; always use the same letter if you cannot eliminate any of the options. (You should have a sequence of letters, e.g. C, D, B, A, and always stick within that sequence for your guess. For example, in a question, you may be able to eliminate options C and A, then your guess would be "D" because that is next in your sequence as "C" was already eliminated).

Generally, if the last option is a "none", "zero change", "all of the above" or similar choice, it is best to avoid it and go to the next lucky letter. Generally, it is not a good idea to select "D" as your lucky letter. This would be of greater importance if the final option "D" is of the type, "None of the Above", "All of the Above", "No Change", etc. On the last AAMC practice test, the test makers have started mixing up these types of options. In that case, you could try "D". My suggestion is always to have "D" as your last guess letter.

It is very important that you do not spend a lot of time determining if a guess question is a guess question; that's the reason for this test skill. Spend only a few seconds and move on. You should leave the answer blank on the answer sheet (computer) in case you have more time than you anticipate to return and maybe spend some time on it. Most likely, you will just mark your lucky letter of

the day in the last few minutes of the test time (MAKE SURE you have the time to enter an answer for each question!!!!!).

A related concept is the value of each question. Remember, time is important. Each of the questions in the science and verbal subtests counts exactly the same. There is no extra credit for getting the more difficult questions correct. Additionally, the questions are not in order from easiest to the most difficult. Even if they were, there would be certain topics you may be better in and a hard question for another student would be an easier question for you. The point is not to get bogged down, especially early, with the harder questions. If a question appears more difficult or more time consuming, then it is best to move on and come back to it later.

Harder questions are also demoralizing and increase negative anxiety and never discount the importance of a positive attitude and confidence. You should learn to recognize what makes a question hard for you and then skip those questions and come back to them later. Use your answer sheet to determine the questions you need to go back to. If you are not sure of the answer to a question, then don't mark an answer. It is OK to mark off incorrect options, if you are sure, on the test booklet (computer) itself; not on the answer sheet! Then after you have gone through the whole test, and hopefully answered most of the easier questions correctly, go back and tackle the more difficult ones. Ultimately, if you still can't figure out the answer, then make your best guess, with your lucky letter of the day;

do not leave questions unanswered at the end of the test.

Some of the question types you may want to pass over in the first pass are:

- questions with Complex Sounding Options **(SB A.2.2)**, questions with a lot of complex data/information/graphs/experiments;
- Multiple Choice **(SB A.1.2)** types;
- Three or More Steps **(SB A.1.4)** Analysis;
- more complex arithmetic calculation questions;
- questions with longer options (the answers); and finally,
- questions that just "seem hard."

Again, if too many of the questions appear to be guess questions, you may need more preparation.

You should not be afraid of unfamiliar passage content passages. Not all, but a majority of the passages on the test will be on topics you have not seen before. It is essential that you do not panic when you see these types of passages. They are used to test one of two skills, like most of the passages.

First, they may test basic knowledge that you should have prepared for. In this case, you will have to recognize the concept being tested and not be confused by the trickiness of the question.

Second, they may test some new knowledge that is present in the passage. Some of these will be straightforward and others will require some effort. No question will test you on anything other than the content outlined in the AAMC student manual other than information in the passage as Passage Knowledge. A key skill to eliminate options is to recognize options that fall outside of these two arenas. These passages can come in many forms. Some may be on a topic you have never seen, such as "rail guns." Other passages may have a topic you are familiar with but may present it in a different format or manner, such as acid-base concepts discussed as acid rain.

Still others may present an experiment or research project. Others will present a whole new concept that was not required of your basic study but that extends your Study Knowledge and you will have to integrate it with your basic study. Others will present medical school topics that may make you think you should have taken more advanced courses. Yet, each of these are only testing Basic Knowledge **(SB A.2.2)** that you should have brought to the test, some use of information from the Passage Knowledge, or a combination of basic information and passage interpretation. Also, the passage interpretation is most often straightforward or one or two steps at the most.

A.2.5 Internal Inconsistency of Options

This is one of the Option Elimination Analysis **(SB A.2)** techniques (has links for CBT questions for Internal Inconsistency of Options). It occurs when the option itself contains components that cannot be true together. To recognize this will require application of Study Knowledge or, less likely, information from the Passage Knowledge. For example, if an option contains the phrase "will increase OH^- and lowers pH," this would be an internal inconsistency because you should know that OH^- is basic and this will increase the pH. This technique does require some level of knowledge. An example from the AAMC practice tests:

Stem: In the titration of ammonia, why does the pH drop sharply near the equivalence point?

Option A - The concentration of NH_3 increases sharply near the equivalence point.

Option B - The concentration of OH^- increases sharply near the equivalence point.

Option C - The concentration of NH_4^+ decreases sharply near the equivalence point.

Option D - The concentration of OH^- decreases sharply near the equivalence point.

This problem was supposed to be solved in relation to a passage and a graph, but certain options may be eliminated because they have internal inconsistencies. You should know that NH_3 and OH^- have basic properties from your Study Knowledge **(SB A.2.2)**. This means that as either increases, the pH should increase also. Options A and B then cannot be correct, because of the inconsistency of a base increasing with pH decreasing; the opposite has to occur. You would then know the answer has to come from C or D. Either use your knowledge or guess the answer. Likewise you would know that option D is a consistent statement as decreasing OH^- would cause a pH drop. Then if you remembered that NH_4^+ is acidic, you would know that Option C cannot be correct. The only option left is option D.

A.2.6 Mutually Excluding Options

This is a test skill technique of Option Elimination Analysis **(SB A.2)** (has links to CBT Questions for Mutually Excluding Options). These do not arise often.

When two different options have the same effect relative to the answer, then they are the same and mutually exclude each other; neither can be correct. To recognize the similarity, you must have a solid understanding of Study Knowledge **(SB A.2.2)** and concepts or use information from the Passage Knowledge. An example:

Stem: The solution will precipitate out the product when the pH is lowered. Which of these changes will result in the increased precipitation of the product?

Option A - Bubbling CO_2 through the solution
Option B - Increasing pK_a of the component

Option C - Decreasing the pK_b of the conjugate of the component
Option D - Bubbling O_2 through the solution

This problem actually needs information found in the passage, but you can still eliminate two options. In this example, options B and C are essentially the same because of the definitions of pK_a, pK_b, conjugate acids and conjugate bases; the effect of moving them in opposite directions is the same. As the effect is the same, neither can be correct. To make this assessment requires a good solid basic knowledge of these concepts.

A.2.7 Similar Pair Options

This is a test skill of Option Elimination Analysis **(SB A.2)** (has links to CBT Questions for Similar Pair Options). Similar Pair Options should not be confused with Mutually Excluding Options **(SB A.2.6)** or with Dichotomy of Options **(SB A.2.3)**. Similar Pair Options are two options that are similar in some manner. They may be similar on the basis of your Study Knowledge, Passage Knowledge **(SB A.2.2)**, or some other characteristic. It is best only to use Similar Pair Options when there are only two options that are similar. Some questions will have pairs of similar appearing options; you should not use this technique when this occurs.

An example of Similar Pair Option from the AAMC practice tests is:
(Information from passage - not provided)

Stem: Of the following procedural alterations, which would be required if a researcher wanted to isolate a thermophilic species of Bacillus?

Option A - higher incubation temperatures
Option B - lower incubation temperature
Option C - longer incubation periods
Option D - longer 100 °C steam treatment

Of the four options, A and B are very similar. They both deal with incubation temperatures. This makes them similar and distinguishes them from the other two options. For this question, you must have the passage available to answer it, but you have narrowed the possible answers down to A and B without the passage. This is what guessing is all about. This is when you would use the technique, when you have to guess. Your chance for a correct guess just doubled from 25% to 50%; a 100% increase. In fact, the correct answer is either A or B. This is also a Three Out of Four **(SB A.2.8)** type skill. Options A, B, and D all deal with temperatures of some sort, but A and B are still a similar pair within this set (go to that discussion for a more detailed explanation).

Another example of Similar Pair Option from the AAMC practice tests is:
(Information from passage - not provided)

Stem: According to Table 1, which of the following variables are significantly affected by heat but NOT by pineal gland secretions?

Option A - Testes and seminal vesicle weights
Option B - Body and liver weights
Option C - Adrenal and pituitary weights
Option D - Testes and pituitary weights

It may be dangerous to use the Similar Pair Option technique on this problem because there is more than one similar pair. Options A and D both contain testes, and options C and D both contain pituitary; each of these sets is a similar pair, but which is correct? You could take your answer from one of these as B is not in either; if you're truly guessing, why not? Or you could guess D since this is in both. In this problem, the correct answer does not come from A, C, or D; so, you would guess wrong. This is why I would not use the Similar Pair Option if more than one similar pair is present.

An often good similar pair to guess from is a mirror, or opposite pair type. This occurs when the structure is similar but the two options are in contrast, or opposite, of each other.

An example from the AAMC practice tests:

Stem: As a result of being a weaker base than ammonia, hydrazine:

Option A - has a smaller acidity constant (K_a) than does ammonia.
Option B - has a smaller basicity constant (K_b) than does ammonia.
Option C - can be protonated twice to form $N_2H_6^{+2}$.
Option D - forms hydrogen bonds in aqueous solution.

Options A and B are similar and are contrasting. They are distinctly different from options C and D. They would make a good guess for similar pair options.

To summarize, it is NOT a good idea to use Similar Pair Option when:

1. There is more than one obvious similar pair present.
2. A dichotomy of options is present.
3. The similar pair conflicts with an obvious three out of four type options.
4. The similar pair is simple word(s) that can be inclusive or exclusive allowing another similar pair to be created simply using "NOT" or some equivalent.

An example will be given:

In a passage dealing with Puritans and science, the following were the options:

A) Many of its early members rose to prominence during Chromwell's rule.
B) Charles II took an amateur's interest in science.
C) Over a third of its charter members had remained Royalists.
D) It received nothing from Charles II but its charter.

Options B and D could be a similar pair because of "Charles II". But, options A and C are also a similar pair by NOT having "Charles II". So, this becomes a multiple similar pair due to the simplicity of looking at the word(s) "Charles II".

Similar Pair Options have increasing value in this sequence:

1. There is only one similar pair present.

2. The similar pair is part of a Three Out of Four Options **(SB A.2.8)**.

3. The similar pair is of the mirror image/ opposites structure. An exception seems to be if the similar pair is not part of a three out of four. In this situation, the whole similar pair may be incorrect; you have to exert more care in this situation.

4. The similar pair is based on study knowledge or passage knowledge. The second group of positive reasons can outweigh the first group of negative reasons. However, you should have practice in applying these concepts.

During the most recent AAMC practice tests, there has been an increasing number of similar pairs which are incorrect. Whether this trend is significant or not remains to be seen. If they are using this as a response to the analysis is uncertain. But, it can be a bad trend if they want to eliminate two options because of this suggestion. At any rate, be more cautious in the use of this technique.

A.2.8 Three Out Of Four

This is a test skill of Option Elimination Analysis **(SB A.2)** (has links to CBT Questions for Three Out of Four questions). Questions of this type appear very frequently on the AAMC MCAT practice tests. This technique directs you to select three out of four options that have some similarity with each other and are distinct from the fourth. Usually, the correct option will come from the group of three you select. You go from a 25% guess to a 33% guess for the correct answer; this is approximately a 33% increased chance of guessing the correct answer, which is still a significant increase in your guess percentage.

In general, nothing is always true, but when three out of four of the options center around a specific concept, data, etc., the answer is probably one of those three. This is especially the case when the stem of the question is more of a positive and inclusive type question and not a Negative Question (**SB A.1.2**).

There will be three options that are related in some manner, and there will be a fourth option that is an outlier. In general, that outlier will be incorrect and can be eliminated when the question is positive or inclusive. It will be rare for a question to have three outliers and one correct option in the possible answers, but it does happen sometimes. So, if you are not sure, go for one of the three similar options.

An example from the AAMC practice tests:

(Information from passage - not provided)

Stem: According to the Bronsted-Lowry acid-base theory, which of the following species is the conjugate acid of ammonia?

Option A - H^+
Option B - H_3O^+
Option C - NH_3OH
Option D - NH_4^+

This is a passage question but if you had to guess cold you could use the Three Out of Four technique and select options A, B, and D as the three and option C as the fourth, or outlier. A, B, and D all are positive ions, giving them a similarity. So, if you had to guess, you would choose from A, B, or D. The answer does come from A, B, or D.

An exception is when the question asks for exclusion of others, for the one most likely, or is a Negative Question (**SB A.1.2**). For these questions, you can use the Three Out of Four technique, but realize you have a reversal and the answer may well be the outlier.

An example from the AAMC practice tests:

(Information from passage - not provided)

Stem: According to the passage, bremsstrahlung will NOT be produced by collisions between electrons and:

Option A - He
Option B - He_2^+
Option C - Li^{1+}
Option D - protons

As the passage is not available, you have to guess on this question. This has a Three Out of Four pattern with options B, C, and D being the three similar options; all are ions and all are positive. Option A is the outlier as it is a neutral molecule. If this was a positive question, without the negative qualifier "NOT," then the answer would most likely come from B, C, or D. But, because this is a negative or exclusion question, you have to be more careful. There will be enough times when the answer is the outlier in a negative question that is Three Out of Four. In this problem, the answer is A.

Another exception, which is not rare, is when the outlier option is a "no change" type. Most of the time, the question will result in a change of some type and the outlier of no change, zero, etc. will not be correct; but again, be careful in these questions. This may take multiple different forms such as "no-change", "zero", "all of the above", "none of the above", and similar options should never be your guess. Always consider these as the outlier in a Three Out of Four type question. This is also true for absolute type options with words like "all," "never," or similar phrases; treat the absolute option as the outlier. These will occasionally be correct, but you should choose them by elimination or analysis and not by guessing; you only select them when you are sure this type of option is correct.

Sometimes there will be double Three Out of Fours or even triple Three Out of Fours. In the rare situation where three Three Out of Fours can be identified, the remaining option is potentially the correct answer. In general, always be very cautious where you start to identify multiple Three Out of Fours.

Finally, there is the situation where you will have a Three Out of Four and a Similar Pair Option. With these problems, you should first have one set of Three Out of Four and then within that set you will have a similar pair. The rules of Similar Pairs and Three Out of Fours should both be followed.

An example from the AAMC practice tests was discussed in Similar Pairs (SB A.2.7) and is:

(Information from passage - not provided)

Stem: Of the following procedural alterations, which would be required if a researcher wanted to isolate a thermophilic species of Bacillus?

Option A - higher incubation temperatures
Option B - lower incubation temperatures
Option C - longer incubation periods
Option D - longer 100 °C steam treatment

The Three Out of Four is the A, B, and D options, as all relate to temperature. Options A and B are a similar pair because both relate specifically to incubation temperatures. You can either take your Three Out of Four guess from A, B, or D for your 33% chance. Or, you can take your guess from A or B for your 50% chance of being correct. Generally, go with the similar pair when you can identify this type of problem. But, options A, B and C are a second Three Out of Four and option D is the outlier. These two Three Out of Fours eliminate options C and D and you are left with the similar pair previously discussed.

A.2.9 Illogical Sequence of Options

This is a type of Options Elimination Analysis (SB A.2).

In a few questions, you will notice there is a sequence of options that does not follow a logical order of presentation. This may be a clue as to which options may be incorrect and which may be correct. A logical sequence would relate to numbering of some form, primarily. There may be other logical or illogical sequences that will vary greatly. An example of an illogical sequence from one of the AAMC practice tests is (the stem is omitted):

A. $Pb(NO_3)_2$ by threefold
B. $Pb(NO_3)_2$ by twofold
C. $C_2H_6O_2$ by twofold
D. $C_2H_6O_2$ by threefold

The illogical sequence is options A and B. Why should 3 come before 2? This is especially noticeable because options C and D are in a logical sequence of 2 followed by 3. This should suggest to you that option A is probably correct. Why? Because the

only reason for the illogical sequence is to maintain the "randomness" of the answers. Often test makers will use a set of random numbers to determine the answers so they will not unconsciously bias the sequence of answers, which can happen. However, this is a sign of "doggedly" sticking to that sequence when it makes the sequence of answers illogical. You would have logically expected option A and B to be reversed, which would be a "logical" way to present these. Why present them in any other way? Why are options C and D not in the same sequence? Because of symmetry? Doubtful. This is easy to correct for the test makers. But, when you see it, you might as well take advantage of it, but with caution. The correct answer is A.

A.2.10 Analysis of AAMC Tests For Option Elimination Analysis

Option Elimination Analysis is a method of increasing your guess percentage on the MCAT. There are eight specific methods you should study and learn as efficiently as possible. How you fare with questions that involve each method is found in the Test Report for the CBT; click "Test Report" on the bottom menu, click "CBT", click the subtest you want, and then scroll down the leftmost panel to find the "Option Elimination Analysis" breakdown. The use of these methods is found in the CBT Solutions section in the Study Center. When "guess correctly" is used in this concept, it means you have eliminated incorrect options and

the remaining options contain the correct answer.

Complex Sounding Options (SB A.2.2)
A Complex Sounding Option is an option that goes beyond your Basic Knowledge. You should study this concept and fully understand what Basic Knowledge means and how you can apply it to solving MCAT problems. This is a frequently applied method that is especially important for the Sciences.

Dichotomy of Options (SB A.2.3)
Dichotomy of Options is a very frequently

found method applicable to Verbal Reasoning and especially to the Science subtests. You will be taught to recognize the Dichotomy of Options questions and how to apply your Basic Knowledge to choose the correct half of the dichotomy.

Guess Questions (SB A.2.4)

There are certain questions that you just will not be able to answer; this is true for everyone at one time or another. The faster you can recognize these questions and move on, the better. This concept discusses how to recognize these questions and how to manage them.

Internal Inconsistency of Options (SB A.2.5)

Internal Inconsistency of Options questions usually involve situations where the option has some statement that conflicts with or contradicts Basic Knowledge. You use your Basic Knowledge and logic to apply this method. It is most commonly used for the Sciences, but it may be occasionally applicable to Verbal Reasoning.

Mutually Excluding Options (SB A.2.6)

This occurs infrequently. It is characterized by two options having essentially the same meaning. If both options are the same, then neither can be correct; only one option per question can be correct. When you come across it, you will have a 100% chance to guess correctly.

Similar Pair Options (SB A.2.7)

Similar Pair Options questions are very common. It occurs when two of the options are similar. This method has a number of subtleties that you have to learn, and which will increase your correct guess rate. It can be used for both Verbal Reasoning and for the Sciences.

Three Out of Four Options (SB A.2.8)

This is the most frequently encountered of all of the methods. Three Out of Four Options can be used with Basic Knowledge or as a pure guess. It is equally applicable to Verbal Reasoning and to the Sciences.

Illogical Sequence of Options (SB A.2.9)

Illogical Sequence of Options is a very infrequently encountered method. What is found is a sequence of options that is illogical, for example, sequences that are not in alphabetical or numerical order. On the most recent CBTs, the test makers are making the option sequences more logical and this technique will be less and less available.

Detailed Analysis of AAMC Practice Tests: Option Elimination Analysis

Description	Verbal Reasoning		Physical Sciences		Biological Sciences		Total	
	#	%	#	%	#	%	#	%
Complex Sounding Options	1	0.1	25	1.9	47	3.7	73	5.7
Dichotomy of Options	18	1.4	100	7.8	82	6.4	200	15.6
Guess Question	3	0.2	4	0.3	4	0.3	11	0.9
Illogical Sequence of Options	0	0.0	1	0.1	0	0.0	1	0.1
Internal Inconsistency of Options	5	0.4	52	4.0	40	3.1	97	7.5
Mutually Excluding Options	1	0.1	9	0.7	5	0.4	15	1.2
Similar Pair Options	74	5.8	44	3.4	53	4.1	171	13.3
Three Out of Four Options	186	14.5	160	12.5	131	10.2	477	37.1
None	72	5.6	68	5.3	100	7.8	240	18.7
Total	360	28.0	463	36.0	462	36.0	1285	100.0

Lessons from the analysis of Option Elimination Analysis:

• The Most Frequently Found Techniques

- Three Out of Four
- Dichotomy
- Similar Pair

You should study each of these thoroughly

and learn how to apply them by studying the CBT Solutions in detail.

• The Frequency of Questions with Techniques Applicable in Each Subtest

- Biological Sciences - 86.0%
- Physical Sciences - 91.1%
- Verbal Reasoning - 82.3%

• The Frequency of Correct Guesses Using the Techniques in Each Subtest

- Biological Sciences - 89.1%
- Physical Sciences - 89.3%
- Verbal Reasoning - 86.3%

• Although the most uses of Option Elimination Analysis were found in the Physical Sciences, over 80% was found in both Biological Sciences and Verbal Reasoning. This shows these option types are very common and widely applicable.

• When the techniques were applied, you would have selected the correct options

to guess from in 86 to 89% of the guesses. This is extraordinary.

• Note that Three Out of Four is fairly evenly scattered across the subtests, but is found the most in Verbal Reasoning.

• Dichotomy of Options is found most heavily for Biological Sciences and Physical Sciences.

• Similar Pairs is also fairly evenly distributed but with a clear preponderance in Verbal Reasoning.

• Complex Sounding Options are more commonly found in Biological Sciences.

• Internal Inconsistency of Options is more likely to be found in the science subtests.

Use this analysis to help you guide your study and what to be thinking about as you take each subtest.

DrFlowersMCAT.com

MCAT-Prep.com

Section-B
VERBAL REASONING

AAMC REAL PAST MCAT TESTS

Section B

AAMC REAL PAST MCAT TESTS

Explanations and Analysis for
the new MCAT VR

MCAT-Prep.com

B.1 General Thoughts on Verbal Reasoning Preparation

It is an unfortunate fact that performance in the Verbal Reasoning (VR) section is more difficult to improve compared to the Science section. This is because performance in VR is largely determined by your reading background. Those who have been reading as a hobby for pleasure and instruction for several years are best placed to tackle VR questions. Generally, the MCAT VR passages are taken from scholarly writing from fields as diverse as literary criticism, psychology, social science, natural science, etc. Therefore, a strong and eclectic nonfiction reading background is the best possible preparation for the VR section.

However, even a diet of thrillers, Westerns, pulp and romantic fiction, or popular magazine articles will be helpful, because any kind of regular reading would automatically result in a greater reading speed. Given that an average of only 9 minutes can be devoted to a passage, reading speed is a critical factor. Reading is a skill, like swimming and cycling, and regular practice is necessary to maintain the skill at a high level. Therefore, any kind of regular reading is better than no reading activity. If you are not a reader, you will have a harder time, but it is not too late to begin now. Magazines such as The New Yorker, The Economist and The Atlantic have well-written essays, and you should make it a point to read them regularly. Try and absorb words in chunks rather than letter by letter, to increase your reading speed. You should easily be able to do this initially with articles (a, an, the), prepositions (in, on, over, around, etc.), and conjunctions (and, but, or). Later, try chunking shorter words not in the above categories. When you chunk a word, you "swallow" it whole, so to speak.

B.1.1 MCAT Essentials

Carefully read the parts of MCAT Essentials and Preparing for the MCAT Exam, at www.aamc.org (and follow the MCAT links) that deal with VR. This was previously found in the MCAT Student Manual. The manual is packed with information and also has many practical tips. In the MCAT you will have to tackle 7 passages consisting of 40 questions in 60 minutes, which works out to about 9 minutes per passage. The manual suggests four passage-reading methodologies. You will have to determine in advance which method works best for you, and stick to it. Otherwise, you may waste time thrashing around wildly from paragraph to paragraph, which could produce feelings of panic and loss of control. You should note another important nugget of information in the manual: passages in the exam are not of uniform difficulty. The easier passages are to be found at the beginning and the toughest passages at the end. So, some performance fluctuation is natural; it is not something to get worried about. Your scores will be lower on the harder passages.

B.1.2 Key Elements

There are two key elements to VR performance: comprehension and time. A useful suggestion in the manual is a diagnostic exercise to help you identify which area you should concentrate on. The manual suggests that you first take a sample test without imposing time constraints on yourself. Try and answer the questions correctly. Now, if your score is satisfactory but you took longer than 60 minutes, you need to work faster. If your score is low and you took longer than 60 minutes, the problem is more serious: you will have to improve your comprehension skills first, and then work on your speed.

One characteristic of all the MCAT passages was mentioned earlier: they are taken from scholarly writing. Another important attribute all of them share is that they present arguments. An MCAT passage presents the author's point of view on a specific topic, and other opposing points of view will also occur in the passage. However, because the writing is scholarly, formal, and often full of jargon, the lines dividing an argument from a counterargument will not usually be clearly drawn. The author will never come out and say directly, "I believe in ... " You will have to read between the lines, so to speak, and clear away the details strewn on your path like obstacles to arrive at the author's thesis. What is he or she trying to say in the passage? Why did the author invest time and energy in writing this piece?

Personalize the passage: How does he or she want to influence me? What kind of effect is the passage having on me? Do I find myself agreeing or disagreeing? Also, watch out for give-away (clue, transition, or emphasis) words and phrases like however, but, on the contrary, clearly, obviously, etc.; the first three words signal transitions, and the latter two indicate which way the argument is blowing, so to speak. These words will help you track the argument as it winds and wends its way down the course set for it by the author. It is absolutely critical to avoid getting distracted by details and facts; your immediate goal is to identify the author's thesis, after which you have to understand how that thesis is supported by the paragraphs in the passage.

Look at the big picture. Imagine yourself in an airplane flying over a forest looking down: major features like clumps of trees, herds of animals, open spaces, rivers, etc., will be clearly visible, whereas details like blades of grass and even individual trees will not. Aim for this kind of bird's-eye view of the passage when you read. Maybe you can imagine that you are suspended in midair over the desk, or that you are a fly on the ceiling. Do whatever it takes to gain that perspective. Don't give the details and nuances individual attention; rather, observe how they contribute to the overall argument. You can read faster than usual, because you do not have to understand every detail and every nuance in the passage; you only need to identify the thesis of the passage and how the details support the thesis. Try and identify the author's thesis after reading the first paragraph. When reading the subsequent paragraphs, relate what you read to this thesis. Pause after every paragraph and ask yourself: How does this paragraph reinforce the author's thesis?

As you would have grasped by now, you do not have to understand every niggling detail to answer the passage questions. You do need to closely follow the thread of the author's argument. This is only logical; the MCAT paper setters are not interested in playing cat-and-mouse games with you in a setting that is alien enough with jargon-filled scholarly writing from some esoteric branch of knowledge. They do, however, want to know if you can cut to the chase and discern the contours of the author's argument.

B.1.3 Passage Comprehension Skills

This brings me to another step you can take to improve your passage comprehension skills. Get hold of a college-level text on rhetoric (e.g., The Elements of Argument by Annette Rottenberg). You will find the various standard forms of argument analyzed threadbare. Do not try and read the book from cover to cover; read just enough to understand the different types of arguments. Skim through (or omit if time is a problem) the theoretical parts, but do work through as many illustrative passages as possible and the exercises based on them; this will sharpen your critical thinking skills. After working for some time with such a book, you should see at least a modest increase in your MCAT VR performance.

You should also work through the MCAT practice tests. As a learning exercise, I suggest that you begin with passages V and VIII from 6. These are passages that we have analyzed from the point of view of a student in the examination hall (login to The Study Center—>MCAT Solutions—>MCAT Practice 6). Attack either of these two passages first and give it everything you've got. Next, study our analysis of the passage and see if you understand where you went wrong in your answer selection. Then study the MCAT solutions for the passage. The solutions are excellent and clearly explain why a particular option is right and the rest are wrong. Repeat this exercise for the second of the two passages mentioned earlier. Taking two passages apart in great detail like this and seeing what makes them tick is excellent preparation for tackling the MCAT VR section.

A point to keep in mind when answering passage questions is this: answer questions from passage knowledge alone. For example, you may know from outside reading that Winston Churchill liked his brandy; however, if it is not mentioned in the passage, do not be tempted to go for an option that says Churchill liked his daily tipple. For an MCAT examinee, the VR passage represents gospel truth, and outside knowledge is illicit knowledge. The questions have to be answered based on passage content. Of course, as you undoubtedly have seen, this does not mean that only direct questions are asked. Critical thinking skills are tested, so you will be asked to extend the author's argument, apply it in hypothetical situations, etc.; however, if something is not mentioned in the passage, do NOT use it as a basis for choosing or eliminating an option. Sometimes, an option will consist of a self-evidently true statement; however, if the statement is not mentioned in the passage, do NOT pick that option. There will be another option that can be picked from passage knowledge, so look around.

B.1.4 Arguments

I will end with a suggestion you can begin using immediately. I have already emphasized that MCAT passages invariably present arguments supporting a point of view. These arguments are not like the arguments that husbands and wives have; they are expressed in scholarly language and often employ sophisticated reasoning. Nevertheless, they are arguments, and I believe an argument is something every human being can identify with. We have all participated in arguments. Argument is a part and parcel of human activity. Most of us find arguments interesting, if only because of the gaming aspect: most arguments have winners and losers. Yes, arguments are fun. Preparation for the VR section should be an enjoyable and exciting business. So, to help you on your way, I invite you to join in the mother of all arguments: Does God exist?

Buy and read the 2006 best seller The God Delusion by the British biologist Richard Dawkins. Then buy and read the counter to this book, The Dawkins Delusion, written by British biochemist-theologian Alistair McGrath. List and compare the main arguments and counterarguments. Look for holes in arguments. Write reviews of both books comparing their methodologies and describing their strengths and weaknesses. If you do not want to buy the books and cannot find them in a library, I give some links below this article to get you started. The idea is to immerse yourself in a complex argument during your run-up to the MCAT, so that you become familiar with the complete repertoire of weapons deployed in an argument conducted through the medium of formal writing.

Web Links

The God Delusion

http://en.wikipedia.org/wiki/The_God_Delusion

Section B: Verbal Reasoning Analysis

http://www.randomhouse.com.au/Downloads/
News/GodDelusion_extract_revised.pdf

http://www.dwillard.org/articles/artview.
asp?artID=52

Criticisms of The God Delusion

http://en.wikipedia.org/wiki/The_Dawkins_
Delusion%3F

http://www.reasonablefaith.org/site/
News2?page=NewsArticle&id=5493

http://www.nytimes.com/2007/03/03/
books/03beliefs.html?ex=1182571200&en=3
1333ad7ea00d52f&ei=5070

http://www.christianitytoday.com/
bc/2007/002/1.21.html

B.2 Verbal Reasoning: Phases of Preparation

B.2.1 Phase: Prior to Beginning Actual Study

Many have weighed in with their opinions regarding how to best prepare for the Verbal Reasoning test. Following are some comments found on the Internet regarding the Verbal Reasoning on the MCAT:

- All passages are long/extensive/dry.
- Many passages are esoteric/unfamiliar.
- Many questions are long/extensive.
- Many new terms are introduced/not explained explicitly.
- Passages are well written and organized.
- Sequence of information does not always begin at the beginning.
- Passages are condensed from longer articles but retain details and eliminate extras.
- Three major areas: Humanities, Social Sciences, Natural Sciences.
  No best method to approaching passages.

Following are some general suggestions to do even before you start your formal study:

- Study/review concepts from high-yield subjects.
- Study/review vocabulary from high-yield subjects.
- Read articles in mid/high sources on high-yield subjects (e.g., New York Times editorials, Time essays, etc.)
- When reading articles/materials, do the following to read actively:

  - Anticipate or generate questions like on the MCAT (comprehension, evaluation, application, new information).
  - Identify and decipher unknown word/phrase definitions from contextual information.
  - Determine credibility of information.

- Determine how it relates to known information/facts/theories.
- Determine implication of "if's".
- Determine what would enhance/ prove or diminish/disprove.
- Look for transition/clue/cue words and phrases.
- Identify the central thesis or theme.

- Identify secondary contentions/ themes.
- Identify how theses/contentions are supported, the evidence for them provided by the author.
- Identify examples/explanations used by the author to support the theses/ contentions.

B.2.2 Phase: MCAT Preparation

Following are general suggestions to follow/ do when you are studying for and actually taking the test:
From general Internet sources:
- Always read for the Central Thesis **(SB B.8, B.9)**
- Underline or Highlight **(SB B.6, B.7)** key words/phrases/concepts.
- Speed reading is a mistake (the passages are too condensed for effective speed reading; speed reading is most effective when you are familiar with the material - not the case for the MCAT).
- Read first and last sentences of every paragraph (*see* VR:Answer Location Analysis).
- Do not read questions first. Other Comments (examples are from AAMC 9): *See* Passage Highlighting **(SB B.6, B.7)**.
- Other contentions/theses more important than Central Thesis (based on absolute number of questions).
- If not sure of Central Thesis, note more than one (sort out later if needed). (This is contrasted to the approach of Examkrackers which may be better for some students - you should try their approach).
- Examples/supporting evidence very important to read for.
- Look for any of these:
  - Words in quotations or italics (e.g., "female fiction," "female experience," Jane Eyre)
  - Unfamiliar words/phrases/concepts (ice-crystal theory)
  - Transition or emphasis words or phrases (e.g. This term we may define ..., An example ..., There is, I feel, no male ..., More specifically ..., There are two general theories ..., We must find ..., According to this theory ..., We are therefore led ..., Next)
  - It is not these words/phrases themselves that are important but what follows them.
- Learn and practice effective underlining/ highlighting skills.

B.2.3 Phase: Taking the MCAT

Time Is Important
Don't let anyone fool you; time is a critical component of this test. When you take the Verbal Reasoning subtest, be prepared to maximize your concentration and focus every second you have available for this test. Make sure all of your skills are sharp. The ability to scan or read rapidly is also important. Use Timing to push yourself to optimize your skills. If you study any of the approaches by Kaplan, Princeton Review, Examkrackers or others, they require "time" for you to get ready to answer the questions. You have to decide which approach you can do effectively. Anyone who tells you time is not important either does not appreciate the test fully or has developed a skill to automaticity through fortunate genetics or practice.

Sacrifices
Because time is a critical factor, you may need to sacrifice either questions or a whole passage. As you do the AAMC CBTs, you should determine if you can complete the 40 questions and 7 passages in 60 minutes. If you are finding this impossible, and you are not getting good scores, it may be wise to consider the "Sacrifice." The Sacrifice means nearly completely ignoring certain questions or passages. It would make more sense to do this for questions, but not always, because nearly all passages have a few simpler questions. If you choose to do this, you will have difficulty getting double digit scores, but should be able to get an 8 or 9 or possibly 10. For higher double digits, you

cannot sacrifice passages.

Sacrificing questions: questions that should be considered for sacrifice are those with the following characteristics:
1) Negative Questions (SB A.1.2);
2) Multiple Choice Questions (SB A.1.2);
3) Questions that focus on the whole passage instead of specific location or reference. For example, these are the ones that use the wording "according to the passage," "using information only in the passage," and generally questions that require you to have a gestalt or understanding of the whole passage (see Answer Location Analysis; SB B.6, B.7);
4) Questions that introduce new information or concepts;
5) Questions that want the author's viewpoint "challenged" in some way;
6) Questions with very long stems compared to others;
7) Questions with very long options compared to others;
8) Guess Questions (SB A.2.4).

However, you will find that a great number of questions fall into these categories. What you should do is use your Test Report to determine your strengths/weaknesses for those categories assessed. Then practice these so they become easier questions for you. Also, you can focus on the other question types as previously discussed to increase your efficiency in answering them. It will be difficult to neglect more than

7 questions (usually the most in any one passage) on the test and achieve the score you desire. However, remember that the goal is to get more of the 33 questions correct, because you are ignoring the 7 questions and have more time to concentrate on them.

Sacrificing passages may be a better option because you do not have to read the passage fully. If after the first paragraph, the passage seems like one that is difficult for you, you can skip it entirely.

Don't forget to use Option Elimination Analysis **(SB A.2.10)** for your sacrificed

questions. This may allow you to go from a 25 percent guess rate to over a 33 percent guess rate. These small percentages can mean valuable increases in your overall score.

Also, when you do not fully assess a question, always guess your lucky letter of the day if you cannot eliminate any options.

If you choose to sacrifice a passage or questions and have time left over, you can go back and tackle that passage or questions. Remember not to spend a lot of time on any sacrificed passage or question.

B.3 AAMC Student Manual Suggestions for Verbal Reasoning

B.3.1 General Topics

The AAMC Student Manual (at www.aamc.org) provides a number of good suggestions to prepare for the Verbal Reasoning passages. The Verbal Reasoning passages are taken from the following general topics: Social Sciences, Humanities, and Natural Sciences. The specific subjects from the AAMC Manual are:

Humanities
  Architecture
  Art and art history
  Dance
  Ethics

Literary criticism
Music
Philosophy
Religion
Theater

Social sciences
  Anthropology
  Archaeology
  Business
  Economics
  Government
  History
  Political science

Section B: Verbal Reasoning Analysis

Psychology	Computer science
Sociology	Ecology
	Geology
Natural sciences	Meteorology
Astronomy	Natural history
Botany	Technology

B.3.2 Basic Study Tips

The AAMC Student Manual gives some basic study tips, which you should follow for the verbal passages:

1. Take a variety of classes in college in the General Subject areas **(SB B.3.1)**.

2. Courses with critical thinking and reasoning **(SB B.1.3)** requirements are valuable.

3. Review with someone, a study or tutorial center, about argument as a form of writing **(SB B.1.4)** (purpose, content, and structure of argument)

4. Read a variety of general materials **(SB B.3.1)** (books, journals, magazines, newspapers, etc.) and analyze them critically.

5. There are suggested ways to Attack Passages **(SB B.4)** (you have to determine which is best for you):

   a. Read the passage, and then answer questions going back to passage as needed.
   b. Skim through passage, then read it,

and finally answer questions.
   c. Skim through the passage only, then read the questions, next read the passage, and finally answer the questions.
   d. Read the questions, next read the passage, and finally answer questions

6. Practice marking the passages **(SB B.6, B.7)** to determine which is the best method for you. The options are:

   a. Underline words or phrases;
   b. Make notes in the margin;
   c. Both underline and make notes in the margin.

7. You have about 9 minutes per passage.

8. Comprehension and evaluation type questions are directly based on the passage.

9. Application and new information type questions **(SB B.7.4)** require you to extend the information in the passage.

B.4 Verbal Reasoning: How to Attack Passages

B.4.1 How to Attack Passages — Read, Study, or Skim?

Reading
• Not suggested.
• Passages are condensed.
• Speed reading is ineffective because "extras" are already eliminated. But, you should have a good reading speed, so practice on it is not unreasonable.

Studying
• Absolutely not to be done.
• Much of the information in the passage is not required to answer the questions.

Skimming/Reading
• Most reasonable/effective approach.
• This is a mixture of skimming but reading enough to get the overall feeling/gestalt of the passage.
• The purpose is to get the "gestalt" and where information is located.
• To make efficient the back and forth trips between questions and the passage, use Highlighting **(SB B.6, B.7)**.

B.4.2 How to Attack Passages by Attacking the Questions

Factors to consider:

• Number of questions

 - If more than 5, don't skim questions; go over passage.
 - If 5 or fewer, skimming questions may help, but generally not recommended.

• Length of questions

 - Long or complex questions — little value in skimming.
 - For short, simple, or direct/specific references, there is possible value in skimming.

Section B: Verbal Reasoning Analysis

B.4.3 What to Focus on when Skimming Questions

- To make back and forth trips between question and passage efficient, use highlighting.
- Look for direct references: specific line, paragraph, chart, table, etc.

- Look for specific references: specific person/place/thing/event noted.
- Look for "according to passage/author," etc.
- *See* examples under Answer Location Analysis **(SB B.6, B.7)**.

B.5 Inferences

B.5.1 Example of Drawing Inferences

Inferences are important for the MCAT because many questions directly or indirectly test the students' ability to work with inferences. This is only to be expected, because the MCAT Verbal Reasoning section (and to some extent, the Writing section) is designed to test critical thinking skills, and the ability to draw inferences is probably the most important critical thinking skill. We all work with inferences daily, although we may not be aware that we are doing so. Let me give you a simple example of inferences at work in an everyday context.

It is around 7:30 am, and I'm accompanying my two sons, aged 4 and 7, to school in a taxi. On the way, we see a big puddle of water on the road, and this triggers a logical question from the kids: "Where did that water come from?" Three brains swing into action. "Maybe it rained at night," the younger son suggests. "But the rest of the road is dry," objects his brother. He's right; everything else in sight is bone dry, except for that mysterious puddle. "Perhaps a water pipe burst," I suggest. As we mull over this, the driver, who obviously has been following the conversation keenly, volunteers: "The water is from the gas station. They wash a lot of cars." His tone is authoritative, and I realize he must be right. There is a gas station next to the puddle. The clincher for me is that the driver must have personal knowledge of the operations of gas stations on account of his profession; indeed, he may even have had his car washed at that very station, and observed the puddle forming.

This is a typical example of how we work with inferences. On the basis of a known fact, namely, the puddle on the road, we hypothesize about something unknown, namely, the cause of the puddle. All of us perform this kind of thinking dozens of times daily; indeed, we couldn't get through life without drawing inferences.

B.5.2 Definition of Inference

Let us now look more closely at inferences. The best definition of an inference is given in an excellent book on semantics by S.I. Hayakawa, Language in Thought and Action: "An inference, as we shall use the term, is a statement about the unknown made on the basis of the known." He then goes on to give examples of inferences in a wide variety of contexts: "We may infer from the material and cut of a woman's clothes her wealth and social position; we may infer from the character of the ruins the origin of the fire that destroyed the building; we may infer from a man's calloused hands the nature of his occupation; we may infer from a senator's vote on the armaments bill his attitude toward Russia; we may infer from the structure of the land the path of a prehistoric glacier; we may infer from a halo on an unexposed photographic plate its past proximity to radioactive materials; we may infer from the sound of an engine the condition of its connecting rods.

Inferences may be carefully or carelessly made. They may be made on the basis of a broad background of previous experience with the subject matter or with no experience at all. For example, the inferences a good mechanic can make about the internal condition of a motor by listening to it are often startlingly accurate, while the inferences made by an amateur (if he tries

to makes any) may be entirely wrong. But the common characteristic of inferences is that they are statements about matters which are not directly known, made on the basis of what is observed."

Another important characteristic of an inference is that an inference is not a directly stated fact. Here is how Annette Rottenberg puts it in her Elements of Argument (third edition): "By definition, no inference can ever do more than suggest probabilities. Of course, some inferences are more reliable than others and afford a high degree of probability. Almost all claims in science are based on inferences, interpretations of data on which most scientists agree. Paleontologists find a few ancient bones from which they make inferences about an animal that might have been alive millions of years ago. We can never be absolutely certain that the reconstruction of the dinosaur in the museum is an exact copy of the animal it is supposed to represent, but the probability is fairly high because no other interpretation works so well to explain all the observable data — the existence of the bones in a particular place, their age, their relation to other fossils, and their resemblance to the bones of existing animals with which the paleontologist is familiar. Inferences are profoundly important, and most arguments could not proceed very far without them. But

Section B: Verbal Reasoning Analysis

an inference is not a fact."

To illustrate this point, let us return to the puddle of water of the **SB B.5.1** example. Three inferences were made as to the cause of the puddle: rain, a burst water pipe, and effluent from a gas station. We decided that the last inference was most likely true. Nevertheless, it is not a fact, merely an inference with a high probability of being true. Now, imagine that we stop the taxi and ask an attendant at the gas station about the puddle, and he confirms that the puddle is indeed due to washing cars at the station. At this point, our inference is no longer an inference; it has become a fact (assuming that the attendant is telling the truth, which would be a reasonable assumption in everyday life but perhaps not in a court of law). This is an important point to remember when answering inference questions on MCAT passages: an inference cannot be a directly stated fact. Therefore, an inference cannot be anything directly stated in the passage. You must logically extend the information provided by the author in the passage to arrive at a conclusion, or inference. In other words, consider what the passage implies, not what it directly states, when asked to draw an inference. There are various ways of inferring the author's opinions as expressed in the passage. The passage could be one-sided in that opposing viewpoints are not mentioned at all or dismissed after a cursory examination. In other cases, the author's true feelings could be betrayed by loaded words.

B.5.3 Drawing Inferences

Let us look more closely at the mechanics of how we draw inferences. We have seen that an inference is a statement about the unknown based on what is known. What is known, or observed, is called the premise. The link between inference and premise is called the argument. In a passage, words and phrases such as since, because, given that, if, assume, suppose, in case, etc., signal premises. Inferences are signaled by words such as therefore, thus, hence, etc. Inferences may be either deductive or inductive. A deduction is an inference that has to be true if all the premises are true. For example: (1) All Americans are good-natured; (2) Jones is an American; (3) Jones is good-natured. Statements 1 and 2 are premises, and statement 3 is the inference.

It is clear that if both premises are true, then the inference must be true. However, if either premise is untrue, the inference is undermined.

In an inductive argument, it is likely (but not certain) that the inference is true if the premises are true. Here is an inductive argument: (1) Americans are usually good-natured; (2) Jones is an American; (3) Jones is good-natured. If both premises are true, it is likely, but not certain, that the inference (statement 3) is true. All this suggests that one way of tackling questions that ask one to select an option that invalidates an argument is to show that the premises of the argument are false.

B.5.4 Inductive Arguments

A final point should be made here regarding inductive arguments: the most common definition of an inductive argument is that an inductive argument is one that draws a general conclusion from a limited number of observations. For example, from past observation that the sun rises daily in the east, we conclude that the sun will continue to rise daily in the east in future. Is the conclusion justified from this observation alone? Strictly speaking, only additional evidence — astronomical evidence — can enable us to categorically conclude that the sun will continue to rise in the east and set in the west on a daily basis, barring some catastrophe in outer space.

We lean heavily on this type of inductive reasoning — in which we arrive at general conclusions from specific observations — in our daily lives, which is why the previous definition of inductive reasoning (forming a general conclusion from specific instances) is common. However, it is important to understand that this definition is not accurate, and that the earlier definition is the correct definition, namely, that an inductive argument is one in which the conclusion is supported — but not ensured, as in deductive reasoning — by the truth of its premises. (Recall that the first example of an inductive argument given earlier, dealing with good-natured Americans, moved from the general to the specific.)

B.6 Highlighting: Basic Approaches and Skills

(*see* Highlighting: Advanced; **SB B.7**)

B.6.1 Definition of Highlighting

It is important to develop the skill of concisely and effortlessly highlighting certain words and phrases as you Skim **(SB B.1.2, B.3.2)** the paragraph. The point of this process is to be able to quickly refer back to the paragraph and find the key words or phrases that might appear in the questions. You do NOT want to try to read carefully or remember everything in the paragraph … this would be time consuming and wasteful. But, the ability to pick out a limited number of phrases or words so that they can be

Section B: Verbal Reasoning Analysis

found rapidly is critical. You should practice on each paragraph and test to enhance these skills. The following is done on the first skim of the paragraph without looking at the questions. You can then compare what was underlined for yourself and what was eventually asked. There should not be a 1:1 correspondence. You should have highlighted phrases or words that are not important in the questions. There will be questions relating to areas of text you may not have highlighted. The process will be for you to learn what has the greatest probability of being used in a question by committing yourself first, and then looking at the words/phrases you selected, noticing which words/phrases you missed, and, then over time, trying to make them converge.

B.6.2 How to Highlight Effectively

Again, you want to do this quickly, because you are SKIMMING and not studying the passage. Some pointers for highlighting all passages:

1) New words, ideas or concepts: If these occur repeatedly, underline each occurrence and place an asterisk, underline, or other marking available at the site where it is explained or defined (if it is).

2) The statements after transitions, clue words or phrases (such as "but," "on the other hand," "I emphasize," "I feel," "I believe," "therefore," "because," "yet," etc.); sometimes these transitions or clue words will follow the key phrase/word.

3) Italicized words or phrases.

4) Words or phrases in quotes.

5) The central thesis (the same as the author's general point of view), if you can easily identify it:

For the central thesis, remember that the whole passage centers around it. Each example, each secondary thesis or contention, relates back to the central thesis. You will find statements that seem important or critical, but they are not the central thesis; they are contained within themselves. Also, the central thesis will appear in multiple locations and the use of the examples and secondary contentions will relate to it and not vice versa.

It is very important that you develop a good idea of the central thesis and the author's viewpoint as you go about your skimming and highlighting. It is noteworthy that ExamKrackers, one of the few commercial prep companies with suggestions that have value, focuses entirely on understanding the author and the central thesis without highlighting. If you are able to do this, it can be a good approach to many, but not 90 percent, of the questions. You should determine if you are a "gestalt" person, being able to pick out the central thesis and author's point of view easily, or if you need highlighting, or if you function better with a mixture of both. We do recommend understanding and trying their approach if highlighting per se is not effective for you. See the detailed discussion of Central Thesis Analysis **(SB B.8, B.9)** to develop this critical skill.

6) Secondary contentions or theses, if you can easily identify them (*see* VR: Answer Location Analysis).

7) Examples or data to support ideas and contentions (*see* VR: Answer Location Analysis).

8) Notice that equations, graphs, or charts, which are easily found, do not need to be underlined (mainly for science passages).

B.6.3 Special Instructions for Science Passages

You should practice highlighting the science passages, but you should use some additional techniques:

1) Do not highlight charts, graphs, reactions, equations, etc. proceeded by/attached to a specific label, for example, "Equation 1," "Reaction 1,"

or similar specific description. These are "obvious" in terms of their locations in the passage.

2) Pay special attention to specific pieces of data such the $c = 3.0 \times 10^8$ m/s^2.

B.6.4 How to learn by Highlighting (Underlining)

1) Highlight the science and the verbal passages.

2) Do your highlighting prior to reading the questions.

3) Because the test on the computer will not allow you get your highlighting easily, you may want to print it out,

and highlight and take the test on paper so you can have it intact to refer to. Go back over what you highlighted and compare that to actual questions asked and how you answered them.

4) Alternatively, you can highlight on the site, use your "Print Screen" or "Prt Srn" or some variation (you will need

to determine this on the basis of your keyboard), then paste the screen to a Word document (or other equivalent document) that you can refer to (note: to enlarge the image, use your "View" and then "Zoom" function from your top menu of your Word document).

5) Determine how many of the questions were helped by your highlighting/ underlining, and try to determine what you did and how that underlining helped.

6) Determine which of the questions were missed by your highlighting/ underlining and why, and try to correct this on the next passage.

7) Compare your highlighting to the sample highlighting in the CBT Solutions (notice this was not made by an expert nor were the questions looked at prior to the highlighting). You should then go back to the sample highlighting provided, and determine how it could have been more efficient, streamlined, and accurate. For example, what words could have been excluded without your losing the information in that phrase. In a passage on Frankenstein, the following was highlighted, "longing for his forbidden knowledge" and "Ellen Moers has pointed out". It would have been just as effective and efficient to highlight "forbidden knowledge" and "Ellen Moers" only. You would have still found the area by these key words/

phrases. You want to learn to highlight only critical information that helps you locate the area of the passage you need to answer a question.

8) Remember a question may use a phrase or word that you have highlighted, but may also use a related concept or idea (an example is "deleted" in the question, and "removed" in the passage).

9) You can compare your highlighting to those found in the CBT Solutions.

10) As you practice, you will need to realistically time yourself. We suggest you purchase a timer (*see* Timing; **SB B.2.3** for a free online stopwatch), such as that used for chess matches. One that you can click on as you start and will go "ding" after a set time, or one you can click to stop the timer.

Your goal should be to complete your highlighting within 40 seconds for each half column of the passage. For example, if a passage runs for 1.5 columns, then you want to complete your skimming and highlighting within $3 \times 40 = 120$ seconds. As you practice more and more passages, this goal should become achievable. If not, then set your goal at 50 seconds per 1/2 column. Generally, you should NOT take more than 180 seconds (3 minutes) per passage for skimming and highlighting and determining the central thesis. Taking 3 minutes to skim will allow you about 1 minute per question on the average six-question passage.

Nearly all passages will have from five to seven questions per passage. Time is critical on the Verbal Reasoning test. You have to practice, practice, practice to optimize your skills to be able to complete all of the passages.

11) Also, remember that the actual test may not allow the retention of the highlighting if you leave the passage. This may change, but ask about the current ability to retain your highlighting if you leave the passage. Otherwise, you will have to factor this into your test-taking strategy.

12) As you are answering questions and skimming over your highlighting, you will find that you will gradually develop a better comprehension of the passage. In effect, you have internally organized the passage. This is just a by-product of good and effectively highlighting. You will find that your scanning over your highlighting to answer one question may help you when you go to the next question.

13) When you study the CBT Solutions we provide, you will find that multiple areas of highlighting may be shown and each option may be discussed in some detail. This is for learning only.

During the real test, you will need to have developed the skill and confidence to know when you have found the correct option and can move on, because time is of critical importance.

14) View highlighting as your secret plan to speed reading. One of the tenets of speed reading is that you "see" the print in chunks. Good highlighting will accomplish this. So, when you go through the passage to find the solution to a problem, you are able to take in large portions of the passage simply by using your highlighting. Then using the suggestions here and in the advanced highlighting discussion, you can rapidly and efficiently locate the answer.

15) Finally, learn to trust your highlighting. Once you have fully practiced, and only after you have done this, then it is time to trust what you have highlighted. This means if something in a question or option is not found in your highlighting by a rapid scan, then assume it is NOT in the passage. The time it will take you to find something which is not highlighted will result in too much wasted time. If your highlighting skills are good, then this will rarely happen. Time conservation will be most positively affected by assuming the option is incorrect and moving on.

B.7 Highlighting: Advanced Concepts and Skills

(*see* Highlighting: Basics; **SB B.6**)

These additional skills are developed as a result of the study and analysis of the application of the Basic Highlighting techniques to actual AAMC CBT questions.

You should study and practice these suggestions to further understand and improve your highlighting.

B.7.1 A true and pertinent statement from the passage

These are the statements which have direct or a close indirect link to information found in the passage and will help answer the question correctly. For example, the following question was asked in a passage on partisanship: "According to the passage, one drawback of partisanship is that it can:". Then one of the options was "distort voters' views of reality." An underlined phrase was "distort their picture of reality." So, this was nearly the same phrasing, and it was the correct answer.

B.7.2 A true but nonpertinent statement from the passage

These are the statements which are directly or indirectly tied to information in the passage and are true. However, they have no relevance to the question. They are a misdirection. If you do not fully understand their context, because you have read them, and they seem true, you may think they are correct; yet they are not. For example, a CBT question presented a study related to economic conditions and then asked how that information would impact the author's assumptions. One option was "they cooperate only with other jurisdictions within the same state." That subject is, in fact, in the passage and is a true statement. But it is completely unrelated to the issue involved with "economic conditions," which is discussed in a different paragraph and has no connection to one on state cooperation. In fact, in the pertinent paragraph, intrastate cooperation is explicitly discussed.

Another variation on this type is the true statement as a specific reference, and often an example, found in a completely different paragraph, but the question attempts to use it to explain something referenced in a totally different paragraph. But there is no reference or discussion of it in the totally different paragraph. For example, in a passage dealing with the history of scientific thoughts and laws and the public acceptance of them (a real AAMC CBT passage and question), the stem states, "According to the author, our social, political and moral beliefs:". One option is "grew out of the acceptance of Darwinism and Marxism among educated people in the late nineteenth century." The reference in the stem was found by indirect highlighting located in paragraph 5 nearly stated word for word.

The reference to "Darwinism and Marxism" was found in paragraph 2 as an example.

In paragraph 2 they do state that Darwinian and Marxist beliefs were eventually accepted, and that ""nonscientific" beliefs of reflective people" were eventually modified. But this was not specifically tied to "social, political and moral" as was specifically done in paragraph 5. Also, what is meant by "nonscientific beliefs"? Are these supposed to be "social, political, moral" beliefs, or just that the beliefs were NOT scientific? The Darwinian/Marxist answer was incorrect. So, be careful of the location and the specific use of examples and keep them at one location unless there are really compelling reasons not to do so.

B.7.3 Rephrasing of a statement from the passage

An example of a rephrase from the passage is found in a passage dealing with human learning as: "The author asserts that children can infer the rules of their language without explicit instruction. Yet, the speech of older children is often ungrammatical by adult standards. Can these two assertions be reconciled by the author's argument?"

In some of these, you will need to use logic to arrive at the answer and may not need to refer to the passage. In others, such as this one, by finding the rephrased statement, which was easily found by the highlighting, it led to the location where the answer was easily found.

B.7.4 Introduction of new information or apparently new information

(Not found in your highlighting)

Some will appear to be from the passage but are not. A real example is a passage which discusses "schemas" and how these

are used in memory and recall. One option in a question states "scripts cannot be partially activated." Were "partially activated" schemas discussed? Certainly "activation" of schemas was discussed in multiple locations. Would you have highlighted "partially activated" or "incompletely activated" or some other related description? Since the stem asked if the statements in the options "would best support the assertion," this means that statement, or a simple inference from it, must have been in the passage. Highlighting did not pick up anything close to this. So, again, did you miss it? A review, for learning purposes, showed that the phrase "partially activated" was not anywhere in the passage. The phrase was an attempt to make you think it was. Good and confident highlighting could have worked for you by your knowledge that you would have picked that phrase up as important. Since you did not, it was probably not there.

Overall, the options in the questions have some connection to the passage, and it is critical to appreciate and capitalize on this. There are very few options which are not connected to the passage directly, by a one step inference, by simple rephrasing, or by similarity of meaning of some type. Effective highlighting is critical in this time-limited test to make your navigation back and forth between questions, options, and the passage as efficient and effective as possible.

　　i. Some will appear to be "great-sounding" options but have no connection to the passage and are Complex Sounding Options **(SB A.2.2)**. In the passage on "schemas," the stem asks you to determine which option "would best support the assertion that." An option given is "schemas are instantiated subconsciously." The

word "instantiated" is highlighted twice. In neither location is there any reference to "subconsciously" or "consciously." In fact, there is no place in the passage where this is found. The connection of "subconsciously" to "instantiated" is similar to the prior discussion. But it "sounds good" that these "schemas" found deep in the brain are pulled out "subconsciously." And, in fact, they probably are "instantiated" subconsciously. But there is no such statement or discussion in the passage. This is why they are Complex Sounding Options and cannot be correct.

　　ii. Some will be new-information options with a simple inference to connect them to the passage and may be correct. Some will be totally new information with no connection to the passage. In these, you will often have to use logic to determine if the option is correct or not. For example, a question regarding Neanderthals was, "The statement that stone tools "signal the pace of change in human prehistory" means that:". The part in quotes is directly from the passage and has simply been pulled out and placed in the stem. Sometimes this will mean that you do not even have to refer back to the passage; other times you will. This phrase was not highlighted, but "stone tools" was, which allowed rapid location of the discussion and review to determine the answer.

Typical of the options is, "changes in tools indicate changes in the toolmaker." This option has no connection to the passage. So, there is NO need to try to find it. Part of your ability to recognize this will come as your practice. If you do not immediately recognize it, you can do a quick scan, and you will find nothing you can use to connect it to the passage. So, you have to rely on pure analysis and logic to answer the question. You may want to rescan the paragraph to get a feeling for the gestalt of the passage and the concept being discussed. In this paragraph, they were discussing changes over time, and your logical analysis should focus on this idea.

B.7.5 Quickly Locating the Answer in the Passage

Quickly locating the correct answer becomes important and your ability to quickly arrive at the best option. Normally, you will go through the options A to B to C to D. If A is the correct option, and you determine that with confidence, then you can move on rapidly. But, if D is the correct answer, how should you handle the other options.

E.g., a passage on red tides had the question "The author implies that the reason red tides are difficult to control is that:". Option A was "phytoplankton can multiply rapidly, covering extensive areas."

The highlighting had noted in paragraph 3 that "photosynthesize and multiply", "increase rapidly", "spectacular and catastrophic". Reading in this area, it is evident that this is considered a problem. In fact, the passage highlighting was consistent with the option and appears to be a reason that "red tides are difficult to control". If you are confident in your highlighting and analysis skills, you could stop here and move on to the next question. This option was the correct option. This question was rated as a "hard" question, but the effective highlighting rapidly found the answer and saved a lot of time.

E.g., the same passage on red tides had the following question and options: "Assume that a committee of environmentalists who are aware of the information in the passage is appointed to advise Congress on ways to reduce the problem of red tides. The members would probably recommend that:

A) fisheries release their products only in areas that are free of algae.
B) whales and other important marine life be driven away from affected areas.
C) herbicides be used to destroy all toxic species of algae
D) plant nutrients be removed from wastewater before it is released into waterways.

Using a combination of highlighting, rapid scanning and logic, you will find that options A, B and C have no specific highlighting related to the statements. There is highlighting relating to "fisheries' products", and "whales", but nothing on "herbicides". And these are somewhat vague and raise questions as you think about them. Remember if an option starts to generate more and more questions that are difficult to answer, more importantly have no answer readily apparent in the passage, it is most likely incorrect.

What you can do with these vague or out there options is to rapidly categorize them as such, then skip over them until you find an option that is definitely in your highlighting and may address the question. In the last paragraph, "rich in plant nutrients" is found. A quick read of the area tells you this is a

problem with wastewater and can set steps in motion that result in red tides. Logically, this is something that is achievable, but more importantly for your MCAT score, it is found directly in the passage. So, by rapidly skipping over vague options or misdirected options, you can arrive at the correct answer rapidly. This also was classified as a "hard" question.

B.7.6 Passage Evidence

a. A statement regarding facts present in the passage which is supported by direct/indirect evidence in the passage.

b. A statement which gives a direct clue to which highlighting may be important. There are many of these. In a passage on learning and memory, a question was, "To judge whether instantiation has occurred, a researcher would need to determine:" Because "instantiation" is an unusual term, the suggestion of highlighting it for each occurrence should have been done. It was in this case, and the student could rapidly find the locations to contextually define the word, understand and then answer the question.

c. A statement which gives an indirect clue to which highlighting may be important. For example, a CBT stem is, "The passage suggests that economic competition

between subnational units of government provides." The highlighting had found "effect of interjurisdictional competition." The stem is, in effect, asking about "competition" which is "subnational," which is equivalent to "interjurisdictional." So, this effective highlighting rapidly directs you to the correct paragraph. But you have to make some mental adjustments to realize that "subnational" and "interjurisdictional" mean the same thing; your vocabulary must be good. In this particular question, this highlighting "effect of interjurisdictional competition" does not provide the answer. But it directs you to the paragraph that does contain the facts to assess the option. You can then rapidly skim the rest of the paragraph and, in fact, you will find the details which can determine if the option is true or false.

B.7.7 Rephrasing the Stem

You must learn how to rephrase or make an inference and relate what is in the stem or option to what is in the passage. For example, a real CBT option states, "an increase in efficiency for the competing governments." But there is nothing in the passage dealing with "efficiency." However, the highlighting had "no overall increase" and this was, when fully reviewed, "no overall increase in national productivity." Then you can rephrase "efficiency" into "national productivity." Then, the option would be false, because you also can make the inference that "efficiency" and "national productivity" would be congruent; i.e., if one increased, so would the other.

The highlighting is to rapidly get you to the correct area by connecting key words or phrases, but you must then read in the area, and make other connections and inferences to arrive at the correct answer. For example, in the previous example, "increase" found in the option and "increase" found in the passage could have been enough to quickly visually connect the option and the passage. Then you quickly scan/read the area and you will find "national productivity," which should connect to "efficiency"; you can then infer that the passage is stating there is no increase in "national productivity," so there is probably no increase in "efficiency" and the option is a false statement. Time is of critical importance on this test. You need an effective method to navigate back through the passage; highlighting effectively is that method.

B.7.8 Rephrasing Information in the Passage

Often you will only need to use logic to answer this type of question. Sometimes you will need to use your highlighting to find the answers to these. For example, a question regarding Neanderthals was, "The statement that stone tools "signal the pace of change in human prehistory" means that:". The part in quotes is directly from the passage and has simply been pulled out and placed in the stem. Sometimes this will mean that you do not even have to refer back to the passage; other times you will. This phrase was not highlighted, but "stone tools" was, which allowed rapid location of the discussion and review to determine the answer.

Some stems may appear to require only logic or inferences to answer the question, but may really require good highlighting to find the exact answer. E.g., a passage on retirement communities had the question: "New arrivals at one retirement community were told by its director: 'You are like pilgrims crossing the ocean to take up a new life.'

Section B: Verbal Reasoning Analysis

This simile implicitly supports the author's assumption that those moving to retirement communities feel:"

So, you are asked to recall your understanding of "Pilgrims" and apply it to the passage. Option A was "ambivalence about the wisdom of breaking with the past". This may have been a concern with the pilgrims, but was it an assumption of the author? A scan of highlighted phrases/words showed no "ambivalence" raised by the author. Option B was "satisfaction at becoming independent of their families". Certainly, the pilgrims wanted their independence, but did the author assume this? Again the highlighting did not justify this statement.

Option C was "relief at leaving situations that had become difficult". Certainly, this was one of the reasons for the pilgrims' journey, but again the highlighting did not support this in the passage. Option D was "optimism about being among those with similar goals." The highlighting had found "friendships and endless pleasures", "new adventure", "traditions of their own", and "found in their segregated lives the advantages". These are more related to option D and are in the passage. So, even though you may first think that logic can answer the question, it still may depend on information in the passage that was rapidly found by good highlighting.

B.7.9 Clue Words and Phrases

To move through questions more rapidly, if you can use a clue word/phrase in the stem to find a key highlighting, then use the info in the area to rapidly scan the options to locate the correct option. The following is a question from a passage dealing with myths:

"A reasonable expectation for someone who accepts Freud's views on religion would be that:"

The highlighting and scanning of the location in paragraph 5 found the following: "Freud, religion was the obscessional neurosis of children, destined to be outgrown as humanity evolved."

What you want to do is scan the options to

see if anything is close to this statement. The options were:

" A) the religious will increasingly be considered mentally disturbed.
B) conversions form cults to the major religions will increase.
C) membership in nonreligious organizations will increase.
D) attendance at religious services will decline."

You can see that option D, "religious services will decline" is consistent with "destined to be outgrown". If religion is outgrown, fewer will attend. So, option D is the best option based on the highlighting. So, once you have found the highlighting and scanned the area around it, a quick glance and comparison to the options may reveal the answer.

B.7.10 Highlighting Context

As you are skimming the highlighting for a specific subject/phrase/word/idea, etc., quickly look at the words/phrases just before and after the highlighting for relevance. This is because you do not highlight everything initially, and some of the specifics for a particular stem/option may be just outside of the highlighting. Also, in a stem, there may be multiple possible connectors to the passage, but you may not have highlighted the key one, but you can use secondary words/phrases to get to the correct location. For example, a question on the AAMC CBT dealing with ethics is, "Which of the following actions is an example of what the author probably means in implying that giving can be an assertion of power?" In the passage highlighting, nothing related to "assertion of power" or neither of these words was individually highlighted. However, checking giving, "giving could be a minor" was found. Then quickly scanning the non highlighted sentences surrounding this, "assertion of his power" was found. This was the exact location where the answer was found.

You must be confident about your highlighting skills. The only way to get good at highlighting is to practice, practice, practice, and learn from your practice. You need to study the CBT Solutions to the Verbal Reasoning passages which we provide. This is because there will be a number of options which sound good but have nothing to do with the passage and which have no reasonable inference, on your part, to be true. For example, a real CBT question was, "According to the passage, to whom might one look to foster cooperation rather than competition between jurisdictions?". One option was "Academic researchers." With good highlighting skills, "academic researchers" could have been highlighted; there was no highlighting present. However, "academic" and "researchers" are always a good option to look to for help.

So, did you miss the highlighting? This is when you have to be confident that you would have highlighted this, or something close/similar to it. Since there was no highlighting, the passage did not discuss this. Whether it sounds good or not, if it's not in the passage and if you can't make a simple inference to get to it, it cannot be true. You assess it as false because it is a Complex Sounding Option **(SB A.2.2)**.

Section B: Verbal Reasoning Analysis

B.7.11 Word Repetition

Unusual words which are repeated may need to be highlighted with each occurrence. If an unusual word, phrase, concept, idea, etc., appears in multiple locations, it is probably going to be significant in the passage. Because you don't know which location will become a question, you should probably just underline it with each occurrence. If there is a location where it is defined/explained, you should put an asterisk (or other mark available on the computer) at that location. For example, in a CBT passage, "instantiated" was used multiple times. So, it should be highlighted each time, and an asterisk placed at the location it is explained (if it was).

If the word is a key idea and is repeated over and over or referred to, then it may not be necessary to highlight every occurrence. For example, in a passage on memory and learning, "instantiation" was listed twice and was highlighted. In the same passage, "schema" was repeatedly used and referred to, and there was no need to highlight it every time. "Instantiation" came up in more than one question, as did "schema."

Even if you do not highlight everything that is present in the questions, if you have highlighted most of the pertinent words and passages, then this will give you time to scan the whole passage once or twice for some issue that you may not have highlighted. For example, in a real CBT question, the option stated, "scripts cannot be partially activated." There was no underlining of "partially activated" or anything close. So, you could just assume it wasn't there. If your highlighting has become skilled, then this is not an unreasonable assumption. However, if you are not fully confident, then you can scan the whole paragraph just to be sure. The whole passage was scanned and there was no direct or indirect reference to "partially activated." So, good highlighting had been done.

B.7.12 Key Words

You will want to highlight the general example or contention, but it is advisable to highlight some of the key details which follow the general point. For example, in a real AAMC CBT question dealing with partisanship, the stem queried why a republican, in a presidential election, had so many democratic votes. The highlighting pointed to "strengthen or weaken" as a general contention as to why individuals may go outside of party lines to vote for a candidate. If only that was highlighted, it may have been visually difficult to quickly locate the specifics of the question. However, "attractiveness of the candidates" and "foreign and domestic policy" were also highlighted as specifics of the general contention. This made it very easy to locate these, and they did point to the correct answer.

When reading the stem or options, you need to be able find key words or phrases which can direct you to your highlighting. For example, in a passage dealing with linguistic evolution, the following stem and options are found (this is an actual AAMC CBT):

Stem: "The passage suggests that creationists dislike the idea that certain biological structures may be:"

The key word here is "creationists". When the passage is scanned, these are found highlighted: "creationist opponents" and "argument of creationists." These highlighted areas pointed rapidly to the answer.

This is a simple example. Other key words may be in longer phrases or sentences. However, the point is that if you recognize them in the stem and options, you then rapidly search for them in the passage. For example, in a passage on an AAMC CBT dealing with partisanship, the following option is found: "personal qualities that made Eisenhower an especially attractive candidate."

The key phrase was "attractive candidate." Highlighted in the passage was the following: "attractiveness of the candidates." This was the location of the answer. Other phrases or words are possible such as "Eisenhower" or "personal qualities," but none of these were highlighted or found in the paragraph. You would have to realize that "Eisenhower" was a new-information example and was not expected to be found in the paragraph.

B.7.13 Gestalt Questions

Some stems and options will have fairly specific highlighting points which will help you arrive at the answer. These will be direct. Some questions will require a general gestalt for the passage. You are advised to practice recognizing those questions which will be answered by specific highlighting and those questions which will require a gestalt for the passage. Practice and experience and attention to the questions will help you develop these skills. For example, a passage dealt with Mary Shelly's Frankenstein. A stem of one of the questions was as follows:

"Apparently, the author's preferred approach to the interpretation of a novel is to concentrate on:"

The options were:

"A) the social attitudes of the intended readers.
B) the unconscious motives of the characters.
C) the socio-historical context of the plot.
D) correspondence between the characters and the novelist."

This was a "gestalt" question. There is no specific highlighting which would have helped answer the question. After reading and answering the other questions, and after repeated scanning of the passage and the highlighting that was done to answer those questions, it became evident that this was a "psychoanalysis" type discussion. There was no discussion of "readers," there was no "sociohistorical" commentary, there was some, but very little, relating characters to the "novelist." The "gestalt" was clearly one of "unconscious motives." And questions relating to "Oedipal Complex" and related thoughts and feelings of characters clearly pointed to the best answer to this question.

The general or gestalt type questions, those requiring information from multiple parts of the passage and deeper inferences, are questions that may be skipped over or placed into the Guess Question **(SB A.2.4)** category. The key is to recognize these rapidly so you don't waste time trying to solve them. Time is critical on this test.

B.7.14 References

When a specific reference is made, you must carefully read the information around it and that just preceding it. Look for any connections in the area of the reference. Be careful about information that is distant from the reference but appears correct. For example, in a passage dealing with Cezanne, a question was, "The author's suggestion that reality in art before Cezanne had been a "will-o'-the-wisp" can most reasonably be interpreted to mean that artists before Cezanne had not:" One option was "been able to perceive reality."

In the first paragraph, a statement was made, "penetrate to the reality that did not change." This was in reference to the other artists not doing this. So, this was a true statement and could possibly be correct. But, the "will-o'-the-wisp" had been highlighted and was rapidly found in the fourth paragraph. In the third paragraph, there had been a discussion of how the prior artists tried to depict reality using a technique, and a highlighting had noted "no more an accurate representation." This meant the artists had not succeeded in representing reality.

Then reading in the highlighted area of paragraph 4, you find "One might conclude from the history of art that reality in this sense is a will-o'-the-wisp." This transition directly ties this to the prior paragraph. Then the correct option of "not ... found a way to depict reality effectively" becomes the correct option. This was a moderately difficult question as only 65 percent of students got it correct.

SECTION B

B.7.15 Use of General Knowledge

Occasionally, you will be required to use some general knowledge that is not found in the passage to answer a question. This is rare, but always be aware of the possibility. It will not be the focused or deep knowledge or understanding that you need for the Physical Sciences or Biological Sciences. For example, a question dealing with a passage about "Spiritual History of the Living World" had the following question:

"The author seems to be trying to understand:

A) the beliefs of primitive peoples from the perspective of an anthropologist.
B) the interactive balance among species from the perspective of an ecologist.
C) the orderly recurrence of natural forces from the perspective of a poet.
D) the genetic regulation of behavior from the perspective of a biologist."

Even though the passage focused on natural occurrences, much as an ecologist may view them, the answer was option C. Highlighting was not particularly helpful. The AAMC solution included this statement: "The poetic qualities of the passage occur in the emphasis on vivid physical descriptions and imagery that appeal to the senses or the emotions rather than reflect scientific accuracy." The test makers have the belief that scientists cannot write in expressive or beautiful prose. So, you would have to know the difference in how scientists write and how poets write to distinguish between options B and C.

B.7.16 General Idea of the Stem

Glance at the options, after reading the stem, to get an idea of the general area of concern of the stem. A stem can lead in multiple different directions. By looking at the options, you can determine the general direction which should become the focus of your highlighting search. For example, in a passage dealing with nations becoming economically competitive in a technological age, the question, the stem, was "Which of the following findings is most clearly contrary to the reported influence of the use of computers in the workplace?"

The options were:

"A) Office workers can follow computer-generated schedules with less training than they need to devise their own schedules
B) Executives who correspond with customers by letter generate more business than those who rely on e-mail alone

C) Workers using non automated production processes are more efficient than workers on automated assembly lines

D) Mechanics who use computerized diagnostic methods earn less than mechanics who use traditional methods."

The highlighting had found "computer-based methods" and "use computers." This was focused on because of the "use of computers" in the stem. Notice the exactness of the phrasing for the second highlighting. Reading in this area, you find, "Workers who use computers on the job also earn more than do those of the same education level who do not use computers at work." Can you determine the correct option using this statement from good highlighting (remember the "contrary" term)?

By a quick survey of the options, and then scanning in the area of good highlighting, you may be able to rapidly find the answer as in this example.

B.7.17 Secondary Thesis

Do not confuse secondary contentions, or theses (ST), with the central thesis (CT). The same is true of confusing the examples with the CT, e.g. in a passage discussing how to study literature, a question is "What is the main idea of the passage?"

The options are:

"A) Those who create literature understand it more completely than do those who only study it.

B) The methodologies of science and the study of the literature have many features in common.

C) There are valid methods for studying literature that differ from the methods of science.

D) The achievements of the humanistic disciplines have been obscured by the achievements of the physical sciences."

Each of these options had a specific reference in the passage (this was the actual highlighting chosen for this passage):

Option A is found in paragraph 1 as "distinction", "literature and literary study", "distinct activities", "one is creative, an art", "science, is a species of knowledge". This paragraph argues that it is not necessarily those who create the literature who can best study or analyze it. Yet, this is a secondary contention and not the central thesis.

Option B is found in paragraph 3 as "done with methods developed by the natural sciences", and in paragraph 4 as "overlap". So, there are statements by the author that "methodologies of science and the study of literature have many features in common". But, these are secondary contentions and not the central thesis. This is used to develop the central thesis. See discussion of option C.

Option D is found in paragraph 5 as "obscured by the theoretical and practical triumphs of the modern physical sciences". Again, this is a secondary contention provided to support the central thesis (see option C). Notice how the stem is nearly word for word from the passage.

Option C is found in paragraph 4 as "Literary scholarship has its own valid methods",

"not always those of the natural sciences", "intellectual". This is a succinct statement of the central thesis. All of the secondary contentions mentioned support and lead into this central thesis.

This example illustrates the difference between CT and ST and you should attempt to make this distinction as you read/skim/highlight the passage.

B.7.18 Phraseology

Sometimes you have to pay attention to the phraseology used in the question and options. Unless you have overwhelming reasons not to, try to be true to the phraseology of the question, e.g. a passage dealt with women writers:

"According to the passage, if women who write are labeled women writers, then eventually:

A) these women will become classical feminists.
B) these women will become political.
C) the human component of literature will disappear.
D) only male writers will be called writers."

One highlighting was of "write as women". This could be construed to be "women writer". Reading in this area, you find "Women who write with an overriding

consciousness that they write as women are engaged not in aspiration toward writing but chiefly in a politics of sex." This is a pretty strong connection between "write as women" and "politics". If you interpret "women writers" as "women who write," and that is not at all unreasonable, then this becomes a very good option. But, another highlighting found in another paragraph had the following: "born into one of two categories, women writer or writer" and "expected to be male". Reading in this area, you find "Writers will very soon find themselves born into one of two categories, woman writer or writer, and all of the writers will be expected to be male". This specifically indentifies "woman writer" and that "all of the writers will be male". This is identical to option D which turns out to be the best option. So, exact phrasing may be important sometimes. But, also see the previous discussion in **SB B.7.7** about similar meanings.

Section B: Verbal Reasoning Analysis

B.7.19 Guessing

It is equally important to know when to use highlighting as when it will probably be ineffective and time consuming. Also, you need to recognize the Guess Questions (SB A.2.4). An example from a passage dealing with the evolution of flowers:

Stem: "The ideas in the passage seem to derive primarily from:"

This was one of the most difficult questions on this particular test as only 30% of students got it correct; in essence, they all guessed. There are red flags regarding this question which should put it in the guess category and you should NOT spend a lot of initial time on it or maybe not any time at all. First, the stem "ideas in the passage seem to derive primarily from" contain a lot of warning words which portend problems on a timed test. The words "seem" and "primarily" are very nonspecific. They are warning you that this is a nebulous question.

There is no definitive answer to be easily found in the passage. The phrase "in the passage" is telling you that you have to consider the whole passage. All of these are telling you that you will have to do a lot of thinking and comparing of everything in the passage. There is no easy highlighting here, there may be a central thesis here, but this is not about the central thesis. It's about how the ideas, which would be the central thesis, came about. The bottom line is that this should have been a Guess Question (SB A.2.4), in its purest form. You could use some Option Elimination Analysis (SB A.2.1) techniques or simply choose your Lucky Letter of the Day and move on.

B.7.20 Information Found in the Question

On occasion, you will be able to determine the central thesis from a question itself. While this is not directly an application or technique of highlighting itself, the observation is very important. Sometimes they will actually state the complete Central Thesis (SB B.8, B.9) in the stem of the question. Another presentation is found in the following passage example dealing with the evolution of flowers:

Stem: "The passage discussion most clearly suggests the hypothesis that as flowers evolve they increasingly form reproductive structures that:"

The correct answer was the option "exclude insects not of a particular type." When you combine the part in the stem of "As flowers evolve they increasingly form reproductive structures that" and the answer of "exclude insects not of a particular type", you effectively have a good statement of the central thesis as "As flowers evolve they increasingly form reproductive structures that exclude insects not of a particular type." This

answer could be arrived at by highlighting but also more quickly by understanding the Central Thesis **(SB B.8, B.9)**.

B.8 Determining the Central Thesis of a Passage: Part I

B.8.1 Definition of Central Thesis

One useful skill you will need to acquire to tackle the Verbal Reasoning (VR) section successfully is the identification of the central thesis (CT) of the passage. The CT of a passage is the main theme of the passage. It is what the author is trying to convince the reader of. Most MCAT passages present a point of view, or slant, on some topic. If you can identify this point of view, you are well on

the way to identifying the CT of the passage. The CTs of some passages are harder to identify than others. In some passages, all the questions may be based on the CT. In other passages, no question may be asked that involves the CT. Nevertheless, the ability to identify the CT of a passage is crucial to improving your score in this section.

B.8.2 Active Reading

Let us take a closer look at the act we are engaged in when we tackle the VR section: the act of reading. Most of us think of reading as a passive process, in contrast to activities such as jogging and working out at the gym. Get rid of that notion now. Reading, at least reading the kind of passages that are set for the MCAT exam, should be an active process. One must actively engage with the passage in order to understand it. Effort is

required because the ideas presented in the passages are, typically, complex. Unless the passage is actively read, confusion rather than comprehension will likely be the result. Therefore, do not be deceived by the apparent external simplicity of the act of reading. Appearances are deceptive. Beneath the calm and placid exterior, under the hood, the reader's brain should be humming with activity.

Section B: Verbal Reasoning Analysis

Almost anyone can "read" aloud an MCAT passage, even a student in primary school. Most words would be familiar, and the unfamiliar words can be pronounced in analogy with the pronunciation of familiar words. However, this robotic exercise does not constitute reading. Reading is concerned with extracting meaning from the author's sentences. Extraction of meaning from text operates at two levels. At the first level, we read individual sentences and understand what they individually convey. Almost any reader is capable of performing this task.

At the second level, we put together the individual meanings of individual sentences and try and synthesize from them a unified meaning. This is what makes reading a demanding activity: we have to see the individual trees (the sentences), and we also have to see the forest (the paragraph or passage as a whole). It is almost as though we have to see with a microscope and a telescope simultaneously. This dual nature of reading has to be clearly understood for optimal performance in the VR section of the MCAT examination.

As stated earlier, the first task in reading is to understand the individual sentences that make up a paragraph or passage. If the sentences are clearly worded and include no unfamiliar words, this task is usually simple. The second task — which is what separates the men from the boys — is to combine the individual ideas expressed by sentences into broader, more general ideas. The sentences may be well written, but the task of organizing them into a meaningful, unified whole has to be performed by the reader. This organization requires skill and a more than superficial level of comprehension. The writer's job is to write clearly; however, it is the reader's responsibility to distil, combine, and organize the writer's sentences into coherent units of meaning. This is why you should read actively.

While you read, your mind should be humming like the well-oiled engine of a well-maintained car. You will have to develop the skill of combining ideas expressed in sentences into larger overarching units of meaning. It is this reorganization of meaning that the reader must achieve if he or she is to formulate the central thesis of a passage, which is really a summary statement of the passage.

B.8.3 Extracting Information

Let us now see how this process of reorganizing meaning works in practice. To do so, we start at the very beginning and ask a fundamental question: How do we extract meaning from a sentence? A sentence conveys meaning by naming something and then making an assertion about what was named. The "something" named in the sentence is called the subject of the sentence. The assertion about the subject is called the predicate of the sentence. As an example, consider the following sentence:

"The sky was cloudy." The subject, that is, the part of the sentence about which something is said, is sky. The predicate, that is, the part of the sentence that says something about the subject, is was cloudy. Thus, a sentence is a group of words that expresses a single idea, the idea being embodied in an assertion about a subject. As stated earlier, it is relatively easy to understand the meaning of a sentence if it is clearly worded and contains no unfamiliar words.

A paragraph is a collection of sentences. A well-written paragraph is a group of related sentences. (MCAT passages are excerpts from articles or books authored by professional writers, so the paragraphs in such passages will almost always be well-written. Exceptions, however, do exist!) We can extract meaning from paragraphs similar to how we extract meaning from sentences. Since a paragraph consists of related sentences, every paragraph is governed by one main thought, the controlling idea. The controlling idea of a paragraph is expressed in a sentence called the topic sentence. Just as the subject of a sentence tells us what the sentence is about, the topic sentence of a paragraph tells us what the paragraph is about. Just as the predicate of a sentence tells us something about the subject, the remaining sentences in the paragraph support the topic sentence by developing its controlling idea further.

B.8.4 Topic Sentence

How does one identify the topic sentence of a paragraph? When we read a paragraph, two questions should be uppermost in our minds: What is this paragraph about? How is this idea being limited or qualified? Once these two questions have been answered, the topic sentence of a paragraph can be identified by asking another question: Which sentence in the paragraph best expresses this idea? It is clear that these questions are not trivial questions, which again underlines the importance of active engagement with the text while reading. It is necessary to understand the relationship between the topic sentence and the developmental sentences in order to understand what the paragraph means, that is, what the paragraph is driving at. The topic sentence of a paragraph is usually found at the beginning or end of a paragraph. It is rare that a paragraph will not contain an expressed topic sentence. In this case, we will have to draft a topic sentence ourselves to express the purpose of the paragraph.

Now, a passage, just like a paragraph, will have a clear controlling idea. The controlling idea of a paragraph is the topic sentence. The controlling idea of a passage is the central thesis (CT) or thesis statement. The CT is a statement of the controlling idea of the passage. The CT will usually be found in the passage, but in rare cases, the CT may not be directly expressed in the passage.

Section B: Verbal Reasoning Analysis

In such cases, we will have to frame the CT ourselves in our own language. The CT of a passage will usually be found toward the beginning or end of the passage.

B.8.5 Finding the Topic Sentence

Now that we have familiarized ourselves with the previous theoretical framework, let us test ourselves with some practical exercises and see how the principles explained previously are applied.

Pick out the topic sentences in each of the following paragraphs:

(a) Repealing the drug prohibition laws promises tremendous advantages. Between reduced government expenditures on enforcing drug laws and new tax revenue from legal drug production and sales, public treasuries would enjoy a net benefit of at least ten billion dollars a year, and possibly much more. The quality of urban life would rise significantly. Homicide rates would decline. So would robbery and burglary rates. (Source: CBT3, Passage I)

(b) State and local governments have reacted to this situation by taking actions intended to make themselves more attractive to new and relocating enterprises. If a business firm is unhappy with conditions in a community, it may seek a new location, and it is likely to find other communities waiting with open arms. When the Mack Truck Company announced its intention to relocate its manufacturing facility from Allentown, Pennsylvania, it had an array of communities from which to choose. To make themselves more enticing, the beckoning jurisdictions (and their state governments) offered a panoply of incentives, including property tax abatements, below-cost land, infrastructure, and training programs for potential employees. Mack Truck decided to relocate to South Carolina. (Source: CBT5, Passage I)

(c) The standard story told of Picasso is that his precocious talent enabled him to surpass, without effort, all other artists in his milieu. It is worth considering Picasso's own opinion that what is often considered early genius is actually the navet of childhood. "It disappears at a certain age without leaving traces." It is possible that a young child who shows unusual flair will one day become an artist, but he or she "will have to begin again from the beginning. I did not have this genius. For example, my first drawings could not have been hung in a display of children's work. These pictures lacked childlikeness... At a youthful age I painted in a quite academic way, so literal and precise that I am shocked today." At an exhibition of children's art, Picasso once quipped, "When I was their age, I could draw like Raphael, but it has taken me a whole lifetime to learn to draw like them." (Source: CBT3, Passage V)

(d) Thus, there are very different levels of friendship, levels which are understood in moral terms, in terms of how fully one cares for the other. Friendship always involves a giving of self to the other and a valuing of the other for his or her own sake. Friendship is an expression of moral activity on our part. (Source: CBT3, Passage VII)

B.8.6 Answers

(a) The topic sentence is the opening sentence of the passage: "Repealing the drug-prohibition laws promises tremendous advantages." The other sentences in the paragraph develop this controlling idea.

(b) Again, the topic sentence is the opening sentence of the passage: "State and local governments have reacted to this situation by taking actions intended to make themselves more attractive to new and relocating enterprises." The other sentences in the paragraph describe a concrete example illustrating the idea contained in the topic sentence. (Note: Topic sentences of paragraphs, if they exist in the paragraph, are usually found at the beginning or end of the paragraph.)

(c) The ideas expressed in this paragraph are complex. Therefore, it is difficult to pick out a single topic sentence that can stand on its own; more than one sentence is required for clarity. Here is

one attempt: "Picasso contrasts children's art with the academic art of adults. According to him, the best art has to resemble the art produced by children, which has a special quality made possible by the navet of childhood. Picasso himself painted like an adult as a child, and had to work hard to paint like a child as an adult." However, under the time constraints of the MCAT examination, clarity can be dispensed with; brevity is the key. Thus, the following paradoxical sentence could be framed as expressing the key idea of the paragraph: "Picasso himself painted like an adult as a child, and had to work hard to paint like a child as an adult." Clarity is sacrificed, true, but you should internalize the supporting detail. The skilled reader need only underline the somewhat cryptic last sentence of the paragraph: "At an exhibition of children's art, Picasso once quipped, 'When I was their age, I could draw like Raphael, but it has taken me a whole lifetime to learn to draw like them.'" The supporting explanation would be internalized.

(d) This is a very short paragraph. Why? A clue is that it begins with the word "Thus." Actually, this paragraph summarizes the argument of the passage. The topic sentence of the paragraph is the first sentence: "Thus, there are very different levels of friendship, levels which are understood in moral terms, in terms of how fully one cares for the other." Not surprisingly, this sentence also happens to be the central thesis of the passage.

B.8.7 Argumentative Topic Sentences

Most MCAT passages have an argumentative edge. Topic sentences and thesis statements in such passages will usually clearly express the author's attitude about the subject under discussion. Pick out the key words in the following topic/thesis sentences that reveal the author's attitude to the subject.

(a) Alcohol consumption is a form of escapism.
(b) Religious beliefs are necessary for a person to lead a moral life.
(c) Abolishing the death penalty will increase crime.
(d) Nuclear weapons testing should be suspended.
(e) Medicine has become so technology-oriented that it is no longer a "caring" profession.

Answers:

(a) The key word is escapism. The author's attitude to alcohol can be expected to be negative.
(b) The key words are necessary and moral. The author's attitude to religion is positive.
(c) The key words are increase crime. The author wishes to retain the death penalty.
(d) The key word is suspended. The author is against nuclear weapons.
(e) The key words are no longer. The author believes that reliance on technology has dehumanized modern medicine.

B.9 Central Thesis Analysis: Part II

B.9.1 Analyzing a Passage

Let us now analyze a passage from CBT6 in light of the previous information, paragraph by paragraph (indented paragraphs are from the passage):

Paragraph 1:

> Words provide clues about their history when etymology does not match current meaning. Thus, we suspect that emoluments were once fees paid to the local miller (from the Latin molere, to grind). Evolutionists have always viewed linguistic change as a fertile field for meaningful analogies. Charles Darwin, advocating an evolutionary interpretation for such vestigial structures as the human appendix and the embryonic teeth of whalebone whales, wrote: "Rudimentary organs may be compared with the letters in a word still retained in the spelling but become useless in the pronunciation but which serve as a clue in seeking for its derivation."

Which is the topic sentence in the opening paragraph? Here it is: Evolutionists have always viewed linguistic change as a fertile field for meaningful analogies. The other sentences in the paragraph serve to support this statement.

Paragraph 2:

> Scientists who study history, particularly an ancient and unobservable history, must use inferential rather than observational or experimental methods. They must examine modern results of historical processes and try to reconstruct the path leading from ancestral to contemporary words, organisms, or land forms. Once the path is traced, we may be able to specify the causes that led history to follow this, rather than another, route. But how can we infer pathways from modern results? In particular, how can we be sure that there was a pathway at all? How do we know that a modern result is the product of alteration through history and not an immutable part of a changeless universe?

Which is the topic sentence in the previous opening paragraph? Here it is: Scientists who study history, particularly an ancient and unobservable history, must use inferential rather than observational or experimental methods. The other sentences in the paragraph serve to support this statement. Note how the paragraph ends in a cascade of questions, an effective rhetorical device that underlines the difficulty of the problems of studying "unobservable history."

Section B: Verbal Reasoning Analysis

Paragraph 3:

This is the problem that Darwin faced, for his creationist opponents did view each species as unaltered from its initial formation. How did Darwin prove that modern species are the products of history? We might suppose that he looked toward the most impressive results of evolution, the complex and perfected adaptations of organisms to their environments: the butterfly passing for a dead leaf, the bittern for a branch, the superb engineering of a gull aloft or a tuna in the sea.

Note that this paragraph does not make sense by itself. The very first word of the paragraph (this) makes it clear that this paragraph continues the line of thought begun in the previous paragraph. A passage, after all, is a unified whole. With that point out of the way, let us once again ask: Which is the topic sentence in the opening paragraph? Here it is: How did Darwin prove that modern species are the products of history? Note that this question is not answered in the paragraph; the stage is only set for the answer in this paragraph. This is because the answer is so surprising, so paradoxical, that the author decided to dedicate a full paragraph to it (the following paragraph). Remember, writing is not an exact science; writers are entitled to artistic license.

Paragraph 4:

Paradoxically, he did just the opposite. He searched for oddities and imperfections. The gull may be a marvel of design; if one believes in evolution beforehand, then the engineering of its wing reflects the shaping power of natural selection. But you cannot demonstrate evolution with perfection because perfection need not have a history. After all, perfection of organic design had long been the favorite argument of creationists, who saw in consummate engineering the direct hand of a divine architect. A bird's wing, as an aerodynamic marvel, might have been created exactly as we find it today.

Which is the topic sentence in the opening paragraph? Here it is: Paradoxically, he did just the opposite. He searched for oddities and imperfections. Our topic sentence is made up of two sentences. That's perfectly alright. You can use as many sentences as are needed to express the controlling idea of the paragraph. Here, the two sentences express a single idea, which is why both sentences effectively begin with the word He. It may even happen that the paragraph does not contain a topic sentence. That would be an opportunity for you to be creative and manufacture the topic sentence yourself.

Paragraph 5:

But, Darwin reasoned, if organisms have a history, then ancestral stages should leave remnants behind. Remnants of the past that do not make sense in present terms — the useless, the odd, the peculiar, the incongruous — are the signs of history. They supply proof that the world was not made in its present form. Why should a general word for monetary compensation refer literally to a profession now virtually extinct, unless it once had some relation with grinding and grain? And why should the fetus of a whale make teeth in its mother's womb only to resorb them later and live a life sifting krill on a whalebone filter, unless its ancestors had functional teeth and those teeth survive as a remnant during a stage when they do no harm?

Which is the topic sentence in the opening paragraph above? Here it is: Remnants of the past that do not make sense in present terms — the useless, the odd, the peculiar, the incongruous — are the signs of history. They supply proof that the world was not made in its present form. Again, two sentences are needed because the controlling idea is complex. However, the two sentences express a single idea. Note that the subject of the second sentence (they) merely renames the subject of the first sentence, remnants of the past that do not make sense in present terms. The two sentences make assertions about the same subject, and therefore can be grouped together as a single unit of thought.

Paragraph 6:

No evidence for evolution pleased Darwin more than the presence in nearly all organisms of rudimentary or vestigial structures, "parts in this strange condition, bearing the stamp of unutility," as he put it. "On my view of descent with modification, the origin of rudimentary organs is simple," he continued. "They are bits of useless anatomy, preserved as remnants of functional parts in ancestors."

The final paragraph winds up the paragraph with a flourish, hammering the point home with a quote from Darwin himself. Now, what is the topic sentence of this final paragraph? Take a look at the final sentence of the passage. What does "They" stand for? Obviously, "rudimentary organs." Therefore, a possible topic sentence is, "Rudimentary organs are bits of useless anatomy, preserved as remnants of functional parts in ancestors". This statement is the climax that the argument has been inexorably building up to.

B.9.2 Topic Sentence Overview

Let us now line up the topic sentences one below the other:

"Evolutionists have always viewed linguistic change as a fertile field for meaningful analogies. Scientists who study history, particularly an ancient and unobservable history, must use inferential rather than observational or experimental methods. How did Darwin prove that modern species are

Section B: Verbal Reasoning Analysis

the products of history? Paradoxically, he did just the opposite. He searched for oddities and imperfections. Remnants of the past that do not make sense in present terms — the useless, the odd, the peculiar, the incongruous — are the signs of history. They supply proof that the world was not made in its present form. Rudimentary organs are bits of useless anatomy, preserved as remnants of functional parts in ancestors." We have here an outline from which a passage summary can be written. The outline does not read smoothly, but it can be fleshed out into a passage summary.

B.9.3 Finding the Central Thesis Using Topic Sentences

Now, where do you think the CT of the passage can be found? Usually, you will pick one of the previous topic sentences. Remember, the CT will usually be at the beginning or end of the passage. In our case, the CT, or thesis statement, is clearly the topic sentence of the last paragraph: Rudimentary organs are bits of useless anatomy, preserved as remnants of functional parts in ancestors. To this we add one key phrase that occurs in the last paragraph: evidence for evolution. The thrust of the passage is that rudimentary organs are evidence for evolution, which, with some elaboration, is the CT of the passage:

Rudimentary, or vestigial, organs such as the appendix in humans are evidence of evolution. They are remnants of organs that were once functional in ancestors. The second sentence of the CT was included for clarity; it is optional.

Additional Comment: You should note a key idea of this passage that follows directly from the central thesis: "Poor design is a better argument for evolution than good design." Also, it is difficult for creationists to account for poor design. Good design, on the other hand, can be explained satisfactorily by both evolutionists and creationists.

B.9.4 Central Thesis in Other Texts

You may wonder why every essay, article, or passage does not begin with a clear statement of the CT. Well, writing is not an exact science. Writers have different styles, and there are many ways of handling the same topic. Imagine how predictable reading would become if the CT were always to be found at the beginning of the text! Some authors delight in obscurity, and literary critics disagree even after decades of It is analysis. The passage selected is noteworthy for it's crystal-clear logic and faithful adherence to its thesis. Not all passages will be such models of clarity, because not all writers have a direct style. Some paragraphs may not have clear-cut controlling ideas. Jargon may get in the way of comprehension. Topic sentences may not be present in the paragraph. The CT of a passage may not be present in the passage. In such cases, be prepared to draft topic sentences and CTs in your own words. After all, MCAT passages are excerpts from articles and books, and not all excerpts read as well as the original.

It is important to know that you should not read an MCAT VR passage as you would read an MCAT science passage. As you read a VR passage, try and figure out what the author is driving at. Why did the author take the trouble to write the passage? What is he or she trying to say? How am I as a reader reacting to the author's persuasion? Do I find myself in agreement with the writer? Do I violently disagree with the writer? What is the purpose of this sentence or paragraph? (These are questions you do not need to ask when reading a science passage.) Engaging

with the passage in this way will help you grasp the contours of the author's argument. (Most MCAT passages present arguments.)

Look out for key words such as obviously, clearly, on the contrary, nevertheless, thus, however, further, but, also, etc. These words are clues to the writer's thought processes. Your goal should be to view the passage as a unified argument, not a bunch of facts. So, do not try and remember details; rather, understand how details contribute to the overall argument, how they relate to a central point. Also, you do not have to understand everything in the passage to understand the passage argument. Try and get the big picture. Remember, the central thesis of a passage simply captures the big picture in words.

Sources:
1. Reading to Discover Organization by Joseph Fisher, McGraw-Hill
2. Writing Clear Paragraphs by Robert Donald et al., Prentice Hall
3. From Thought to Theme by William Smith and Raymond Liedlich, Harcourt Brace Jovanovich

Chapter 1
PHYSICAL SCIENCES

Chapter 1

AAMC MCAT PRACTICE TEST 3

Explanations and Analysis for
Physical Sciences

MCAT

MCAT-Prep.com

Q01 — Pre-Study Suggestions

Review the following if needed:
1) Chemical Equations **CHM 1.5**
2) Three Out of Four Type Question **SB A.2.8**
3) Internal Inconsistency of Options **SB A.2.5**
4) Similar Pair Options **SB A.2.7**
5) What is the key piece of information from the passage required to answer this question?
6) Solve the problem.

Solution Discussion

The key piece of information is found in the description of Reaction 4:

"The PbCO$_3$(s) was removed … dilute HCl."

If you have to analyze a reaction, one skill you should have is to determine what are the reactants and the products. You are told some molecules react to release a gas. All of the equations have a gas on the product side, so this will not help distinguish between the choices. The stem (the question itself) gives you the reactants as PbCO$_3$ and HCl. These two compounds must appear in the reactant part, the left side of the equation. This means the only possible answers are A or C.

Option B is incorrect. The reactants are PbCO$_3$ and HCl and not Na$_2$CO$_3$ and HCl as shown in the option. So, there is no way this can be correct.

Option C is incorrect. The reactants are correct, but the chemical equation is totally unbalanced (*see* Stoichiometry **CHM 1.5**). It doesn't make a lot of 'chemical sense' either! The main way you determine this option is wrong is simply by doing a mass/atom balance. The oxygens and carbons are not balanced and there is no legitimate chemical means of getting them balanced.

Option D is incorrect. This is the same as option B. The correct reactants are not used. The PbI_2 is not the reactant of Reaction 4.

Option A is correct. It uses the correct reactants. The equation is balanced and makes chemical sense.

CHAPTER 1

Test Taking Skills Comment

A general understanding of chemical formulas and equations is needed as shown. With this knowledge, you should have eliminated options B and D immediately as neither had the correct reactants. You also eliminate option C because it is not balanced. Usually, but not always, it is necessary to have balanced chemical equations - to be safe (in order to get the right ratios), always make sure the equations are balanced or can be balanced.

In general, the MCAT does not expect you to be able to know reactions as in this example. When you are faced with a chemical reaction that you are not familiar with, look for other ways to eliminate options such as found in this one.

This question fits Three Out of Four/Similar Pair **(SB A.2.8)**. Options A, C and D all have Pb, in some form as a reactant - this is the three out of four. Then options A and C are similar in that both have $PbCO_3$ and the similar pair **(SB A.2.7)**. This suggests the correct option is from A or C. If you did not have an idea of the correct answer by applying your knowledge, then you would use this Option Elimination **(SB A.2)** technique to narrow down your options.

The molecular mass (MM) of a gas is what a cat does outdoors: "Dirt over pee"

$$MM = dRT/P$$

d = density, R = ideal gas constant, T = temperature, P = pressure; derived from $PV = nRT$, the ideal gas equation.

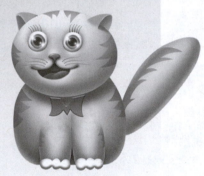

Internal Inconsistency of Options **(SB A.2.5)** is another Option Elimination technique useful here - option C has internal inconsistencies as described previously.

Options B and D are internally inconsistent because you are told the reactants are $PbCO_3$ and HCl - any equation that does not have these on the reactants side cannot be correct. Option C is also internally inconsistent because it is a non-sensical equation as discussed previously.

Q02 — Pre-Study Suggestions

Review the following if needed:
1) Solubility **CHM 5.3**
2) Common Molecules and Ions **CHM 5.2, 5.3.3**
3) Chemical Equations **CHM 1.5**
4) Three Out of Four Options **SB A.2.8**
5) Internally Inconsistent **SB A.2.5**
6) What is the key piece of information from the passage required to answer this question?
7) Solve the problem.

Solution Discussion

The key piece of information is the details of Reaction 1:

"$Pb(NO_3)_2(aq)$ was mixed with ... $Na_2SO_4(aq)$ ... All the $Pb(NO_3)_2$ reacted to ... precipitate"

From the key piece of information, you should determine that $Pb(NO_3)_2$ and Na_2SO_4 are the reactants. Since Pb^{+2} and Na^+ are positive (cations **CHM 5.2**), and NO_3^- and SO_4^{-2} are negative (anions **CHM 5.2**), and the product must contain a cation and an anion, this means the only possible products are $PbSO_4$ and $NaNO_3$ or option C or D as the only possible answer. Also the passage states that Compound A produces PbI_2 when reacted with KI, and so we know that Compound A must contain Pb.

Option B is incorrect. Where did the iodine come from? This is not some type of nuclear reaction **(PHY 12.4)** or radioactive decay **(PHY 12.4)** as these are the ways one element is changed to another. In chemical reactions, (*see* bond breaking mechanisms **CHM 3.3.3, ORG 1.1-1.6** and valence electrons **CHM 3.5**), the elements retain their individual identities, as it is the electrons that are rearranging and not the nuclei.

Option A is incorrect. The $Pb(NO_3)_2$ is a reactant and not a product and not a solid product even if it was a product because it is soluble in water as noted in the passage (it formed a solution).

Option C is incorrect. $NaNO_3$ is a theoretical product of the reaction, but it is a soluble compound. It is soluble on two counts. All sodium salts are soluble in water and all nitrates are soluble in water - (*see* solubility rules **CHM 5.3.2**).

Option D is correct. Sulfates are soluble except for a few which includes the lead. The reaction proceeds as follows:

$$Pb(NO_3)_2(aq) + Na_2SO_4(aq) \rightarrow Pb(SO_4)_2(s) + 2NaNO_3(aq)$$

Compound A reacts with KI to produce PbI_2 as follows:

$$PbSO_4 + 2KI \rightarrow PbI_2 + K_2SO_4$$

• this is a double displacement reaction **(CHM 1.5.1)** with the cations **(CHM 5.2)** switching and the anions **(CHM 5.2)** as well

• the complex ions **(CHM 5.2,**

5.3.3), nitrate and sulfate, exchange as a unit

• in oxidation-reduction reactions **(CHM 10.1)** and some others the complex ion may be broken apart

• the sulfate of lead forms a precipitate **(CHM 5.3)** which drops out of the water solution

• the nitrate of sodium is soluble in water and remains in the solution

• notice the charges on the atoms and the complex ions and charge balance and mass balance.

Test Taking Skills Comment

Solubility **(CHM 5.3)** can be a complicated concept (even beyond MCAT requirements). This question shows that you should have some understanding of the general solubility of compounds and ions.

This question is a Three Out of Four Options **(SB A.2.8)** question. Options A, B and D all contain Pb compounds. If you did not know

how to answer this question, you should make your guess from these options.

You could also determine that this is a Similar Pair Options **(SB A.2.7)** question because A and C both contain NO_3^-, but remember to only use the Similar Pair Options when Three Out of Four Options is not available and when there is only one similar pair.

Option B is eliminated because of Internal Inconsistency of Options (**SB A.2.5**) because I⁻ (iodide) is not a reactant in Reaction 1 which is where Compound A is formed.

Q03 — Pre-Study Suggestions

Review the following if needed:
1) Solubility **CHM 5.3**
2) Le Chatelier's Principle **CHM 9.9**
3) Acids and Bases **CHM 6.1, 6.2**
4) pH **CHM 6.5, 6.6.1**
5) Ion Product of Water **CHM 6.4**
6) Three Out of Four Options **SB A.2.8**
7) Camouflage and Distractions **SB A.1.3**
8) Solve the problem.

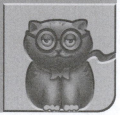

Solution Discussion

There is no information needed from the passage other than the equation which is given in the stem (**SB A.1**). The key is to recognize this is a Le Chatelier's problem (**CHM 9.9**) - there is a dynamic equilibrium and the change in pH would affect that established equilibrium. The equilibrium is given by the equation for the dissolution of $Pb(OH)_2(s)$ in water:

$$Pb(OH)_2(s) + H_2O(l) \rightleftharpoons Pb^{+2}(aq) + 2OH^-(aq).$$

The pH of pure water is 7.0. The new pH is 9.0, this increase in the pH corresponds to an increase in the concentration of the OH^-. If OH^- increases, in order to reestablish the equilibrium, a shift to the left will occur, and as a result less $Pb(OH)_2$ will dissolve (*option A is correct*).

Option B is incorrect. If any substance in the equation changes, then other substances in the equation will also change. If the pressure was increased or decreased, then the amount would not change. This is because gases, and hence pressure, are not factors in the equation and are not found in the equation. Also, a catalyst, if any, increased or decreased would not change the equilibrium of the equation.

Option C is incorrect. To get more of the $Pb(OH)_2$ to dissolve, the equilibrium would have to shift to the right. This would occur by increasing any substance on the left, other than $Pb(OH)_2$ or by decreasing any substance on the right of the equation. So, if OH^- would decrease, or if pH would decrease, then more $Pb(OH)_2$ would dissolve.

Option D is incorrect. See discussion in <u>Test Taking Skills Comment</u> which follows.

CATions are **PAWS**itive. An **ANION** is **A N**egative **ION**.

Test Taking Skills Comment

Usually, options which show no change or effect are incorrect as option D (mentioned previously). If you don't know the answer, it is better not to choose this type of option.

In chemical questions like this one, you might find it easier to conceptualize and solve if you write out the balanced equation as we have shown previously. The process of dissolution **(CHM 5.3)** is one in which the solvent surrounds each of the ions holding them in solution. The dissolution equation will then show this as done above. This is also an equilibrium equation **(CHM 4.3)** as the solid will move into the solvation phase and back to the solid phase.

Anytime you have an equilibrium, you may have the opportunity to apply the Le Chatelier's Principle **(CHM 9.9)** to solve the problem. The process of dissolution is an equilibrium process. Next, you must fully understand pH **(CHM 6.5, 6.6.1)** and pH changes and what they mean in terms of changes in the H^+ and OH^- which

are the acid and base **(CHM 6.1, 6.2)**, respectively, in all water solutions.

Since the pH of pure water is 7, which you must know, and the 'new' pH is 9, this means the pH will be increased and this is the direction of the comparison. To go from pH of 7 to a pH of 9, OH^- must be added or H^+ must be removed. Knowing these various pieces of information allows you to solve the problem. If you simply remembered that bases tend to be insoluble in bases **(CHM 5.3)**, the $Pb(OH)_2(s)$ is basic, then this compound would be less soluble in the higher, more basic pH.

This is a Three Out of Four **(SB A.2.8)** type question. Options A, B and C relate to the substance dissolving. Option D is an outlier and related to no change. Outlier options will usually be incorrect and can be ignored. This is also a Camouflage/Distraction **(SB A.1.3)** type question because you had to identify the need for the concept of Le Chatelier's Principle.

Q04   Pre-Study Suggestions

Review the following if needed:
1) Solubility **CHM 5.3**
2) Three Out of Four **SB A.2.8**
3) Three or More Steps Options **SB A.1.3**
4) Guess Questions **SB A.2.4**
5) What information is needed from the passage to solve the problem?
6) Solve the problem.

Solution Discussion

The following information is needed from the passage to solve the problem:

Reaction 1: $Pb(NO_3)_2$ reacted with Na_2SO_4 to form a white precipitate (Compound A).

> *Interpretation*: Compound A is $PbSO_4$

Reaction 2: KI is added to the $PbSO_4$ and PbI_2 is formed as a yellow precipitate.

> *Interpretation*: $PbSO_4$ is more soluble than PbI_2. The least soluble compound will precipitate out of the solution.

Reaction 3: PbI_2 was added to Na_2CO_3 and a precipitate of $PbCO_3$ formed.

Interpretation: PbI_2 is more soluble than $PbCO_3$.

Overall Interpretation: This then means $PbCO_3$ is more insoluble than $PbSO_4$ as well. The sequence of solubility would be $PbSO_4 > PbI_2 > PbCO_3$ (from more soluble to less soluble)

Reaction 4: not needed to answer this question.

When the Pb^{+2} is added to the solution, those compounds that are least soluble will precipitate out first. For the three ions above this means the precipitation order will be: 1 = CO_3^{-2}, 2 = I^-, 3 = SO_4^{-2}.

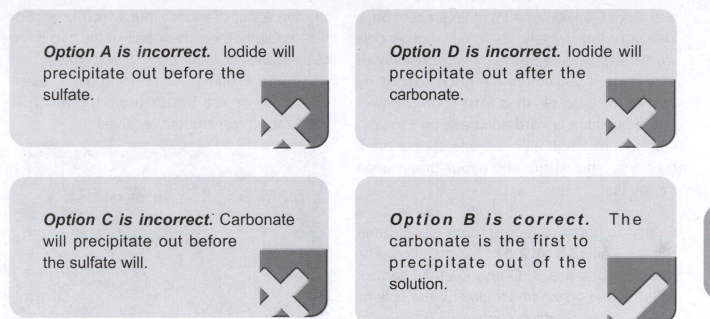

Option A is incorrect. Iodide will precipitate out before the sulfate.

Option D is incorrect. Iodide will precipitate out after the carbonate.

Option C is incorrect. Carbonate will precipitate out before the sulfate will.

Option B is correct. The carbonate is the first to precipitate out of the solution.

CHAPTER 1

Test Taking Skills Comment

This is rated as an extremely difficult problem as only 25% of students got it correct. A class of first graders would get the same percentage correct by guessing! Only a general understanding of solubility **(CHM 5.3)** is required to solve this problem. This requires in-depth analysis of the passage as I have shown previously. This is one of those very difficult and time consuming questions, Guess Questions **(SB A.2.4)**, which is best left to the end of the test. This is a guess question because of the level of reading and interpretation required.

You have to read and interpret nearly every reaction in the passage. Also, it is a Three

or More Steps Options **(SB A.1.3)** 1) you have to read each reaction involved to determine when the ion precipitates, 2) you have to then compare the two ions to determine if the option is true or false **(SB A.1.2)**, and 3) you then have to determine which option is correct **(SB A.1.2)** type question which means you have go through extra steps beyond those for the typical question. Valuable time, which may be used on questions you may have a better chance on, may be wasted trying to figure out this question.

Since only 25% of students got this correct, your guess would be just as likely to get you into this 25% without a lot of time spent on it. Use your time wisely. Each question is only worth one point whether it is very easy or very hard. If you've done a good solid study to prepare yourself, then trust your judgment that a question is hard and pass on it in your first go through. If all questions appear hard, then you should question your preparation for the test.

Finally, to guess, this is a Three Out of Four/Similar Pair **(SB A.2.8)** type question. The three options are B, C and D as all contain CO_3^{-2} in the option and another three options are A, B and D which contain I^-. The Similar Pair Options **(SB A.2.7)** is then B and D both of which contain I^- and CO_3^{-2}. So, if you had no idea, you could increase your guess rate, using your lucky letter **(SB A.2.4)**, by guessing from B or D for an increase to 50%. If you are less sure, you could select one of

the three out of fours - but which one? For this problem, the similar pair of the two three out of fours is a very good bet. Notice that whether you guess 1/3 or 1/2, both of these percentages are better than 1/4 which is what the typical student received.

A 'chemical' is a substance that:

An organic chemist turns into a foul odor.
An analytical chemist turns into a procedure.
A biochemist turns into a cycle.
A chemical engineer turns into a profit.

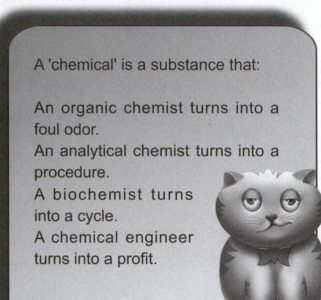

Q05 — Pre-Study Suggestions

Review the following if needed:
1) Chemical Formulas and Structures **CHM 1.2**
2) Concentration Units **CHM 5.3.1**
3) Moles **CHM 1.3**
4) Equation Interpretation
5) Similar Pair Options **SB A.2.7**
6) What information from the passage is needed to solve the problem?
7) Solve the problem.

Solution Discussion

The key information needed from the passage is:

"...mixed with 15.0ml of 0.300M Na_2SO_4(aq)."

The molarity (M) **(CHM 5.3.1)** (moles per liter = 0.300 M) is given as well as the volume (V)(15.0 ml = 0.0150 L). For each molecule of the Na_2SO_4(aq) in solution there will be 2 atoms of the Na^+. The moles of the Na_2SO_4(aq) in the solution is found by:

MV = moles in solution
= (0.300 M)(0.0150 L)
= (0.300 moles/L)(0.015 L)
= (0.300)(0.015) moles of Na_2SO_4.

The moles of Na^+ are then twice this number to give:

Number of moles of Na^+
= moles of Na_2SO_4(aq) x 2
= (0.300)(0.0150)(2) moles
= (0.300)(0.0300)
= 0.00900 moles.

This means the **correct option is B**.

Test Taking Skills Comment

This is rated as a difficult problem as only 40% of students got it correct. This is actually a study knowledge **(SB A.2.2)** problem of your understanding of moles **(CHM 1.1)**, chemical formulas **(CHM 1.2)**, concentration units **(CHM 5.3.1)** and solution chemistry **(CHM 5.3)**.

Don't make an arithmetic mistake. There is nothing of substance in the text, other than data (i.e., the numbers) required to solve the problem. Always write out the calculation instead of mentally doing it (unless you are very, very good and good under stress). These days we are so used to doing everything with calculators, mental calculations are becoming more risky unless you are very good at them or do a lot of them. Also, in calculations, it is generally best to hold calculations until all the steps have been completed.

Often numbers will cancel each other out and this will save you time and decrease the risk of errors in lengthy calculations (*see* approximation **PHY 2.6.1, GS A.6**). Editorially, calculators should be allowed as they are part of all of our everyday lives. The issue these days is do you understand and are you able to conceptualize and set up the problem and not just multiply or divide or take a square root in your head or on paper.

Finally, if you had to guess, this is a Similar Pair Options **(SB A.2.7)** type question. The similar pair is options B and D. Both have a '9' in it. So, if you had to guess, and wanted to use similar pairs to increase your guess rate, choose B or D for a 50% chance of being correct which is better than the 40% of students who got it correct. Also, the AAMC had an opportunity to use significant figures **(GS A.6)**, which they did not, but they may use it in the future (the answer on the test does not have the correct number of significant figures).

Q06   Pre-Study Suggestions

Review the following if needed:
1) Quantum Atom **PHY 12.5**
2) Electronic Transitions **PHY 12.5**
3) Photons **PHY 11.1**
4) Electronic Spectra **PHY 9.2.4**
5) Graphs and Charts **GS A.3**
6) Three or More Steps Options **SB A.1.3**

7) Similar Pair Options **SB A.2.7**
8) Complex Sounding Option(s) **SB A.2.2**
9) What information is needed from the passage to solve the problem?
10) Interpret the graph of Figure 2.
11) Solve the problem.

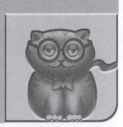

Solution Discussion

The pieces of information from the passage needed to solve this problem are:

Paragraph 2 - "A continuous spectrum is produced by bremsstrahlung ... collisions with ions"

Paragraph 3 - "A line spectrum results when an electron having sufficient ... an X-ray photon."

Last paragraph - "determine the relationship between X-ray... graphed the results of the experiment, as shown in Figure 2."

Interpretation of the graph of Figure 2:

The horizontal axis is the wavelength, λ, of the emitted photons. The wavelength is associated with a certain frequency, not noted, but as given in the equations, wave relationship **(PHY 7.1.2)** and Planck's relationship **(PHY 12.5)**. The vertical axis is I, intensity, of the photons emitted at the wavelength. It is proportional to the number of photons emitted at that wavelength. Since each wavelength represents a certain energy **(PHY 7.1.2)**, the greater the intensity means more photons are being emitted at that particular energy, or wavelength. The lower or curved line represents the bremsstrahlung. The sharp peaks mean there is an abundance of photons being emitted at a certain energy, wavelength value. Peak (1) occurs at a shorter wavelength but higher frequency and energy than does peak (2). Peak (2) has more photons emitted than peak (1).

Then synthesizing all of the above, it should be clear that the bremsstrahlung would have a smooth and continuous curve like the lower part of Figure 2 from which the peaks arise. The sharp peaks would represent a lot of photons of the same energy (frequency, wavelength) such as occur during a specific energy transition.

Option A is incorrect. The bremsstrahlung should occur as a continuous curve and not as peaks.

Option B is incorrect. The absorption of a photon could result in an electron excitation as discussed above. But, the spectrum would be an absorption spectrum **(PHY 9.2.4)** and would decrease the intensity of the electromagnetic radiation **(PHY 9.2.4)** detection and not increase it as shown in Figure 2 (which is specifically for emitted photons).

Option D is incorrect. The acceleration **(PHY 1.5)** of electrons does not produce electron transitions per se. The graph is specifically for emitted photons. This is a 'left field' or Complex Sounding Options **(SB A.2.2)** answer choice. While it is true electrons are affected and may be accelerated by the magnetic field force **(PHY 9.2)**, there is nothing in the passage (passage knowledge **SB A.2.2**) or from your study that could connect this statement and Figure 2; therefore, it must be incorrect.

Option C is correct. The graph depicts emitted photons. You are told that intensity is proportional to the number of photons emitted at a given wavelength. An atom will have specific energies, which correspond to the wavelength, or frequency, the peaks, at which electrons will undergo transitions. These are the transitions that occur as the electron moves from a higher n value to fill the void created when the electron is ejected from the lower n value. This is similar to an emission spectrum **(PHY 9.2.4)**.

A physicist places 2 identical cats on the roof at the same height and lets them both slide down at the same time (*please don't try this at home!*). One of the cats falls off the roof first so obviously there is some difference between the two cats.

What is the difference?

One cat has a greater mew.

P.S. mew (μ) is the coefficient of friction!

Test Taking Skills Comment

The use of Complex Sounding Options **(SB A.2.2)** was discussed in option D previously. This is also a Similar Pair Options **(SB A.2.7)** question. Options (B and D) are similar, because they deal with the transitions or excitations of electrons. If you had to truly guess, you could choose B or D to increase your odds. Similar Pair Options is most effective when there is only one set of similar pairs as in this question. This is also a Three or More Steps **(SB A.1.3)** type question (1) you have to read the passage to understand what Bremsstrahlung and the absorption/emission of photons represent, 2) you have to relate these concepts to the graph as the continuous line or the peak, 3) you have to determine what the line or peaks represent, 4) you have to determine if each option is true or false **(SB A.1.2)** as relates to the peaks or not, 5) then you have to determine if the option is correct **(SB A.1.2)** and this makes the question more difficult than expected because of the time involved.

Physical Sciences PASSAGE 3.PS.II

Q07 — Pre-Study Suggestions

Review the following if needed:

1) Electrical Power **PHY 10.2**
2) Mechanical Power **PHY 9.1.4**
3) Work **PHY 9.1.4**
4) Ohm's Law (V=IR) **PHY 10.1**
5) Equation Interpretation
6) Exponentials and Roots **GS A.4**
7) Camouflage and Distractions **SB A.1.3**
8) Similar Pair Options **SB A.2.7**
9) What are the key pieces of information from the passage?
10) Solve the problem.

Solution Discussion

There is no essential information from the passage.

The formula to use is (which you must know):

$$P = IV$$

P = power in watts (W)
I = current in amperes (A)
= 0.005 A = 5×10^{-3} A

V = electrical potential in volts (V)
= 10^5 V

P = $(5 \times 10^{-3}$ A$)(10^5$ V$)$ = 5×10^2 W.

Option A is correct.

What do you call a politician who writes laws about the output of power plants, but ignores current and resistance?

A voltage regulator.

P.S. P = IV and V = IR !!!
Power output depends on current (I), resistance (R) and voltage (V).
P.P.S. Please keep your cats away from high voltage wires!
PHY 10.1, 10.2

Test Taking Skills Comment

Most students got this correct, so this must be fairly well understood knowledge. Another approach, if the exact formula above was not remembered is a form of dimensional analysis **(GS Part II 2.3 # 16)**. The watt (W) is joules (J)/sec (s). The ampere (A) is coulombs(C)/s. The volt (V) is J/C. There is only one way to combine ampere and volts to get to watts and that is to multiply them:

$$W = J/s$$
$$A = C/s$$
$$V = J/C$$

then,

$$A \times V = (C/s)(J/C) = J/s = W.$$

This is a distraction question **(SB A.1.3)**; it is not a camouflage question because they tell you to find power. You are distracted if you feel you must get some information from Figure 1. There is no information in Figure 1 needed to solve this problem. This is the importance of knowing your Basic Knowledge **(SB A.2.2)** and being secure with it. You are secure in your basic knowledge when you study these materials well.

You might also see this as a Similar Pair Options **(SB A.2.7)** question if you had to guess. You could choose options C or D, both with the coefficient 2, as your similar pair and guess one of them - in this case, it would be incorrect. But, that is going to happen (*see* Option Elimination Analysis, **SB A.2**). The technique is less effective when only numbers are involved, but overall, if you are truly guessing, which you always want as a last resort, it is still better than the 25% uneducated guess.

Q08 — Pre-Study Suggestions

Review the following if needed:
1) Electronic Transitions **PHY 12.5**
2) Ionization Potential **CHM 2.3, PHY 12.5**
3) Exponentials and Roots **GS A.4**
4) Camouflage and Distractions **SB A.1.3**
5) Dichotomy of Options **SB A.2.3**
6) What information from the passage is needed to solve this problem?
7) Solve the problem.

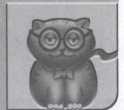

Solution Discussion

Information from the passage:

From the third paragraph:

"For example, if an electron in the n = 1 energy level … will be emitted."

To solve the problem:

Level n = 1: $1{,}400 \times 10^{-17}$ J.

Level n = 2: 240×10^{-17} J.

The energy of the x-ray emitted is the difference between the two levels:

$$
\begin{array}{r}
1{,}400 \times 10^{-17} \text{ J} \\
240 \times 10^{-17} \text{ J} \\
\hline
1{,}160 \times 10^{-17} \text{ J} \\
= 1.160 \times 10^{-14} \text{ J}.
\end{array}
$$

Option C is correct.

Test Taking Skills Comment

If you are not facile with the exponents and the scientific notation **(GS A.4)**, this is a good time to review it. Otherwise the question is straightforward. You do not want to waste time trying to deal with the basic math found on this test - you do not have those seconds and minutes to waste; study these concepts now.

Although the information needed to solve the problem is given in the passage as shown above, this is also basic study knowledge **(SB A.2.2)** which you should know. With good study, you would not have to go to the passage to retrieve this information. Not going to the passage would save you valuable time you could use solving other questions - this is one of the most important

lesions of this very simple but critical concept.

This question has a mild distraction **(SB A.1.3)** if you begin to wonder what the ionization potentials **(PHY 12.5)** are supposed to mean other than giving you the energy levels. They could have left out the ionization potential and just stated energy levels and the question would have been the same.

This could be a Dichotomy of Options question **(SB A.2.3)**, but there is really no easy way to choose between the halves of the dichotomy without solving the problem. Having some logical/knowledge based means of selecting the correct half of the dichotomy is central to the use of this technique.

Q09   Pre-Study Suggestions

Review the following if needed:
1) Three Out of Four Options **SB A.2.8**
2) Negative Question **SB A.1.2**
3) Similar Pair Options **SB A.2.7**
4) Internally Inconsistent **SB A.2.5**
5) What information from the passage is needed to solve this problem?
6) Solve the problem.

Solution Discussion

The piece of information from the passage needed to solve this problem is:

Paragraph 2 - *"A continuous spectrum is produced by bremsstrahlung ...during collisions with ions"*

Option A is correct. He (helium) is not an ion and will not produce bremsstrahlung.

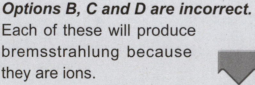

Options B, C and D are incorrect. Each of these will produce bremsstrahlung because they are ions.

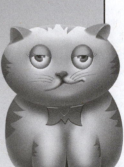

Law of Cat Inertia

A cat at rest will tend to remain at rest, unless acted upon by some outside force - such as the opening of cat food or a running mouse.

Test Taking Skills Comment

This could be a problem on the reading section of the test. This is a Three Out of Four (**SB A.2.8**) type question. Options B, C and D are all charged (you should know that a proton is positively charged, **PHY 12.1**). Option A is an outlier and is not charged. Outlier options will usually be incorrect and can be ignored except in problems like this that are negative questions (**SB A.1.2**). The question is essentially reversed from that usually expected and often, not always, the outlier is the correct answer in a negative type question. This is also a Similar Pair Options (**SB A.2.7**) with options A and B both having 'He'. The similar pair is conflict with the three out of four. Generally, you would ignore the Similar Pair

Options (**SB A.2.7**). But, remember this is a negative question, and often in negative questions, the correct option is the outlier. All of this means you have to be very careful and may not want to use the skills at all if you are in pure guess mode.

What is present here is that options B, C and D are all Internally Inconsistent (**SB A.2.5**) with the Passage Knowledge (**SB A.2.2**) that the bremsstrahlung must be produced by the collision of an electron with an ion. This means B, C and D cannot be correct because they will produce the radiation. Whenever a skill uses Basic Knowledge (study, passage, general) (**SB A.2.2**), you should go with it over a pure guess.

Q10 — Pre-Study Suggestions

Review the following if needed:
1) Velocity **PHY 1.3, 1.4**
2) Acceleration **PHY 1.3, 1.4**
3) Kinetic Energy **PHY 5.3**

4) Potential Energy **PHY 5.4**

5) Conservation of Energy **PHY 5.5**

6) Electric Potential **PHY 9.1.4**

7) Electrical Power **PHY 10.2**

8) Equation Interpretation

9) Camouflage and Distractions **SB A.1.3**

10) Dichotomy of Options **SB A.2.3**

11) What information is needed from the passage?

12) Solve the problem.

Solution Discussion

The information needed from the passage is:

Paragraph 5 (second from the bottom) - *"Another power supply (HV) regulates electron acceleration."*

The formula for kinetic energy (K) **(PHY 5.3)** is:

$$K = mv^2/2$$

m = mass

v = velocity **(PHY 1.3, 1.4)**.

The formula for acceleration (a) **(PHY 1.3, 1.4)** is:

$$a = \Delta v/\Delta t$$

Δt = time elapsed

Δv = change in velocity.

This means acceleration and kinetic energy are related through the velocity:

$$K \propto v^2$$

$$a \propto v$$

then,

$$K \propto a^2.$$

The kinetic energy of the electrons arises from the electrical energy, of

CHAPTER 1

the HV power source. As the potential energy **(PHY 5.4)** or power **(PHY 10.2)** increases, this will increase the acceleration and then the velocity and the kinetic energy of the electrons. The voltage **(PHY 9.1.4)** is related to the energy and power. Increasing voltage increases electrical potential energy and power, and this is converted proportionately to kinetic energy by accelerating the electrons.

Options C and D are incorrect. The LV has nothing to do with the acceleration, and therefore the kinetic energy, of the electrons per the passage.

Option B is incorrect. If the HV is decreased, this means 'a' is decreased and K will decrease.

Option A is correct. As the HV is increased, the acceleration will increase, the velocity of the electrons will increase and the kinetic energy will increase as discussed earlier.

Test Taking Skills Comment

This is a Dichotomy of Options **(SB A.2.3)** question. You should immediately eliminate options C and D (one half of the dichotomy) from reading of the passage. Then you must make the connections as discussed previously to get the correct answer. In a dichotomy question, you can usually pick the correct half of the dichotomy based on your study knowledge **(SB A.2.2)** or passage knowledge **(SB A.2.2)** (as in this case).

The key concept of the relation of velocity (part of kinetic energy) and acceleration are not clearly stated. This is a type of Camouflage and Distraction **(SB A.1.3)**.

Q11 — Pre-Study Suggestions

Review the following if needed:

1) Wave Equation ($v = \lambda f$; $v = \lambda / T$) **PHY 7.1.2**

2) Wavelength (λ) **PHY 7.1.2**

3) Frequency ($v = \lambda f$; $f = 1/T$; $f = 1/s = Hz$) **PHY 7.1.2**

4) Energy of Waves **PHY 7.1.2**

5) Graphs and Charts **GS A.3**

6) Probability **GS A.1**

7) Camouflage and Distraction **SB A.1.3**

8) Dichotomy of Options **SB A.2.3**

9) What information from the passage is needed?

10) Interpret Figure 2.

11) Solve the problem.

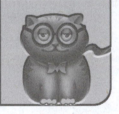

Solution Discussion

The key information from the passage is:

Last paragraph- *"determine the relationship between X-ray ...graphed the results of the experiment, as shown in Figure 2."*

Interpretation of the graph **(GS A.3)** of Figure 2:

> The horizontal axis is the wavelength **(PHY 7.1.2)**, λ, of the emitted photons. The wavelength is associated with a certain frequency **(PHY 7.1.2)**, not noted, but as given in the equations, wave relationship **(PHY 7.1.2)** and Planck's Relationship **(PHY 12.5)**. The vertical axis is I, intensity, of the photons emitted at the wavelength. It is proportional to the number of photons emitted at that wavelength. Since each wavelength represents certain energy **(PHY 7.1.2)**, the greater the intensity means more photons are being emitted at that particular energy, or wavelength. The lower or curved

line represents the bremsstrahlung. The sharp peaks mean there is an abundance of photons being emitted at certain energy, wavelength value. Peak 1 occurs at a shorter wavelength but higher frequency and energy than does peak 2. Peak 2 has more photons emitted than peak 1.

The height of the peak is proportional (**GS A.3**) to the number of photons emitted at a wavelength. This means the wavelength is the event, and the height of the peak is the count of the event. There are two events, λ_1 (corresponding to peak 1) and λ_2 (corresponding to peak 2). Based on the intensity, or height of the peak, each will have a number of photons emitted which may be given by N_1 and N_2, respectively. The total event will then be the sum of N_1 and N_2 (or assume the denominator, number of possible transitions, to be the same for each peak). Then the probability (Pr) of each of the events (only considering these two events!) will be:

$$Pr\,(\lambda_1) = N_1 / (N_1 + N_2)$$

$$Pr\,(\lambda_2) = N_2 / (N_1 + N_2).$$

From this analysis, the second peak is more probable than the first peak because $N_2 > N_1$.

Options A and C are incorrect. Options A and C should be eliminated immediately because the wavelength identifies the events, such as head or tail, and not the count of the events.

Option B is incorrect. The height of the peak corresponds to the count, number of photons emitted, which is the count of the events in question. Since $N_1 < N_2$ based upon the graph, the Pr (λ_1) must be less than the Pr (λ_2). With a lower intensity, the probability would be less.

Option D is correct. See the discussion of option C and above. The higher intensity means more events and a greater probability of them.

Test Taking Skills Comment

This is a difficult question as only 50% of students got it correct. It actually only requires the simplest understanding of probability **(GS A.1)**. The approach to solving and understanding probability is outlined previously and at **GS A.1** and should be reviewed for solid understanding.

This is a Camouflage and Distraction **(SB A.1.3)** question because the events are disguised as explained above. But, you are given the clue of 'probability'. From your study of probability, you should think 'count' of some 'event' and then assess your task is to uncover, rephrase the question if necessary, those events and the count of them as explained. You will usually need a numerator and a denominator as discussed above.

This is also a Dichotomy of Options **(SB A.2.3)** question. Your dichotomy is 'wavelength' versus 'intensity'. You are not counting the wavelengths, so there is no way it can be the probability. The intensity is a count, of photons emitted, and is the candidate for determining probability. So, you should eliminate A and C and realize your answer must come from B or D.

Q12 Pre-Study Suggestions

Review the following if needed:
1) Work **PHY 9.1.4**
2) Equation Interpretation
3) Camouflage and Distraction **SB A.1.3**
4) Three Out of Four Type Question **SB A.2.8**
5) Solve the problem.

Solution Discussion

The formula for work is **(PHY 5.7)**:

$$W = F \times d = F\,d\,\cos\theta$$

W = work in Joules (J)
F = force **(PHY 2.2)** in newtons (N) = 20 N
d = displacement **(PHY 1.3, 1.4)** in meters (m)
　　= 10 m
θ = angle between the force

and the displacement.

Since the θ = 0° as the force and displacement are in the same direction, $\cos(0°) = 1$ **(PHY 1.1.1)**.

Then,

$$W = Fd\cos\theta = (20\ N)(10\ m)(1)$$
$$= 200\ Nm = 200\ J.$$

The **correct answer is C.**

Test Taking Skills Comment

Notice the mass of the object is not needed to solve the problem. Data will be presented which is not needed in the solution - be aware of this. This is a distraction **(SB A.1.3)** type problem because of this. The problem is not camouflaged because you are told to determine the work. You should go directly to your basic knowledge of work and apply what you have learned as shown above. The MCAT does not require you know the cosine factor in the equation above for work **(PHY 9.1.4)**, but it does require you to know that the force and displacement must be along the same direction in the equation W = Fd. This is the same as knowing that $\cos(0)$ is 1 as explained.

You could go out on a limb, if you're truly guessing, and classify this question as a Three Out of Four **(SB A.2.8)** with B, C and D being the three as they are all in the hundreds.

Q13 Pre-Study Suggestions

Review the following if needed:

1) Kinetic Energy **PHY 5.3**
2) Potential Energy **PHY 5.4**
3) Resonance in Physics **PHY 7.1.4**
4) Surface Tension **PHY 6.1.5**
5) Vapor Pressure **PHY 6.1.2**
6) Phase Changes **PHY 6.2**
7) Kinetic Molecular Theory **PHY 5.3**
8) Camouflage and Distractions **SB A.1.3**
9) Similar Pair Options **SB A.2.7**
10) Solve the problem.

Solution Discussion

Evaporation is one of the phase changes **(PHY 6.2)** you should know well. Energy is stored in a phase as potential energy **(PHY 5.4)** in the bonds **(CHM 3.1, 3.2)** or in the intermolecular forces **(CHM 4.2)**. As the kinetic energy **(PHY 5.3)** of the system increases, as heat goes into the system, it exceeds the energy of the bonding and results in the molecules separating. Evaporation is the process of breaking the intermolecular bonds between liquid molecules when the kinetic energy exceeds those intermolecular bond energies.

Option A is incorrect. Resonance has nothing to do with process of evaporation **(PHY 6.2)** of a liquid. The resonance of organic chemistry **(ORG 1.4, 7.1, 8.1)** is simply a means of representing the bonding patterns in molecules which cannot be represented by a single line/dot structure. Resonance in physics **(PHY 7.1.4)** occurs when external frequencies **(PHY 7.1.2)** match natural modes of vibration of the object and energy absorption is maximized.

Option B is correct. The intermolecular forces **(CHM 4.2)**, a type of potential energy, must be overcome. As the temperature of the liquid is raised, the kinetic energy **(PHY 5.3)** of the molecules increase, as in the Kinetic Molecular Theory **(PHY 5.3)** for gases, until molecules have adequate kinetic energy to overcome the molecular forces and escape the liquid phase.

Option C is incorrect. Surface tension **(PHY 6.1.5)** has nothing to do with the evaporation of a liquid. Surface tension results from the imbalance of forces at the surface of the liquid.

Option D is incorrect. The potential energy **(PHY 5.4)** would involve the forces between the molecules **(CHM 4.2)** in the liquid. These must be overcome in order for the molecules to escape to the gas phase.

"**VG PHEST**" (Very Good Festival)

The following are all state functions:

V for volume
G for Gibb's free energy
P for pressure
H for enthalpy
E for internal energy
S for entropy
T for temperature

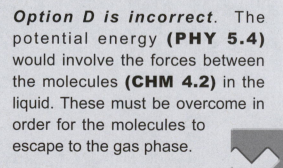

CHAPTER 1

Test Taking Skills Comment

This is a Camouflage/Distraction **(SB A.1.3)** type of question. It is not clear if this is a Physics question or if it is a general chemistry question. This is why you need to understand the concepts as they relate to other concepts. Yet, you are directed to 'evaporation' and 'attractive forces' that you must use to get at your answer.

It is also a Similar Pair **(SB A.2.7)** type question as both B and D are energy related options. If you have to guess, it is not unreasonable to select your answer from these two as there are no other conflicting similar pairs present.

Q14 — Pre-Study Suggestions

Review the following if needed:

1) Uniformly Accelerated Motion **PHY 1.5**
2) Equation Interpretation
3) Camouflage and Distraction **SB A.1.3**
4) Three Out of Four Options **SB A.2.8**
5) Solve the problem.

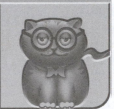

Solution Discussion

Even though the problem does not explicitly state it, the runner is assumed to be running in a straight line. Then the conditions of uniformly accelerated motion (UAM) **(PHY 1.5)** are met. The givens are the acceleration (a) **(PHY 1.3, 1.4)** and the distance (d) **(PHY 1.3, 1.4)**. The best equation to find the time is then:

$$d = d_o + v_o t + at^2/2$$

d_o = the initial distance
v_o = the initial velocity
t = time

$d_o = 0$ $v_o = 0$
$a = 1.5 \text{ m/s}^2$ $d = 3.0 \text{ m.}$

Then solving the equation:

$$3.0 = 0 + 0t + (1.5)t^2/2$$
$$= 1.5t^2/2$$

$$1.5\, t^2 = 6$$

$$t^2 = 6/1.5 = 4$$

$$t = 2 \text{ s.}$$

The **correct answer is C** which is 2.0 sec.

Test Taking Skills Comment

This is a matter of knowing uniformly accelerated motion and recognizing when the problem meets the conditions of it. Whenever the acceleration is constant, non-changing, and the path is a straight line, these equations may be used. Practice using them will help greatly. This is the approach you have to take for many of the problems. You are given some data/information but you are not told this is such and such (in this problem, you are not told it deals with UAM by name, but you are given all the features of UAM and you have to determine that is what you are dealing with). Review Camouflage and Distractions **(SB A.1.3)** for further explanation.

This is a Three Out of Four **(SB A.2.8)** type question. Options B, C and D are all non-exponential numbers. Option A is an outlier being an exponential number. The outlier is often incorrect and should be ignored if you are in the guess mode.

Q15 — Pre-Study Suggestions

Review the following if needed:
1) Torques **PHY 4.1.1**
2) Forces **PHY 2.2**
3) Static Equilibrium **PHY 4.1**
4) Trig Functions **PHY 1.1.1**
5) Vectors **PHY 1.1**
6) Solve the problem.

Solution Discussion

The forces acting on the sheet of material are:

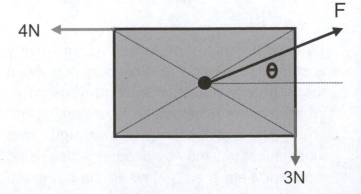

The object must meet both rotational and translational equilibrium **(PHY 4.1)**. You can use either condition to solve the problem. For translational equilibrium, the forces are assumed to be acting at the center of mass **(PHY 4.2)** This problem must assume there is an equivalent effect of the 3N and 4N on the center of mass (shown by the black circle), which is the site of action of the F force. If the 3N and 4N forces **(PHY 2.2)** had no effect on translational motion, the object could not reach translational equilibrium. Choosing the coordinate system **(GS A.3)** as below and showing the forces acting at the center of mass:

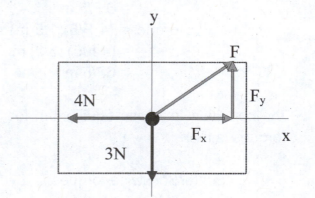

- it should be clear that the components of the F force, F_x and F_y, must balance the other two forces, 4N and 3N, respectively

- this means F_x = 4N and F_y = 3N

- this means the two sides of the right triangle must be 3 and 4; since these two sides are in the ratio of 3:4, the hypotenuse by Pythagorean method

must be 5 (*see* the trig discussion, **PHY 1.1.1** and geometry discussion, **PHY 1.1.1**)

- this means the unknown force must be 5N and *option C is correct*.

- the angle θ will then have a tanθ **(PHY 1.1.1)** = opposite/adjacent = 3/4 = 0.75

- this means the arctan (0.75) **(PHY 1.1.2)** = θ.

If the equilibrium was viewed from the rotational viewpoint **(PHY 4.1)**, you must first select an axis of rotation. The simplest axis to select would be one through one of the corners and other forces. Assume the axis of rotation is through the lower right hand corner by the 3N force. The forces acting to cause rotation about this axis would be:

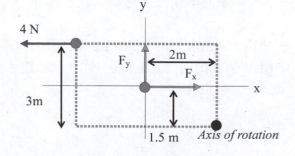

- the components of the F force are shown as F_x and F_y

- the 3 N force is not shown because it is acting through the axis of rotation

• the perpendicular distances from the direction of each force (you may have to visualize an extension of the line of the force) to the axis of rotation is the moment arm **(PHY 4.1.1)** and is shown:

then $F_y = 3F/5$

$F_x = 4F/5$

For each force:

for 4 N: the moment arm is 3 m

for F_y : the moment arm is 2 m

for F_x: the moment arm is 1.5 m.

• the direction of rotation of each torque (for each force) is:

for 4 N: direction is counterclockwise

for F_y : direction is clockwise

for F_x: direction is clockwise

• the F_x and F_y may be substituted for by the F as follows:

arctan $(0.75) = \theta$

$\tan\theta = 0.75 = 3/4$

• this means the triangle is a 3-4-5 right triangle and the ratio of the components are

• the torques are calculated by multiplying the force times the moment arms:

for 4 N: torque = (4 N)(3 m)

= 12 Nm

for F_y : torque = (3 F/5)(2 m)

= 6 F/5 m

for F_x: torque = (4 F/5)(1.5 m)

= (4 F/5) (3/2) m

= 6F/5 m

• the condition for static equilibrium for torques is then

counterclockwise torques

= clockwise torques

12 Nm = 6 F/5 m + 6 F/5 m

= 12 F/5 m

12 N = 12 F/5

N = F/5

F = 5 N.

The answers are the same as they should be.

Test Taking Skills Comment

Whenever there is no motion of an object and there are forces acting on it, one may be able to use the conditions of static equilibrium **(PHY 4.1)**. This problem shows how to approach the issue by translational or rotational equilibrium. It also illustrates to take a moment, when there is more than one option to determine the easiest way to proceed, by the translational approach in this case. If the problem seems to be complicated, e.g. if you only saw the rotational approach, then you may want to give yourself a breather by going on to other problems and come back to this one later.

Q16 — Pre-Study Suggestions

Review the following if needed:
1) Recrystallization and Precipitation **CHM 5.3**
2) Heat Transfer Mechanisms **CHM 7.2**
3) What is the key piece of information from the passage required to answer this question?
4) Solve the problem.

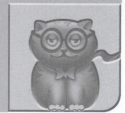

Solution Discussion

No prior information is needed to solve this problem.

From Trial 1:
"The test tube from Experiment (1) was removed …to cool in air at 20 °C."

From Trial 2:
"For this trial, however, the test tube … placed in a beaker of water at 20 °C."

Option A is incorrect. There is nothing to suggest there was any difference in the amount of acetamide used in the two trials.

Option D is incorrect. There is no clear data detailing the melting time for both trials. It may be inferred the melting for Trial (2) was shorter because the water was already boiling. But, is this the most important difference for the trials?

Option C is incorrect. In Trial (2), it does state the water was boiling initially; the exact temperature is not evident from Trial (1) except that it is in excess of 80 °C. This is a difference between the two trials. What is important though is the method of cooling for the crystals to form, and not just the starting temperature which could not be greater than 100 °C - the normal boiling point of water.

Option B is correct. The surroundings used to cool the test tubes are different. In Trial (1), the tube was air-cooled. In Trial (2), the tube was water-cooled. Since the Trials (1) and (2) were evaluating the formation of solid acetamide from the heated water, the rate of cooling would be a significant factor in the crystallization **(CHM 5.3)** process of the acetamide. The difference will be the rate of heat transfer **(CHM 7.2)**. Heat transfer from a tube to air will be slower than the transfer from a tube to a water bath.

Test Taking Skills Comment

This question asks for the most important difference. So, in your analysis, there must first be a difference to even be considered as the correct option. Since option A represents a parameter, the amount of acetamide, for which there is no stated difference in the trials, it must be incorrect. Options C and D both have variables that are different between the trials. Now the question becomes, do they pertain to what is being studied? The trials are looking at crystal formation from a solution. One of the variables important in this is the rate of cooling. Both options C and D are concerned with variables related to the melting, not the freezing of the acetamide. Option B has a pertinent variable which does vary between the trials. "This could be on the Verbal section of the exam."

Q17   Pre-Study Suggestions

Review the following if needed:
1) Laws of Thermodynamics **CHM 7.2**
2) Heat Transfer **CHM 7.2**
3) Energies of Phase Changes **CHM 4.3.1**
4) Dichotomy of Options **SB A.2.3**
5) Camouflage and Distractions **SB A.1.3**
6) What is the melting point of the acetamide?
7) What is the key piece of information from the passage required to answer this question?
8) Solve the problem.

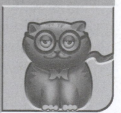

Physical Sciences PASSAGE 3.PS. III

Solution Discussion

There is nothing specifically in the passage to help solve the problem other than the melting point of acetamide. From the Experiment (1), the melting point **(CHM 4.3.1)** of acetamide is found to be 80 °C - this is the temperature which remains constant until all of the acetamide is melted. In Fig 1, there is a curve with square points and one with circular points. You should determine the 'circle curve' represents acetamide melting, and the 'square curve' is the acetamide freezing. For each, there is a flat portion at 80 °C. This flat portion is the freezing (melting) point.

Option A is incorrect. The water does not melt the acetamide. The rise in temperature melts the acetamide. The amount of water per se does not govern whether or not the acetamide melts. The water is used here as a medium to conduct heat and not as a solvent. A solvent may need to be increased in amount to dissolve **(CHM 5.3)** a substance. This is not the purpose of water in this experiment.

Option B is incorrect. Same as for option A.

Option C is incorrect. As long as the temperature, which is given as 90 °C, is above the melting point of acetamide, which is 80 °C, the acetamide would eventually melt.

Option D is correct. Since the boiling point of water is 100 °C, the 90 °C is less than this. This means there is a smaller temperature differential for the exchange of heat to occur. Then to have the needed amount of heat exchanged, it would take longer. This is implied in the discussion on heat exchange

(CHM 7.2): heat exchange, $\Delta H \propto \Delta T$. For 100 $^{\circ}$C vs 80 $^{\circ}$C, the ΔT = 20 $^{\circ}$C. For 90 $^{\circ}$C vs 80 $^{\circ}$C, the ΔT = 10 $^{\circ}$C. Then $\Delta H = q/t \propto \Delta T$, the larger ΔT, the faster (smaller t = time) the exchange and vice versa.

Heat capacity looks like "**MCAT**"!

$$Q = mc\Delta T$$

where Q is heat energy, m is mass, c is the specific heat capacity, and ΔT is the change in temperature.

Test Taking Skills Comment

This question poses a typical dichotomy **(SB A.2.3)** between two sets of answers. One set is options A and B which deals with the amount of water. The second set is options C and D that deal with the acetamide melting or not. Generally, you may be able to eliminate one set as not really pertinent to the solution. In this case, the amount of water is irrelevant, as the water is just a medium of conduction of heat and not a solvent. This leaves options C and D as possessing the correct answer.

A combination of using the passage and prior knowledge **(SB A.2.2)** is needed to solve this problem as discussed. But, by eliminating one half of the options, you have greatly increased your odds of guessing if need be. This is a partially camouflaged **(SB A.1.3)** question as well. There is the strong indication in the options that melting **(CHM 4.3.1)** is important, and it is. But, also, you have to know and understand heat exchange dynamics in this question.

Q18 — Pre-Study Suggestions

Review the following if needed:
1) Experimental Controls **GS C.1, C.2**
2) Three Out of Four Options **SB A.2.8**
3) Dichotomy of Options **SB A.2.3**
4) What is the key piece(s) of information from the passage required to answer this question?
5) Solve the problem.

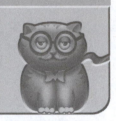

Solution Discussion

A general reading of the passage is needed to solve the problem.

Option B is incorrect. Any experiment must control for some variables - the ones important to the study (*see* Experimental Controls **GS C.1, C.2**). Nothing useful will result in an uncontrolled experiment. Also, it is clear there are controls for melting and freezing and the processes are monitored.

Option C is incorrect. Since there is only one amount of acetamide, 10 g, which is used in the experiment, any question of what it controls and does not control cannot be answered. Also, the passage states freezing, e.g., was controlled by placing the test tube in air or water and not by varying the acetamide.

Option D is incorrect.
Same as option C.

Option A is correct. The important variables must be controlled in an experiment to make it meaningful.

Test Taking Skills Comment

What is needed is the general concepts of the proper construction and running of experiments (*see* Experimental Controls **GS C.1, C.2)**. This is what you should have learned from your lab classes. Again a dichotomy **(SB A.2.3)** in terms of two sets of options is given. The first set is options A and B that deals with melting/freezing in controlled versus uncontrolled conditions.

The second set is options C and D that is concerned about the effect of variable acetamide. Since the acetamide does not vary in the experiments, this set, options C and D, must be wrong. This leaves options A or B and A should be an easy choice since virtually all experiments have some controls as in A. This is also a Three Out of Four **(SB A.2.8)** type question as options A, C and D all have control as the concern and option B has no control and is the outlier-generally, the outliers will be incorrect. This is unusual to have both Dichotomy and Three Out of Four in the same question. Guessing using either method will increase your guess rate success.

Q19 — Pre-Study Suggestions

Review the following if needed:
1) Graphs and Charts **GS A.3**
2) Three Out of Four Options **SB A.2.8**
3) What is the key piece(s) of information from the passage required to answer this question?
4) Solve the problem.

Solution Discussion

The key piece of information from the passage is in Trial (1):

"The acetamide slowly began freezing and was completely solid after 23 min."

The frequency or interval of observation has no effect on when the acetamide became solid. It was going to become solid at the same moment in time regardless of the interval of observation. The number recorded by the observation could vary though. The interval would determine when the observation was made and recorded.

The event will occur between the prior interval and the current one, but will be recorded as occurring at the current interval. For example, if the interval of recording was at 5 minute intervals. At 20 minutes, it would not be solid. At 25 minutes, it would be solid and would be recorded as freezing at 25 minutes. Since the interval in the Trial (1) was 30 seconds or 1/2 minute, the freezing must be recorded upon the 1/2 minute interval. Since the recorded time was 23 minutes for 1/2 minute recording, this means the actual freezing occured at some time after 22.5 minutes but before 23.0 minutes. So, if the interval is now 1-minute intervals, the freezing will still occur between 22.0 minutes and 23.0 minutes. So, when the observation is made at 23.0, the acetamide is frozen and is recorded as such. This means *option B is correct*.

The other time options are just out of the possible range. The temperature choice, *option D is incorrect* because the melting point/freezing point temperature would be the same. Notice that if the observations were made at 15-second intervals, the observed freezing could have occured at 22 minutes and 45 seconds or at 23 minutes even.

Test Taking Skills Comment

No specific knowledge is needed. The reasoning as discussed above will lead to the correct option. This is a Three Out of Four type **(SB A.2.8)** question. Options A, B and C all give specific times. Option D is an outlier relating to temperature. Outliers are usually incorrect.

Physical Sciences PASSAGE 3.PS. III

Q20 — Pre-Study Suggestions

Review the following if needed:
1) Guess Question **SB A.2.4**
2) Negative Question **SB A.1.2**
3) What is the key piece(s) of information from the passage required answering this question?
4) Solve the problem.

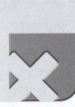

Solution Discussion

The key pieces of information needed are:
   Experiment (1): Melting
"After a period of time, when all the acetamide had melted, the temperature..."

   Experiment (2): Freezing

   Trial (1):
"The test tube from Experiment (1) was removed from the hot water and left to cool..."

"The acetamide slowly began freezing and this process...so another trial was completed."

   Trial (2):
"The same test tube was placed in boiling water until the acetamide completely melted."

Option A is incorrect. The water was boiling in Trial (2) as noted.

Option B is incorrect. This is a true statement, but what does it have to do with the presence of the boiling water in Trial (2) that preceded the cooling?

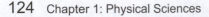

Option C is incorrect. This is probably true also, but what does it have to do with the hot water that preceded this step.

Option D is correct. It should be clear that the test tube used initially in Trial (1) contained liquid acetamide, from Experiment (1), which was allowed to freeze. In Trial (2), since this was the tube used at the end of Trial (1), the acetamide had frozen and had to be re-melted and was re-melted in the hot water.

Test Taking Skills Comment

No specific knowledge is needed. The reasoning as discussed above will lead to the correct option along with careful reading of the selection. This could be considered a Guess Question **(SB A.2.4)** because of the amount of reading and referral back to the passage. Read the link above so you fully appreciate the concept of Guess Question. This is also a Negative Question **(SB A.1.2)**. With negative questions, you have to be more careful in using the test skills and remember for a negative question, the Correct **(SB A.1.2)** may be the False **(SB A.1.2)** option.

Q21 — Pre-Study Suggestions

Review the following if needed:
1) Graphs and Charts **GS A.3**
2) Slope **GS A.3**
3) Three or More Steps Options **SB A.1.3**
4) Dichotomy of Options **SB A.2.3**
5) What are the key pieces of information from the passage?
6) Solve the problem.

Solution Discussion

The key piece of information is:

Trial (1):
"The time for freezing was considered to be excessive, so another trial was completed".

The graph of Figure 1 is a plot as follows:

Both Trial (1) and Trial (2) begins with liquid acetamide at an elevated temperature. The liquid is allowed to cool and freeze. This means the curve will slope **(GS A.3)** downward to the right for both Trials as the temperature is decreasing, to reach the freezing point, the time is increasing. This is the curve in Figure 1 which has the squares

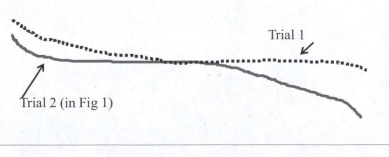

Temperature (°C)

Trial 1

Trial 2 (in Fig 1)

Time (seconds)

marking the curve (which is for Trial (2) - solid line in the graph). This means **options C and D must be incorrect**. Since the cooling and freezing of Trial (1) took too long, this means the curve must reach the flat portion much more slowly as shown above for Trial (1) (the dotted curve). The curve for Trial (1) would then slope downward more slowly, less steeply, than that of Trial (2). This means **option A is correct**. Additionally, because the freezing is slow, all the data points for Trial (1), i.e., the flat freezing portion, may extend out beyond the 270 seconds shown.

Test Taking Skills Comment

No specific knowledge is needed. The reasoning as discussed above will lead to the correct option along with careful reading of the selection. This is a Dichotomy **(SB A.2.3)** type question. As discussed above, you should eliminate the options C and D because the slope has to be downward. This is what you do with Dichotomy questions, you use your Basic Knowledge **(SB A.2.2)** (from the passage or your study) to eliminate one-half of the options and then you do not have to consider them - read the discussion of Dichotomy and Complex Sounding Options **(SB A.2.2)** carefully so you fully grasp and can use this concept).

This is a Three or More Step Analysis **(SB A.1.3)** and this makes it more difficult: 1) the first decision is the slope of the graph, 2) then you have to determine if the reason given in the second part of the option corresponds to the first part regarding the slope, 3) then you have to determine if the option is True or False **(SB A.1.2)**, 4) then you have to determine if the option is Correct or Incorrect **(SB A.1.2)**.

Q22 — Pre-Study Suggestions

Review the following if needed:
1) Wave Characteristics **PHY 7.1.2**
2) Standing Waves **PHY 7.1.5**
3) Harmonics **PHY 7.1.5**
4) Graphs and Charts **GS A.3**
5) Three or More Steps Options **SB A.1.3**
6) Three Out of Four Options **SB A.2.8**
7) Guess Question **SB A.2.4**
8) What is the key piece of information from the passage required to answer this question?

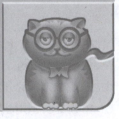

Solution Discussion

Nothing other than the Figure 1a is needed from the passage. A harmonic series **(PHY 7.1.5)** begins with the fundamental waveform that will have the longest wavelength and shortest frequency. The harmonics then increase with each successive harmonic having a shorter wavelength but greater frequency. Musical instruments may have strings, such as the guitar, or use tubes, such as the trombone. Both of these will have a fundamental frequency, wavelength that corresponds to the length of string or tube. This will be the first harmonic. In Figure 1a, this is the wave with the longest wavelength, which is the one that is solid. The second harmonic will then have the next shorter wavelength that fits the requirements of the string/ tube. In Fig 1a, this is the wave with the long dashes. Notice that 2 wavelengths of the long dash match one wavelength of the solid line waveform. The third harmonic has a shorter wavelength that is the short dash line. There are three wavelengths of this for each one of the solid waves in the diagram. This progression is consistent with them being related harmonics in a series. Other relations are also possible, but each will follow a logical series of changes in the wavelength or frequency (PHY 7.1.2).

The relationships of wavelength (λ), and frequency (f), and period (T) (PHY 7.1.2) are:

$$\lambda \propto 1 / f$$
$$f \propto 1 / T$$

then,

$$\lambda \propto 1/(1/ T) \propto T.$$

This means that the shortest wavelength has the shortest period and vice-versa as this is a direct relationship (GS A.3). The third harmonic has the shortest wavelength and will have the shortest period. *Option C is correct*.

Test Taking Skills Comment

Option D should be eliminated just from the reading of the passage as it is clear it is a combination of harmonics and not a pure harmonic. The remainder of the reasoning is as above. This was a difficult problem as only 55% of students got it correct. All of the questions in this section have very low percentages correct reflecting the general lack of confidence or knowledge in problems dealing with waves. I strongly suggest each student carefully review the problems and discussions which are hyperlinked. This is also a Three Out of Four (SB A.2.8) type problem. Options A, B and C all deal with harmonics. Option D is an outlier dealing with waveforms in a specific figure. Outliers, especially in non-negative or non-change questions tend to be incorrect and can be ignored.

This is also a Three or More Step (SB A.1.3) problem (1) you have to know what an harmonic is and then identify each one on the graphs, 2) you have to determine what parameter relates to the period, because it is not given, and then convert this to relative periods, 3) you then have to compare all of the periods and determine which option is correct **(SB A.1.2)** and these tend to be more difficult because of the time involved if not the content and may be a Guess Question **(SB A.2.4)**.

Q23 — Pre-Study Suggestions

Review the following if needed:
1) Wave Characteristics **PHY 7.1.2**
2) Phases of Waves **PHY 7.1.3**
3) Wave Interactions **PHY 7.1.3**
4) Graphs and Charts **GS A.3**
5) Three or More Steps Options **SB A.1.3**
6) Dichotomy of Options **SB A.2.3**
7) What is the key piece of information from the passage required to answer this question?
8) Solve the problem.

Solution Discussion

Waves are displacements of the medium from the equilibrium position. When the wave **(PHY 7.1.2)** passes through the medium, the particles of the medium are disturbed. The disturbance is an oscillation about the equilibrium position. There is no net displacement. The equilibrium position is the position of zero displacement. The solid horizontal line is the zero displacement. So, since the waves cross at that line, each is a zero displacement. You should study the hyperlink to understand clearly the dynamics of waves.

Option A is incorrect. Phase angles **(PHY 7.1.3)** are important for waves of the same wavelength or frequency **(PHY 7.1.2)** and how they may interact **(PHY 7.1.3)** with each other. Since each of the waves is of a different wavelength, the phase angles are not relevant. Even comparing phases, the waves would be at the same position on their cycle which they are not.

LEO the lion says **GER**rrrr

Lose **E**lectrons = **O**xidize

Gain **E**lectrons = **R**educe

CHM 10.1, 10.2

CHAPTER 1

Option D is incorrect. If the displacement were maximum, the amplitude **(PHY 7.1.2)** would be at its greatest above or below the equilibrium line. At the second intersection the displacement is zero.

Option B is incorrect. See the comments for option A. The waves are not at the same position of their cycle and could out of phase, but this is not the best description of what is occurring at the second intersection. Again, for MCAT purposes, phase angle differences will refer to waves of the same wavelength or frequency, but different amplitudes.

Option C is correct. The displacement is zero and the amplitude is zero. This is evident by looking at the corresponding location in Fig 1c. You should try to duplicate the waveforms in 1b and 1c by beginning with the waves in 1a.

Test Taking Skills Comment

This is a dichotomy **(SB A.2.3)** type question. Options A and B should have been eliminated because phase angles are not the issue in this problem. They may still have the same displacement at a given location with the same or different phase angles. The center horizontal line means zero displacement - this leads to option C.

This problem requires three or more steps **(SB A.1.3)** (1) you have to determine if the phase or displacement statement is true or false **(SB A.1.2)**, 2) you have to determine if the option is correct or incorrect **(SB A.1.2)**, and 3) you have to determine if it is the best option **(SB A.1.2)** which is always time consuming.

Q24 — Pre-Study Suggestions

Review the following if needed:
1) Wave Characteristics **PHY 7.1.2**
2) Standing Waves **PHY 7.1.5**
3) Equation Interpretation
4) Ratio and Proportions
5) Dichotomy of Options **SB A.2.3**
6) Three or More Steps **SB A.1.3**
7) nternal Inconsistency of Options **SB A.2.5**
8) What is the key piece of information from the passage required to answer this question?
9) Solve the problem.

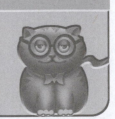

Solution Discussion

The key piece of information from the passage is the fact that the first harmonic (**PHY 7.1.5**), solid wave, has a wavelength twice as long as the second harmonic, long dash wave. This is evident by visual inspection of the Fig 1a.

The frequency (f) and wavelength (λ) (**PHY 7.1.2**) are related as follows:

$$f \propto 1/\lambda$$

Then if the $f_1 (= 100 \text{ Hz})$ of the first harmonic is 100 Hz, the f_2 is found by ratio and proportions using the relationship:

$$\frac{f_1}{f_2} = \frac{1/\lambda_1}{1/\lambda_2}$$

since $\lambda_1 = 2\lambda_2$, the relationship now becomes and substituting for f_1:

$$\frac{100 \text{Hz}}{f_2} = \frac{1/2\lambda_2}{1/\lambda_2} = \frac{1/2}{1} = \frac{1}{2}$$

then,

$$f_2 = 2 \times 100 \text{ Hz} = 200 \text{ Hz}.$$

The relationship of frequency and period (T) (**PHY 7.1.2**) is:

$$f = 1/T$$

then,

$$T = 1/f$$

substituting for f_2:

$$T = 1/f_2 = 1/200 \text{ Hz}$$
$$= 1/200 \text{ s}^{-1}$$
$$= 1/200 \text{ s}$$
$$= 0.005 \text{ s}.$$

Option A is correct.

Another and quicker way to get the answer is by understanding the harmonics are standing waves (**PHY 7.1.5**). Each successive harmonic has a frequency of nf_1 (n =1,2,3...) for if nodes or antinodes (**PHY 7.1.5**) are at each end, and nf_1 (with n = 1, 3, 5....) if a node and antinode are at each end (of the string or tube). The waves shown are of the former form and would use the equation

$$f_i = n_i f_1 \;$$

the second harmonic is

$$f_2 = n_2 f_1$$

where

$$n_2 = 2, f_1 = 100,$$

then,

$$f_2 = (2)(100)$$
$$= 200 \text{ Hz}.$$

And now the problem can be solved as above.

Test Taking Skills Comment

Know the relationships above, know how to use them, and do the arithmetic correctly or take your best guess. There is nothing of substance from the passage that will help you. This problem illustrates a very important concept to do well on this test. Only basic concepts **(SB A.2.2)** are required. In this case the relations $v = f\lambda$ and $f = 1/T$ are basic and simple. Most students would have regurgitated these if they were asked directly. Yet, only 45% (less than 25% excluding guessing) got this question correct. You have to know the basics well, be ready to recognize them and know how to apply them to questions such as this one.

This is a Dichotomy of Options **(SB A.2.3)** question, although it is a difficult one to understand. Recall that for a dichotomy question you must use some basic knowledge **(SB A.2.2)** to determine which half of the dichotomy you must eliminate. The dichotomy here is the decimal options

A and B and the non-decimal options C and D. The basic knowledge is to recall that the frequency and period **(PHY 7.1.2)** are inversely related and since the frequency is 100 Hz, the period must be 1/100 or 0.01 seconds for the first harmonic. Also, your basic knowledge should have reminded you that the harmonics are simple integer multiples of each other and the frequency and hence the period would be some small number multiple of each other and the larger seconds are not possible. A period of 50 seconds would mean a frequency of 1/50 or 0.02 Hz which is long way, not a small integer multiple, from 100 Hz. So, you would eliminate options C and D based on this analysis and take your guess from A and B and this would be better than the 45% that students who tried to solve the problem achieved.

Also, option B is an Internal Inconsistency **(SB A.2.5)** as 0.01 seconds for a period means 1/T = 1/0.01 = 100 Hz for the frequency which is the first harmonic and cannot be correct.

Finally, this is a Three or More Step **(SB A.1.3)** problem (1) first you have locate the first harmonic in the Figure given and know how it relates to the second (see discussion above), 2) you must determine what about the relationship of the two you can use to get to the period of the second, 3) you have to make the calculation to get the period of the second harmonic 4) you have to be sure it is the correct answer). Three or More Step options are difficult because of the time involved if not the content.

Q25   Pre-Study Suggestions

Review the following if needed:
1) Wave Characteristics **PHY 7.1.2**
2) Graphs and Charts **GS A.3**
3) What is the key piece of information from the passage required to answer this question?
4) Solve the problem.

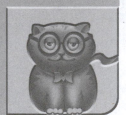

Solution Discussion

Fig 1a and the relative heights of the waves are all that is needed from the passage.

The Fig 1a clearly shows the first harmonic (the solid wave) to have a greater amplitude **(PHY 7.1.2)** (distance from the point of equilibrium to the peak of crest or the bottom of a trough) than either of the other two harmonics. It also shows the second (long dash wave) and third harmonic (short dash wave) to have the same amplitude. This makes **option A correct**. Option A shows the first amplitude the greatest and the second and third harmonics with lower but equal amplitudes. Each of the other options has an incorrect ratio of heights of the harmonics.

Test Taking Skills Comment

This is all a matter of knowing the definition of amplitude of a wave and how to read it from a waveform. It appears this basic bit of knowledge **(SB A.2.2)** is not widespread among students as only 55% got it correct. Study this section carefully.

Q26 — Pre-Study Suggestions

Review the following if needed:
1) Wave Characteristics **PHY 7.1.2**
2) Standing Waves **PHY 7.1.5**
3) Graphs and Charts **GS A.3**
4) Dichotomy of Options **SB A.2.3**
5) Camouflage and Distractions **SB A.1.3**
6) What is the key piece of information from the passage required answering this question?
7) Solve the problem.

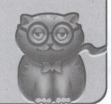

Solution Discussion

Fig 1a and the relative heights of the waves and the relative wavelengths are all that is needed from the passage. The amplitudes of the second (long dash) and third (short dash) harmonics are about the same. The wavelength of the first to second to third harmonics is each decreasing. [The wavelength from the first to the second, as well as the one from the second to the third is decreasing].

Option C is incorrect. Since the wavelengths are decreasing as the harmonics increase, it is expected that the wavelength of the fourth harmonic would be less than that of the others. If the wavelength is shorter, the frequency will be greater or higher and not lower because of the inverse relationship of the frequency and the wavelength.

Options A and B are incorrect. Since the amplitude **(PHY 7.1.2)** of the second and third harmonics is about the same, there is no reason to expect the fourth to be much different. The harmonics relate to frequency, period and wavelength **(PHY 7.1.2)** variations and not the amplitude. The amplitude will depend on the energy applied and not constraints of the object (such as its length, e.g.) which determine the harmonics.

Option D is correct. See the discussion of option C above.

CHAPTER 1

Test Taking Skills Comment

There is a minor Camouflage/Distraction **(SB A.1.3)** here as you should realize what is really at issue is what determines how harmonics relate to each other - if you realize this then you know that amplitude is not important and it is the frequency/wavelengths which distinguish between the harmonics.

This is a dichotomy problem **(SB A.2.3)**. You should eliminate options A and B as not important for standing waves and identify frequency as being important. Since only 55% of students got this correct, you could have did nearly as well as the whole group of students by using this technique to guess.

Q27 — Pre-Study Suggestions

Review the following if needed:
1) Wave Characteristics **PHY 7.1.2**
2) Wave Interactions **PHY 7.1.3**
3) Graphs and Charts **GS A.3**
4) Three Out of Four Options **SB A.2.8**
5) Camouflage/Distraction **SB A.1.3**
6) What is the key piece of information from the passage required answering this question?
7) Solve the problem.

Solution Discussion

An evaluation of the Fig 1c is needed from the passage along with 1a and 1b.

Looking at 1c, you may be able to determine that the summation wave has a complete waveform (PHY 7.1) and is just beginning to repeat itself. By comparing the wave in Fig 1c and the first harmonic in Fig 1a, you will see they begin and end, for a complete wave, at the same points. This would mean they have the same wavelength and the same period. This is not true of the second and third harmonics. Also,

the superimposition (PHY 7.1.3) of the waves cannot be complete until all the waves have completed a full cycle during the summation. Since the first harmonic has the longest wavelength, the summation cannot complete a full cycle until it has summated over its entire wavelength. The summation may require one or some multiple of the wavelengths of the longest wave. This is also why the period, wavelength, of the shorter harmonics cannot be the same as the summation wave. *Option A is correct.*

Test Taking Skills Comment

This is one of the most difficult questions on the test. But, you may have been able to reach the correct answer by carefully looking at the graph and remembering the definition of period and its relation to a wavelength. See the analysis above. Remember waves don't have to be sine waves. The waves in 1b and 1c are waves even though they do

not have the typical sine appearance. The other characteristics of a wave still hold.

This is a Camouflage and Distractions (SB A.1.3) as all you have to determine is that you are just being asked to know what makes a wave (PHY 7.1.2), its characteristics and how do you recognize it.

This is a Three Out of Four **(SB A.2.8)** type question. Options A, B and C all relate to the harmonics individually. Option D is the outlier relating to the sum of the harmonics. Outliers tend to be incorrect and can often be ignored. In this situation, your guess from A, B or C would have given you a 33% chance of success and this compares very favorably to the 30% the whole group of students achieved.

Q28 — Pre-Study Suggestions

Review the following if needed:
1) Wave Characteristics **PHY 7.1.2**
2) Wave Equation ($v=\lambda f$; $v=\lambda/T$) **PHY 7.1.2**
3) Equation Interpretation
4) Graphs and Charts **GS A.3**
5) Three Out of Four Options **SB A.2.8**
6) Camouflage and Distraction **SB A.1.3**
7) What is the key piece of information from the passage required answering this question?
8) Solve the problem.

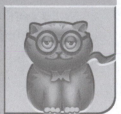

Solution Discussion

The speed of light **(PHY 9.2.4)** in a vacuum is 3.0×10^8 m/s - you are required to know this.

The key piece of information from the passage is the wavelength of the incident light that is:

1.06×10^{-6} m at the conversion efficiency of 0.42 for material B.

The key formula is **(PHY 7.1.2)**:

$$v = \lambda f$$

$v = c = 3 \times 10^8$ m/s
$\lambda = 1.06 \times 10^{-6}$ m
f = frequency in Hz.

Then with the substitutions:

$f = c/\lambda = 3.0 \times 10^8$ m/s / 1.06×10^{-6} m
$\approx 3 \times 10^{8\,-(-6)} \approx 3 \times 10^{14}$ Hz.

This is closest to **option C which is correct**.

Test Taking Skills Comment

This has nothing to do with the passage - only data is required from the passage. The formula is one that should be well known, yet, only 55% got this correct. This again shows the important of a solid understanding of the basic knowledge **(SB A.2.2)** required and not of complex or advanced topics. The wave equation **(PHY 7.1.2)** is very basic and is all that is required to solve this problem.

This problem is also a Camouflage/ Distraction **(SB A.1.3)** question because you may have been distracted by the use of the conversion efficiency. You could have rephrased this question to ask if given the wavelength of light, what is the frequency? This is a Three Out of Four **(SB A.2.8)** question. Options B, C and D all have positive exponents. Option A is the outlier with a negative exponent. Outliers are usually incorrect and can be ignored. Be careful with the Similar Pairs in this problem because more than one set may be visualized (A and D, B and C, and C and D), and when this occurs, it is not a good guess to rely on this method.

CHAPTER 1

Q29 — Pre-Study Suggestions

Review the following if needed:
1) Similar Pair Options **SB A.2.7**
2) Complex Sounding Option **SB A.2.2**
3) What is the key piece (s) of information from the passage required answering this question?
4) Solve the problem.

Solution Discussion

No prior information is needed to solve this problem.

One key piece of information is found in the first paragraph:

"The conversion efficiency (e) of a photoelectric …converted into electrical energy."

and, the second key is in the second paragraph:

"The photoelectric material had a coating that … certain frequencies."

If the coating absorbs more of the light, more of it will be used to excite the electrons and converted to energy. This will increase the conversion efficiency.
The correct option is C.

Option A is incorrect. There is nothing in the passage to suggest this. If it's not in the passage, there is no way you can know it. This is a Complex Sounding Option(s) **(SB A.2.2)**.

Option B is incorrect. Same as for option A.

Option D is incorrect. The current would be expected to increase if more of the incident light is absorbed because more electrons are released. Electron flow is the actual cause of electric current **(PHY 10.1)**.

Test Taking Skills Comment

This is like a reading question as all of the information is found in the passage. Notice that options A and B relate to knowledge. On the MCAT, there are two sources of knowledge (basic knowledge, **SB A.2.2**) as found in Complex Sounding Options **SB A.2.2**).The importance of you fully grasping and applying this concept and skill cannot be overemphasized. One source of knowledge is from your study - study knowledge **(SB A.2.2)**. The other source is from information you glean from the passage - passage knowledge **(SB A.2.2)**. The AAMC Student Manual delineates very clearly what you are expected to know. The knowledge base they require is general and not detailed nor esoteric. When you see an option which requires very detailed, esoteric or medical knowledge, which the general public is not aware of general knowledge **(SB A.2.2)**, it will not be knowledge from anything you were expected to study, know or bring to the test. e.g., options A and B refer to the cooling/warming effect of the absorption coating. This is detailed and esoteric. If the answer is not directly (or clearly indirectly) from the passage, then it is not a correct option **(SB A.1.2)**. There is nothing in the passage which pertains to, or allows you to make inferences regarding, cooling/heating. So, these cannot be correct options. Options A and B could be determined to be Similar Pairs **(SB A.2.7)**, but you use a more powerful skill, which Complex Sounding Options is, when you have this type of situation.

Q30 — Pre-Study Suggestions

Review the following if needed:

1) Electric Circuits **PHY 10.2**
2) Current **PHY 10.1**
3) Voltage **PHY 10.3**
4) Three Out of Four **SB A.2.8**
5) What is the key piece(s) of information from the passage required to answer this question?
6) Solve the problem.

Solution Discussion

The problem is correctly solved by visualizing or drawing the circuits:

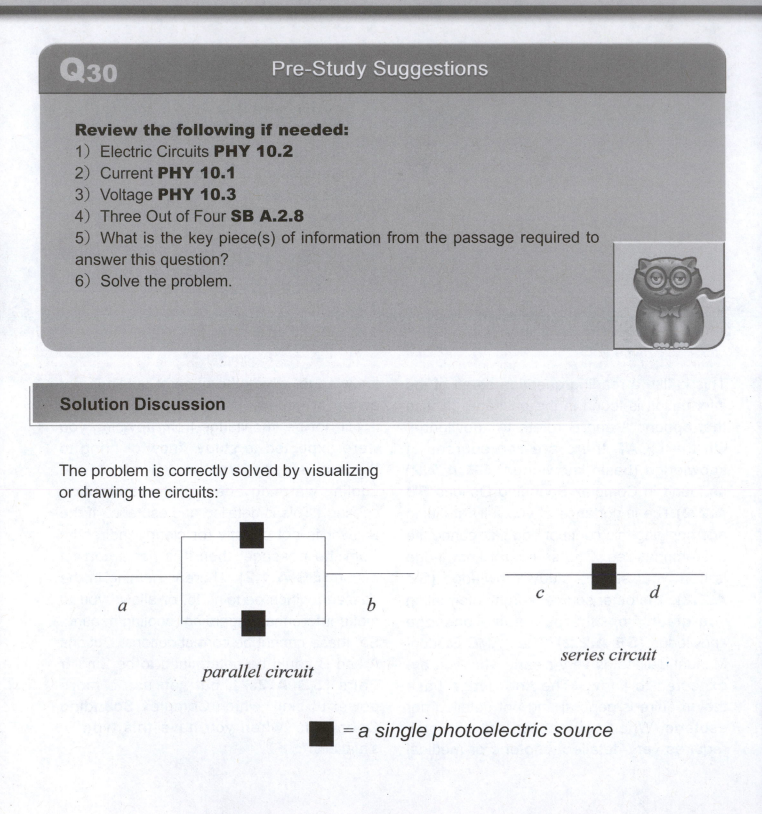

parallel circuit

series circuit

■ = *a single photoelectric source*

The voltage difference **(PHY 10.3)** at points c and d in the series circuit **(PHY 10.2)** of the single device will equal the voltage output of the photoelectric device. For the parallel circuit **(PHY 10.2)**, the voltage at points (a and b) will be the same for each source. This means the potential difference **(PHY 9.1.4)** (i.e., voltage difference) across each will be the same. The voltage difference will then be the voltage output of each of the photoelectric devices. The voltage output will still be the same as for a single device. Because of the parallel arrangement, the voltage is not doubled. ***The correct answer is option D.***

Test Taking Skills Comment

The correct analysis is as given above; it is a matter of understanding parallel and series circuits as discussed above. This is a Three Out of Four **(SB A.2.8)** question. Options A, B and C are all showing some change occurring. Option D is the outlier showing no change. Generally, the outlier will be incorrect and can be ignored. The exceptions are for negative type questions and for change questions. In such exceptional cases, these outliers may be correct. Also, usually the no change or zero option is incorrect. The guess technique did not work in this example but overall it is still very effective (see Test Taking Skills **SB A.2.4**).

Q31 — Pre-Study Suggestions

Review the following if needed:
1) Equation Interpretation
2) Dichotomy of Options **SB A.2.3**
3) What is the key piece(s) of information from the passage required to answer this question?
4) Solve the problem.

Solution Discussion

No prior information is needed to solve the problem.

The key piece of information from the passage is from paragraph 1:

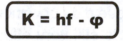

$$K = hf - \varphi$$

K = the kinetic energy of the ejected electron
hf = the energy of the incident photo
φ = the electron energy level (work function).

This means the photon energy, hf, can be written as follows:

$$hf = K + \varphi.$$

The energy of the photon, hf, is used to 'dislodge' the electron, which requires energy = φ. It also needs enough energy to accelerate the electron which is the kinetic energy = K.

Option B is incorrect. If the hf is less than the f, the electron cannot be dislodged.

Option C is incorrect. If the hf is less than K, the electron may not be ejected in the first place. Even if it could, there would be no kinetic energy or acceleration.

The work function must be exceeded by the incoming photon to eject the electron. If the photon's energy is less than the work function, the electron will not be ejected. The **correct answer is option A**.

Option D is incorrect. Same reasoning as C.

Test Taking Skills Comment

This option also has dichotomous sets **(SB A.2.3)** of answers - one set must be the correct set. The kinetic energy is that of the electron after ejection. It is the energy of the incoming photon that is used to accelerate the electron. It has nothing to do with the ejection of the electron itself. So, options C and D are incorrect based on this analysis. Then the choice is between options A and B. From the reading, should be clear; the energy level of the electron, the work function, must be overcome to eject the electron. Remember, the correct half of the dichotomy is determined by basic knowledge **(SB A.2.2)**, in this problem, it is passage knowledge **(SB A.2.2)** which helps you to the correct options.

Physical Sciences PASSAGE 3.PS. V

Q32 Pre-Study Suggestions

Review the following if needed:
1) Graphs and Charts **GS A.3**
2) Relationships of Variables
3) Three Out of Four Options **SB A.2.8**
4) What is the key piece(s) of information from the passage required answering this question?
5) Solve the problem.

Solution Discussion

No prior information is needed to solve this problem.

There is no additional information needed from the passage - the question itself contains all of the information needed.

This is just a relationship between two variables **(GS A.3)**, the conversion efficiency (ε) and the wavelength (γ) of the incident light. The problem states the conversion efficiency is independent of the incident wavelength. This means no matter how the wavelength changes, the conversion frequency will not change. Any graph of the two should show this. The graphs **(GS A.3)** are plotted with the conversion efficiency (ε) on the vertical axis and the wavelength on the horizontal axis. This means the conversion efficiency should have one value. In this case, the graph will be a straight horizontal line that represents one value for the conversion efficiency as the wavelength is changing. If the plot were reversed, with the conversion efficiency on the horizontal axis, the graph would be a vertical straight line. This means *option C is correct*.

Option A, B and D are each incorrect because each shows that the conversion efficiency is changing as the wavelength is changing which means it is not independent. Option A shows a variable relationship where there is peak value of the conversion efficiency at mid wavelengths and a fall off on each side. Option B would show a direct linear relationship. Option D shows an inverse relationship.

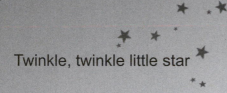

Twinkle, twinkle little star

Power equals I squared R

PHY 10.2

CHAPTER 1

Test Taking Skills Comment

This is really a graph problem to determine if you understand some of the basics of graphs. It is a Three Out of Four (**SB A.2.8**) as options B, C and D all have one general trend of variation. But, it could also be a Three Out of Four for A, B and D because they are changing. In this question, the technique could lead you astray - it is not 100%. Usually the no-change or zero option is incorrect, but in this problem, it is the correct answer - this is why you emphasize knowledge and reasoning and only fall back on the guess techniques when you have to.

Q33 — Pre-Study Suggestions

Review the following if needed:

1) Intermolecular Forces **CHM 4.2**
2) Melting Points **CHM 4.3.2**
3) Colligative Properties **CHM 5.1**
4) Graphs and Charts **GS A.3**
5) Experimental Controls **GS C.1, C.2**
6) Camouflage and Distractions **SB A.1.3**
7) Three Out of Four Options **SB A.2.8**
8) What is the key piece of information from the passage required answering this question?
9) Solve the problem.

Solution Discussion

The information needed from the passage is the Table 1 data.

The relationship between molecular weight and melting point **(CHM 4.3.2)** is a direct one. As the molecular weight increases, the melting point will generally increase. To make comparisons to determine any effect, it is important to change only the variable of concern. In this case, this is the molecular weight. It is very important to control variables that may affect the parameter under study (*see* Experimental Controls **GS C.1, C.2**). In this case, this is the melting point. It is clear that intermolecular bonding **(CHM 4.2)** does affect the melting point just as the molecular weight does. Then to isolate the effect of the molecular weight on the melting point, intermolecular bonding differences should be kept to a minimum. Functional groups **(ORG 1.6)** have differing intermolecular bonding patterns, so, it is important to keep the functional groups as constant as possible.

Option A is incorrect. There is a mass difference between the two acids which is desirable. But, there is also a functional group difference between the variables which is the double bond **(CHM 3.5)** in the crotonic acid. This could skew the evaluation of differences in the melting points being only due to differences in the molecular weights.

Option D is incorrect. This is the same reasoning as in option A.

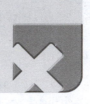

Option C is correct. The only difference between the propionic acid and the butyric acid is the presence of the $-CH_2-$ grouping. This is not considered a functional group and will have the least effect on the intermolecular forces as it is not polar and cannot form hydrogen bonds **(CHM 4.2)**. Its main effect is to add mass to the compound. Since the important variable of intermolecular forces does not change between the compounds, and because the mass does, any differences in the melting point would be reasonable to attribute to the mass differences.

Option B is incorrect. There is a significant difference in the functional groupings between the two compounds in that the oxalic acid has two acid groups to the one of the propionic acid. Since hydrogen bonding affects the melting point, any difference in the melting points could be due to this being present and not just due to the mass differences.

CHAPTER 1

Test Taking Skills Comment

This is a problem in experimental design applied to a specific chemical concept. You could have attacked it from the point of view of experimental design and looked for the least difference between the two compounds other than mass. This should have led you to eliminate option B. You would still have to guess between the others. To really attack the problem correctly, you would have to understand the melting point, factors affecting the melting point and functional groupings (which is really an organic chemistry concept). See the discussion above. This was a difficult question as only 40% of students got it correct. It could have been rephrase (*see* Camouflage and Distractions **SB A.1.3**) to ask what are the factors which affect melting points which could have led to the correct comparison. This can be viewed as a Three Out of Four Question **(SB A.2.8)**. Options A, B and C all contain propionic acid. Option D is an outlier without propionic acid. In general, outliers will be incorrect and can be ignored.

Q34   Pre-Study Suggestions

Review the following if needed:
1) pH **CHM 6.5**
2) Concentration Units **CHM 5.3.1**
3) Acids and Bases Titration **CHM 6.9**
4) Graphs and Charts **GS A.3**
5) Logarithms **GS A.4**
6) Camouflage and Distraction **SB A.1.3**
7) What is the key piece of information from the passage required to answer this question?
8) Solve the problem.

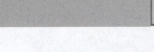

Solution Discussion

The key piece of information is found in Figure 1. At volume of 0 ml, the pH is about 3.

The problem asks for the amount of H_3O^+ (or H^+) present before the titration **(CHM 6.9)** with NaOH begins. This means you must know the equivalents **(CHM 5.3.1)** of acid (same as moles of H^+) present in the solution. The problem tells you there was 0.22g of the acid added to 30.0 ml of water. You could determine the amount of H^+ if you knew which acid was present, which you do not. So, you cannot find the concentration directly. The pH **(CHM 6.5)** is another way (as is the pOH) of finding the concentration of acid, H^+. The pH of the substance being titrated, unknown acid in this case, before any titration begins is the pH at 0 ml of the titrating agent, NaOH in this case, added. This is present in Fig 1 at the 0 ml point of volume (ml), (from the horizontal axis). Since the pH = 3 (approximately), the H^+ may be calculated from it as follows:

$$[H^+] = 10^{-pH} = 10^{-3} \text{ M} = 0.001 \text{ M}.$$

This is directly from the definition of pH and the conversion from pH back to the decimal form as discussed above. *The correct option is A.*

Test Taking Skills Comment

This is a very difficult problem as only 30% of students got it correct. Yet, it deals only with the concept of pH and hydrogen ions. The problem must have been where to get the pH from; this would suggest a deficit in interpretation of titration curves **(CHM 6.9)** that is also required by the MCAT. This section has some very low percentages correct. Acid-base must be another of the areas of general student weakness - this is another section to study carefully. This is a Camouflage/Distraction question. It is really only asking you to understand the relation of pH and H^+ concentration, the camouflage/distraction is forcing you to get the pH from a titration curve.

Q35 — Pre-Study Suggestions

Review the following if needed:

1) pK_a **CHM 6.9.2**
2) Acid Strengths **CHM 6.1**
3) Electrolytes **PHY 6.1.2**
4) Colligative Properties **CHM 5.1**
5) Exponents and Roots **GS A.4**
6) Logarithms **GS A.4**
7) Camouflage and Distraction **SB A.1.3**
8) Internally Inconsistent **SB A.2.5**
9) Dichotomy of Options **SB A.2.3**
10) Three or More Steps Analysis **SB A.1.3**
11) What is the key piece of information from the passage required to answer this question?
12) Solve the problem.

Solution Discussion

The key pieces of information are the pK_a's of the acids in Table 1.

The freezing point depression **(CHM 4.3.2)** depends on the number of particles present in solutions in relatively dilute solutions that are present in this question. Since these are weak acids **(CHM 6.1)**, you must use the pKa's **(CHM 6.9.2)** to determine the number of particles in solution. Since the pKa (3.14 and 4.77) of oxalic acid is lower than the pKa (4.69) of crotonic acid, this means the oxalic acid will be more dissociated in the solution than the crotonic acid. Additionally, there are two dissociable groups for the oxalic acid and only one for the crotonic acid. This means for oxalic acid:

$$HOOCCOOH \xrightleftharpoons{1st} HOOCCOO^- + H^+ \xrightleftharpoons{2nd} {}^-OOCCOO^- + 2H^+$$

1st = first dissociation   *2nd = second dissociation*

for crotonic acid:

$$CH_3CH = CHCOOH \rightleftharpoons CH_3CH = CHCOO^- + H^+$$

The H_o^+ will greatly outnumber the H^+. This means the oxalic acid solution will contain more particles than the crotonic acid solution and have a lower freezing point before the NaOH is added. The NaOH is added to do the following:

$$NaOH + H^+ \rightleftharpoons Na^+ + H_2O$$

- the NaOH is a base and neutralizes the acid

- to reach any common pH higher than that of the original solution, requires more added NaOH for the lower pH solution

- the lower pH solution is the one with the most H^+ which is the oxalic acid solution

- this means more NaOH is added to the oxalic acid solution to raise its pH to 4.7 than for the crotonic solution.

- So, for every molecule of NaOH added, there is the loss of one H^+ in solution and the gain of one Na^+ ion

- this means there is no net change in the number of particles in the solution (the water doesn't count as it is the solvent.

You calculate the pH of the solution by using the pKa of each acid (you do not have to do this to solve this problem):

For oxalic acid: this is too complicated for the MCAT and will be skipped.

For crotonic acid (HA):

Molecule/Ion Present	Start	Equilibrium
HA	0.1M	0.1-x
H^+	0	x
A^-	0	x

using the equilibrium expression **CHM 6.5**

$$K_a = [H^+][A^-] / [HA]$$

$pK_a = 4.69 \approx 4.7$

$K_a = 10^{-4.7} = 10^{-(5-0.3)}$
$= 10^{-5} \times 10^{0.3}$
$= 2 \times 10^{-5}$ M

$10^{0.3} = 2$ by looking up the antilog of 0.3

then,

$2 \times 10^{-5} = (x)(x)/(0.1 - x)$

since the acid is weak, it is assumed the x is small compared to 0.1 M

$2 \times 10^{-5} = x^2 /0.1$
$x^2 = (0.1)(2 \times 10^{-5})$
$= 2 \times 10^{-6}$
$x = 1.4 \times 10^{-3}$ M $= [H^+]$

the pH of the crotonic solution is then
$pH = -\log[H^+] = -\log(1.4 \times 10^{-3})$
$= -\log 1.4 - \log 10^{-3}$
$= -0.15 - (-3) = 2.85$.

You should review this process for your own benefit if it is not familiar to you. The pH of the oxalic acid solution is expected to be lower than this. You do not have to do all of this to solve this problem - it is presented for your overall review.

Option A is incorrect. If there were a lower number of particles, the solution should have a higher freezing point. This option is internally inconsistent **(SB A.2.5)**.

Option B is incorrect. The mass of the solute has nothing to do with colligative properties **(CHM 5.1)**, it is the number of particles in solution which is important. At any rate, since the molecular weight of the oxalic acid is greater than that of crotonic acid (see Table 1), this would not make any sense even if it was true - it is also internally inconsistent. The mass of all acids was the same at 0.22 g and so the percent mass **(CHM 5.3.1)** of all should be the same.

Option D is incorrect. Same as for option B.

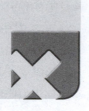

Option C is correct. As discussed previously, this is correct.

Test Taking Skills Comment

Some solid basic information is needed to solve this problem as shown above. You could have solved the problem with a modicum of good knowledge and applying it and would not have to go through the extensive analysis above. If you knew that freezing point depression was a colligative property **(CHM 5.1)** and that colligative properties depended on the number of particles in the solution and not the mass in the solution, you should have been able to eliminate options B and D immediately. Even if you did not know this, and looked at Table 1 and saw that the molecular mass (weight) of oxalic acid was greater than that of crotonic, then options B and D still would not make sense. Then if you further knew that the greater the number of particles, the lower the freezing point depression, and then option A would not be consistent. This analysis would leave you with option D without the complicated review shown above.

This is a Camouflage/Distraction **(SB A.1.3)** question. The real concept being tested is

your understanding of Colligative Properties in general. If you realized this, you would know you only have to determine which solution has the greatest number of particle present to get the correct answer. It also demonstrates internal inconsistency **(SB A.2.5)** of options for options A and B and D. Option A is inconsistent because the freezing point is lowered more for greater molar concentrations and not lower. Options B and D are inconsistent because you are told the mass in the solution is 0.22 g and therefore, the percent mass would be the same for both.

This is a double dichotomy **(SB A.2.3)** problem. The first dichotomy is crotonic / oxalic. Since the molar masses are about the same and since oxalic will dissociate more because of its pka (as seen in Table 1), the oxalic should lower the freezing point more and the correct half of the dichotomy is C or D. Also, if you realized that this is a colligative property question and the number of particles is important and not the mass percent, you would determine that molar concentration is the critical factor and not percent mass and pick options A or C from this second dichotomy. When you have a double dichotomy and properly evaluate both, the answer becomes obvious - C or D from the first dichotomy and A or C from the other dichotomy and the answer must be option C.

This is also a three or more step type question **(SB A.1.3)** (1) for each option, you must assess the second part as true or false, 2) then you must relate the second half to the first half to determine if it is still true or false in relation to the first half, 3) then you must determine if the overall option is true or false, 4) then you must determine if the option lowers the freezing point and how much and 5) you must determine which option is correct.). All of these steps make this a very difficult question.

This question should illustrate well the relative futility of studying simulated MCAT (i.e., made up) questions. These made up questions are rarely, if ever, prepared with the depth found on these MCAT practice tests. This is why this preparation does not rely on made up questions when you have the real tests available.

Q36 — Pre-Study Suggestions

Review the following if needed:
1) Acid Base Titrations **CHM 6.9**
2) Graphs and Charts **GS A.3**
3) Camouflage and Distractions **SB A.1.3**
4) What is the key piece of information from the passage required to answer this question?
5) Solve the problem.

Solution Discussion

The key piece of information is the curve in Figure 1.

When the RCOO⁻ (i.e., A⁻) equals the RCOOH (i.e., HA), this means the pH must be near/at the pK_a **(CHM 6.9)**. This occurs on a titration curve, for the first dissociation, at the point which is 1/2 between the neutralization point and the start of the titration. Note this is for the titration of an acid and for the first dissociation. If the acid had two protons dissociating, the second pK_a would be 1/2 between the two vertical neutralization points. For a base, if the axes are still pH and not pOH, the pK_a would correspond to the pK_a of the conjugate acid of the base **(CHM 6.3)**. For this problem (Fig 1):

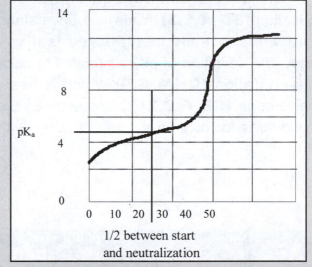

1/2 between start and neutralization

This pH is between 4 and 6 and is near but less than 5. **_The correct answer is A_** as this is the closest one.

Test Taking Skills Comment

This is a problem that requires you have some solid understanding of titrations as outlined above. You could also apply some of your basic knowledge about titrations **(CHM 6.9)** to eliminate some of the answers. If you remember that the vertical line on the titration curve is when the acid, in this case, is completely neutralized, that is, it is converted to its anion form of R-COO⁻ 100%, then you know the pH where there is still some R-COOH left must be prior to this vertical line. In this graph, Figure 1, the onset of the vertical line, or neutralization, is about at pH = 6. This means all the pH > 6.0 cannot be the answer and the only option left is A which is 4.8.

This is also a camouflage/distraction question **(SB A.1.3)**. You must understand that what is really being asked is if you know the definition of pK_a as relates to acid-base titration **(CHM 6.9)** which is basic knowledge **(SB A.2.2)**. You are given the conditions for pK_a on a titration curve with the information from the stem **(SB A.1)** *"concentration of R-COOH equaled the concentration of R-COO⁻"*. You just have to realize, this is a type of camouflage and rephrase the question to the more obvious question of "What is the pK_a?" When something seems very difficult and you are getting the feeling that you just can't possibly know this, try thinking about your basic knowledge as relates to the passage and, specifically, the question and look for camouflages and distractions and then use those techniques to try to reformulate the problem.

Q37 — Pre-Study Suggestions

Review the following if needed:
1) Acid Strengths **CHM 6.1**
2) Three or More Steps Options **SB A.2.8**
3) Internal Inconsistency of Options **SB A.2.5**
4) What is the key piece of information from the passage required to answer this question?
5) Solve the problem.

Solution Discussion

The key pieces of information are found in Table 1:

  • *first, the pK$_a$ of crotonic acid is 4.69*

  • *second, the melting point is 71.6 °C.*

  •*The molecular mass of the unknown was estimated to be 85-92 (last paragraph)*

  • *"... unknown acid that was liquid at room temperature..." (first paragraph).*

Option A is incorrect. Strong acids **(CHM 6.1)** have pK$_a$'s in the 1-2 range or lower.

Option B is incorrect. You are given no clear information to determine this at this time. Although, you are told that the unknown acid is dissolved in water, you don't know if this was crotonic acid. In general, short chain acids, less than 6 carbons, are usually soluble in water **(CHM 5.3)**.

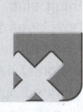

Option D is incorrect. The mass of crotonic acid is in the range of expected molecular weights and it could not be rejected on this basis.

Option C is correct. The molecule, crotonic acid, is a solid at room temperature because the melting point is above 20 °C, the typical room temperature. The unknown is a liquid at room temperature.

CHAPTER 1

Test Taking Skills Comment

This is a reading problem as much as any thing else. The only knowledge required is how does the pK_a relate to the strength of acids or bases. You should have eliminated option D based on reading. You should have affirmed option C based on the phrase noted above about the unknown being a liquid assuming you knew that 20 $^{\circ}$C was about room temperature.

Options A (the pK_a of crotonic acid is inconsistent with it being a strong acid), B (polar organic molecules less than 6 carbons are often soluble in water) and D (the molecular weight of crotonic acid is in

the range projected for the unknown) are all internally inconsistent **(SB A.2.5)** with basic knowledge **(SB A.2.2)**.

This is also a three or more step type question **(SB A.1.3)** (1) first you must determine if the option is true or false for crotonic acid, 2) and this is done by comparing this to your study knowledge or passage knowledge **(SB A.2.2)**, 3) then you must determine if this qualifies crotonic acid to be rejected or not, i.e., is it the correct option). All of these steps make this problem more difficult than expected.

Q38 Pre-Study Suggestions

Review the following if needed:
1) Momentum **PHY 4.3**
2) Conservation of Momentum **PHY 4.4**
3) Nuclear Structure **PHY 12.1**
4) Nuclear Radioactive Decay **PHY 12.4**
5) Equation Interpretation
6) Exponentials and Roots **GS A.4**
7) Approximation **PHY 2.6.1, GS A.6**
8) Camouflage and Distraction **SB A.1.3**
9) Three Out of Four Options **SB A.2.8**
10) Solve the problem.

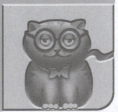

Solution Discussion

This is a conservation of momentum (PHY 4.4) problem. The problem is solved as follows:

- the object (^{226}Ra) is at rest with a velocity (PHY 1.3, 1.4) of zero and a momentum (PHY 4.3) of zero

- when the a particle (PHY 12.1) is emitted spontaneously, the ^{222}Rn (the nucleus loses two protons (PHY 12.1) and is a different element) must recoil because momentum must be conserved as there are no external forces acting

- therefore, the momentum (P_f) of the particles after the collision must equal the momentum before (P_i)

$$\sum P_i = \sum P_f,$$

- this means the following
$M_{Ra}V_{iRa} = M_{Rn}V_{fRn} + M_aV_{fa}$
where M = mass, V = velocity
Ra = for the radium, Rn = radon,
a = alpha particle, i = initial, f= final
M_{Ra} = 226 units (could convert to kg using atomic mass units but why?)
M_{Rn} = 222 (lost two protons and two neutrons)

M_a = 4(the alpha particle is the helium nucleus with two protons, two neutrons)
V_{iRa} = the initial speed of the radium = 0 m/s
V_{fRn} = the recoil speed of the radon (was radium)
V_{fa} = the final speed of the alpha particle = 1.5×10^7 m/s

- then substituting and solving the equation
$(226)(0 \text{ m/s}) = (222) V_{fRn} + (4)(1.5 \times 10^7 \text{ m/s})$

$0 = 222 V_{fRn} + 6 \times 10^7 \text{ m/s}$

$-222 V_{fRn} = 6 \times 10^7 \text{ m/s}$

$V_{fRn} = - (6 \times 10^7) / (222)$ m/s
$= - (6 /222) \times 10^7$ m/s
$= -3 /111 \times 10^7$ m/s
$= 1/37 \times 10^7$ m/s
(111 has a factor of 3 ... why? Approximation PHY 2.6.1, GS A.6)

$V_{fRn} = -0.0270 \times 10^7$ m/s
$= -2.7 \times 10^5$ m/s
$= -2.7 \times 10^5$ m/s.

CHAPTER 1

The correct answer is B. Notice that the sign of the answer depends on the coordinate system chosen. Also, the momentum of the gamma ray should have been included in the calculation but it is said to be negligible in the problem (also its mass is taken to be zero).

Test Taking Skills Comment

This was an extremely difficult problem as only 30% of students got it correct - this is nearly guessing. A student could have been misdirected, camouflage/distraction **(SB A.1.3)**, by thinking this was a spontaneous decay problem **PHY 12.4**. It is just a conservation of momentum **(PHY 4.4)** problem solved as shown above. Another problem could have been lack of knowledge of the particles of decay, because you are not given the mass of the alpha particle **(PHY 12.1)**. Another point is to leave units alone when they will cancel out and are in the correct ratios as for the mass of the radium and alpha particle above (use approximation **PHY 2.6.1, GS A.6** if needed). This appears to be one of those problems that should be skipped for most students until the end of the test and then try again or take your 25% guess. This is the same as a problem of an exploding object, as in a gun recoil, or two objects beginning at rest and moving apart (e.g., two ice skaters on ice pushing off from each other). Each may be solved by the conservation of linear momentum. This is also a three out of four question **(SB A.2.8)** as options A, B and C all are to power of 10^5 and option D is the outlier. Generally, outliers will be incorrect. So, if you just guessed from A, B or C, you would have had a percentage better than the average of those students who tried to do the problem.

Q39 — Pre-Study Suggestions

Review the following if needed:
1) Rate Equations **CHM 9.1**
2) Order of Reaction **CHM 9.3**
3) Kinetics **CHM 9.1**
4) Solve the problem.

Solution Discussion

Since the rate expression is given as rate = k $[NO_2][F_2]$, the order is the sum of the exponents which is 2 and this is second order. The *correct answer is option C.*

Test Taking Skills Comment

The answer is as easy as above - you either know it or you don't. This is a straight-forward study knowledge question **(SB A.2.2)** about kinetics **(CHM 9.1)**. But, only 65% of students got this question correct which suggests a general knowledge deficit. Study the discussion, in the references, carefully.

Q40   Pre-Study Suggestions

Review the following if needed:
1) Enthalpy **CHM 8.1**
2) Heats of Formation **CHM 7.2**
3) Thermodynamics **CHM 7.2**
4) Dichotomy of Options **SB A.2.3**
5) Solve the problem.

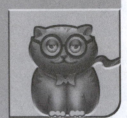

Solution Discussion

The equation is given as:

$$2HCl\ (g) \rightarrow H_2\ (g) + Cl_2\ (g).$$

The only other information given is the ΔH_f of HCl (g) at 25 °C which is -92.5 kJ/mol. The ΔH of the reaction at 25 °C is found as follows:

$\Delta H = \Delta H_f\ (products) - \Delta H_f\ (reactants)$
  $= \Delta H_f\ (H_2\ (g)) + \Delta H_f\ (Cl_2\ (g)) - 2\Delta H_f\ (HCl\ (g))$
  $= (0) + (0) - 2(\ -92.5\ kJ/mol)$
  $= +\ 185.0\ kJ/mol.$

The value of the ΔH_f of the elemental form **(CHM 7.2)** of an atom is 0 kJ/mol. So, the value for the hydrogen and the chlorine are each 0 kJ/mol.

The **correct answer is option D**.

Test Taking Skills Comment

The answer is as discussed previously - you either know it or you don't. Don't forget the units are in kJ/mol, so the number of moles must be accounted for. This is a dichotomy of options **(SB A.2.3)** type question with two sets of dichotomies. The set of 185 vs 92.5 is not of much value as there is no obvious way to select between the two. The set of positive/negative values is not much better. But, if you look at the equation given and remember that the enthalpy is the products minus the reactants, since the HCl is a reactant and negative, it will become positive when subtracting and this suggests the answer is positive and would be C or D. This is a very weak dichotomy and there is no problem with simply ignoring it if you are unsure of the knowledge to select the correct dichotomy.

Q41 — Pre-Study Suggestions

Review the following if needed:
1) Lenses **PHY 11.5, 11.5.1**
2) Lens Equation **PHY 11.5, 11.5.1**
3) Equation Interpretation
4) Dichotomy of Options **SB A.2.3**
5) Solve the problem.

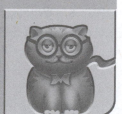

Solution Discussion

The question is solved by using the magnification portion of the lens equation **(PHY 11.5, 11.5.1)**

$$m = -d_i / d_o$$

d_i = the image distance
= 4 f/3 units
d_o = the object distance

= 4 f units

$m = -(4f/3) /4f$
$= -(4f/3) \times (1/4f)$
$= -1/3 = -d_i / d_o$
= ratio of image to the object.

The **correct option is A.**

Test Taking Skills Comment

Answer is as above - you either know it or you don't. The reference discussion is long, but any part of it may be used to test your knowledge. You could try a dichotomy of options **(SB A.2.3)**, but the key to a dichotomy is the application of some basic knowledge **(SB A.2.2)** to select one of the sets in the dichotomy - there is no obvious way to do this.

Q42 — Pre-Study Suggestions

Review the following if needed:
1) Oxidation Number **CHM 10.1**
2) Formal Charge **CHM 10.1, 10.2**
3) Oxidation Reduction **CHM 10.1**
4) Camouflage and Distractions **SB A.1.3**
5) Dichotomy of Options **SB A.2.3**
6) What is the key piece of information from the passage required to answer this question?
7) Solve the problem.

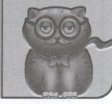

Solution Discussion

The key information is found under the heading, 'Formation of SO_2':

'...sulfuric acids form SO_2 when it reacts with ...SO_2 are formed in hot solutions of Cu(s) in H_2SO_4.'

The reaction would be:

$$H_2SO_4 + Cu \rightarrow Cu^{+1} + SO_2$$
(not all molecules are shown and not balanced).

The sulfur in the H_2SO_4 is (to find **oxidation state CHM 10.1**):

H_2		S		O_4		
↓		↓		↓		
2(+1)	+	X	+	4(-2)	=	0

- the hydrogen is +1 because it is not in a metallic compound
- the oxygen is -2 because it is not in one of the special compounds
- the net charge on the sulfuric acid is zero

then solving this equation,
$$+2 + x + (-8) = 0$$
$$x + 2 - 8 = 0$$

$x - 6 = 0$
$x = +6$ in the sulfuric acid.

In the SO_2, the oxidation state of the sulfur is,

S		O_2		
$\downarrow$		$\downarrow$		
X	+	2(-2)	=	0
X	-	4	=	0

X = + 4 in the sulfur dioxide

So, the sulfur goes from +6 to +4 in the reaction. *Option B is correct.*

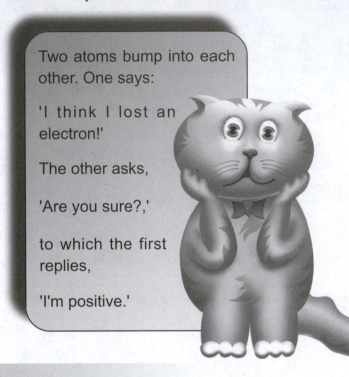

Two atoms bump into each other. One says:

'I think I lost an electron!'

The other asks,

'Are you sure?,'

to which the first replies,

'I'm positive.'

Test Taking Skills Comment

The only information needed from the passage is data which is that sulfur dioxide is the product of the reaction of sulfuric acid with the copper. The rest is all prior knowledge and is analyzed as shown. This is a dichotomy type question **(SB A.2.3)** with the two sets being A/B with 4/6 and C/D with 6/8. There is also a second dichotomy here being options B/C, with the initial oxidation state being +6 and options A/D, with the final oxidation state being +6. There is another dichotomy here which is options A/C, with the sulfur being oxidized **(CHM 10.1)**, and options B/D, with the sulfur being reduced **(CHM 10.1)**. To choose the correct dichotomy, you must use some basic knowledge **(SB A.2.2)**. For the 6/8 vs 4/6 dichotomy, it is very unlikely, but not impossible to have an oxidation state **(CHM 10.1)** of +8. This would mean all eight electrons would have been removed - this is essentially taking all the 8 electrons in s and p orbitals **(CHM 2.2)** from the inert gas configuration **(CHM 2.3)** of the Octet Rule **(CHM 2.3)** - this is highly unlikely. For sulfur, it is also very unlikely because sulfur is in group VIA on the periodic chart **(CHM 2.3)** and this means there are only 6 valence electrons **(CHM 3.5)**, and the last two electrons would have to come from a very stable shell. Based on this knowledge, the options with +8 should be eliminated leaving A and B. The next dichotomy of the initial sulfur being +6 is correct and options A and D are eliminated based on the discussion in the last section. Finally, the reaction in the last section showed the Cu going from 0, its elemental form, to +1 which means it was oxidized. This means the sulfur must be reduced and its oxidation state must decrease. This means options B or D must be correct. Combining all of these, the only possible answer would be B.

Q43   Pre-Study Suggestions

Review the following if needed:
1) Chemical Equations **CHM 1.5**
2) Stoichiometry **CHM 1.1**
3) Combustion Reaction **ORG 3.2.1**
4) Internal Inconsistency of Options **SB A.2.5**
5) Three Out of Four Options **SB A.2.8**
6) What is the key piece of information from the passage required to answer this question?
7) Solve the problem.

Solution Discussion

The key piece of information is found in the paragraph 'Preparation of Sulfuric Acid'
"*...the combustion of elemental sulfur to sulfur dioxide...*"

You are told that elemental sulfur undergoes

a combustion reaction **(ORG 3.2.1)**. This means the sulfur must react with oxygen. The only option which has sulfur, S, and oxygen, O_2, as the reactants is **option D that is correct**. You are told in the paragraph that sulfur dioxide results from the combustion.

Option C is a decomposition reaction **(CHM 1.3)** and *is incorrect*.

Options A and B are combustion reactions, because oxygen is a reactant, but do not involve elemental sulfur and *are incorrect*. These are Internally Inconsistent **(SB A.2.5)**.

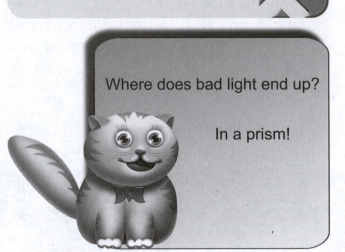

Where does bad light end up?

In a prism!

Test Taking Skills Comment

All this question is asking is do you know what a combustion reaction is. Knowing that a combustion reaction involves the reaction of elemental oxygen, O_2, with a compound or element, this would eliminate option C, which has no elemental oxygen as a reactant. You are told in the question that elemental sulfur, S, is the other reactant - this eliminates options A, B and C which have no elemental sulfur as they are internally inconsistent **(SB A.2.5)**. This leaves option D as the only possible option.

This is also a three out of four question **(SB A.2.8)** as options A, B and D all have oxygen as a reactant. Option C does not have oxygen as a reactant and is an outlier. Outliers are generally incorrect.

You should check to make sure the equations are all balanced if you are having difficulty coming up with the answer - they are.

Q44 — Pre-Study Suggestions

Review the following if needed:
1) Le Chatelier's Principle **CHM 9.9**
2) Camouflage and Distraction **SB A.1.3**
3) Dichotomy of Options **SB A.2.3**
4) What is the balanced equation for the second step of the reaction discussed in the question?
5) What is the key piece of information from the passage required to answer this question?
6) Solve the problem.

Solution Discussion

From the second paragraph is the following:
"followed by the catalytic ... sulfur trioxide."

To get sulfur trioxide from sulfur dioxide, the following must occur:

	Catalyst	
$2SO_2(g) + O_2(g)$	$\rightleftharpoons$	$2SO_3(g)$
Sulfur Dioxide		Sulfur Trioxide

Following the suggestion in the discussion on Le Chatelier's **(CHM 9.9)**, rewrite the equation as:

	Catalyst	
$2SO_2(g) + O_2(g)$	$\rightleftharpoons$	$2SO_3(g)+$ volume
Sulfur Dioxide		Sulfur Trioxide

No information is given as to the energy of the reaction.

Option A is incorrect. There is no information given as to the enthalpy, or free energy **(CHM 8.1)**, of the reaction. You may assume that a combustion reaction would proceed with a negative enthalpy, which is favorable, but the decrease in the number of gaseous molecules suggests that the entropy **(CHM 8.9)** is also negative which is unfavorable. You cannot assess this option with the information given.

Option D is incorrect. If the oxygen is removed, this means the reaction is shifted to the left also decreasing the sulfur trioxide.

Option C is correct. If the sulfur trioxide is removed, this will shift the reaction to the right causing more of it to be produced.

Option B is incorrect. If the pressure is reduced, this means the volume should be increased. If the volume is increased, this means the reaction is shifted to the left as written and this will reduce the sulfur trioxide.

Q: Can you guess the name of a first year chemistry student who scored one "**C**" and **4** "**F**"s in five courses?

A: Carbon Tetrafluoride.
(i.e. **CF₄**)
That was simply awful.

Test Taking Skills Comment

The Le Chatelier's Principle **(CHM 9.9)** is a must when dealing with any system which is at equilibrium and then undergoes a disturbance or change of some sort. You must be able to recognize when it is applicable, as the situations are numerous. Remember the two keys above that are highlighted. Remember, in a camouflage question **(SB A.1.3)**, you are given the conditions or results that suggest what concept/equation/principle you will use. Here you are told what must be done to increase the yield of a reaction. This statement and the disturbances are what occur in the Le Chatelier's - you must recognize this and use it.

This is also a Dichotomy of Options **(SB A.2.3)**, but it is difficult to resolve quickly. The 'reducing' or 'removing' are similar in meaning, and in an equilibrium could cause a shift in either direction depending upon what is affected. When the selection of the half of the dichotomy is not relatively obvious using Basic Knowledge (study, passage) **(SB A.2.2)**, it is best not to use the technique.

CHAPTER 1

Q45 — Pre-Study Suggestions

Review the following if needed:
1) Concentration Units **CHM 5.3.1**
2) Moles **CHM 1.3**
3) Density **CHM 5.3.1**
4) Equation Interpretation
5) Dimensional Analysis **GS Part II 2.3 # 16**
6) Camouflage and Distraction **SB A.1.3**
7) Internal Inconsistency of Options **SB A.2.5**
8) Three Out of Four **SB A.2.8**
9) What is the key piece of information from the passage required to answer this question?
10) Solve the problem.

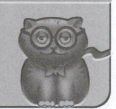

Solution Discussion

The pieces of information needed from the passage are:

- from under 'Properties':
"Concentrated sulfuric acid is 98% sulfuric acid and 2% water by mass."

*"It has a density **(CHM 5.3.1)** of 1.84 g/mL..."*

The formula for moles **(CHM 1.3)** of a substance is:

$$moles = mass / molecular\ mass$$

2(1) + 16 = 2 +18 = 18 g/mole (using the Periodic Table **(CHM 2.3)** that is provided).

The mass of water in the concentrated sulfuric acid is:

- the water is 0.02 (= 2%, a percent mass **CHM 5.3.1**) of the mass of the solution

- one ml of the solution has a mass of

$$\rho = m/V$$

from the density equation above:

$$\rho = 1.84\ g/ml$$
$$V = 1\ ml$$

then,

$$m = \rho V = (1.84\ g/ml)(1ml)$$
$$= 1.84\ g\ of\ mass\ in\ the$$
concentrated sulfuric acid

Since water is 0.02 of this,
mass of water
= total mass x percent of water
= 1.84 x 0.02 g.

Then,

moles of water
= (mass of water)/molecular mass of water
= (1.84 x 0.02 g) /18g /mole
= (1.84 x 0.02) /18   moles in one ml of solution.

This means **option B is correct**.

Option A is incorrect. This is the total moles in one ml of solution. The first part is the moles of sulfuric acid; the second part is the moles of water.

Option D is incorrect. This is the moles of sulfuric acid in one ml multiplied by the molar mass of water - again it is non-sensical.

Option C is incorrect. This is the mass of sulfuric acid divided by the molar mass of water and it means nothing.

Test Taking Skills Comment

This has very little to do with the passage. You must be able to find the key information from the passage that is data only. This question is simply a mole question where you have to determine the moles (CHM 1.3) using densities (CHM 5.3.1) and percent composition (CHM 5.3.1). Analysis for the consistency of dimension (GS Part II 2.3 # 16) will often eliminate options. In this problem, the only elimination would have been option D - all the others do end up with moles as the unit - can you figure this out? The dimensional inconsistency all makes

this an internal inconsistency of options (SB A.2.5). Other inconsistencies are the conflict of the definition of moles with the grams of one substance in the numerator and a different substance's molar mass in the denominator (options C and D).

This is also a dichotomy type question (SB A.2.3) with several possible dichotomies. The one group you should be able to eliminate is any one with 98, the molar mass of sulfuric acid, in the denominator - this eliminates options A and D. You may also be able to determine that you need to use 0.02, the 2% water, to get the mass of water; any option without 0.02 in the numerator would be incorrect - this eliminates options C and D. You should know that the moles of water would have to have only the molar mass of water, 18, as the denominator and this means your answer must come from B or C. This is a double dichotomy and you should end up with the answer, which is B, when you correctly analyze the dichotomies.

This is also a three out of four question **(SB A.2.8)** with several groups of three out of four. One set is A, B and C which all have 18 in the denominator. Then B and C are also a similar pair **(SB A.2.7)** with only 18 in the denominator. So, your answer could come from B or C. But, remember to be careful when using similar pairs when you can identify more than one or when dichotomies are present (they are always two similar pairs). Also, options B, C and D are also a three out of four having only one number in the denominator. Remember, when you use these techniques, you are in a guess mode to increase your guess percentage above 25%. In each of these, you would be above 25% and in several you would be at 50% and with one you would get the correct answer. Only 55% of students got this question correct, so any good guess puts you in their company.

Q46 — Pre-Study Suggestions

Review the following if needed:
1) Oxidation States **CHM 10.1**
2) Oxidation Reduction Reactions **CHM 10.1**
3) Oxidizing Agent **CHM 10.1**
4) Reducing Agent **CHM 10.1**
5) Camouflage and Distractions **SB A.1.3**
6) Internal Inconsistency of Options **SB A.2.8**
7) Three Out of Four Type Question **SB A.2.8**
8) Similar Pair Options **SB A.2.7**
9) What is the key piece of information from the passage required to answer this question?
10) Solve the problem.

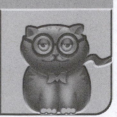

Solution Discussion

The key piece of information from the passage is from the paragraph, 'Formation of SO_2'

"...because most metals react with solutions of H_2SO_4 to form hydrogen gas and a metal sulfate."

The reaction under question then must be (not balanced):

0 losing electrons +2

$$Fe(s) + H_2SO_4 \rightarrow Fe^{+2} + SO_4^{-2} + H_2(g)$$

+1 gaining electrons 0

The numbers show the oxidation states **(CHM 10.1)** of the selected atoms. Notice the oxidation state of the sulfur and oxygen do not change (S is +6, and O is -2). Since the Fe is losing electrons, it is being oxidized **(CHM 10.1)** and must be acting as the reducing agent **(CHM 10.1)**. It is not necessary to know the exact charge of the Fe, only that it goes from neutral to positive. Note it must be positive to form a metal sulfate because the sulfate

is negative. *The correct answer is A*.

Option B is incorrect. The $FeSO_4$ is a product of the reaction per the passage information noted above.

Option C is incorrect. Neither the oxidation states **(CHM 10.1, 10.2)** of the sulfur nor the oxygen has changed.

Option D is incorrect. The hydronium ion, the hydrogen part, is reduced and is acting as the oxidizing agent **(CHM 10.1)**.

CHAPTER 1

First Law of Cat Thermodynamics

Heat flows from a warmer to a cooler body, except in the case of cats, in which case all heat flows to us.

Test Taking Skills Comment

This has very little to do with the passage. You must be able to find the key information from the passage that requires some understanding as shown. If you know the basics about oxidation-reduction, you should be able to eliminate options B and C as discussed above. Notice that whenever you have an acid (CHM 6.1, 6.2) in water solution, you also have H_3O^+. A base (CHM 6.1, 6.2) in water will generate hydroxide ion.

This is a borderline camouflage/distraction (SB A.1.3) type question and you can make it simpler by rephrasing it. It's borderline, because it tells you it wants the reducing agent. You should rephrase the question to 'what agent is being oxidized?' because this is what reducing agents (CHM 10.1) do.

This is also an internal inconsistency (SB A.2.5) of options question. Options B and C are all products and cannot be the reducing agent which must be a reactant. Also, option D, the H part is reduced in the reaction and would be the oxidizing agent.

You could legitimately call this a three out of four (SB A.2.8) or similar pair (SB A.2.7) options. Options B, C and D would be the three as all are multi atom species with A as the outlier. The similar pair would be B and C with the sulfate group. Either of these will lead you to the wrong answer. Remember, the guessing techniques are for guessing - when you have no clue. Overall, the guessing techniques (SB A.2.4) give you a greater than 25% correct rate (the baseline guess rate).

Q47 — Pre-Study Suggestions

Review the following if needed:
1) Acid Strengths **CHM 6.1**
2) Acids and Bases **CHM 6.1, 6.2**
3) Percentage Composition **CHM 5.3.1**
4) Camouflage and Distractions **SB A.1.3**
5) Three Out of Four **SB A.2.8**
6) Solve the problem.

Solution Discussion

The following steps will occur:

1) $H_2SO_4 + H_2O \rightleftarrows H_3O^+ + HSO_4^{-1}$

2) $HSO_4^{-1} + H_2O \rightleftarrows H_3O^+ + SO_4^{-2}$

The first reaction would ordinarily go to completion. But, there is only 2% (percentage composition **CHM 5.3.1**) water by weight. So, not all of the H_2SO_4 can react

with the water. This means a lot of H_2SO_4 will remain undissociated in the solution. There will be no free water molecules in the solution. The second reaction, which would normally proceed well to the right, also, cannot do so because there is so little water in the solution. This means there will be very little of the SO_4^{-2} present. **Option A is correct.**

Test Taking Skills Comment

In the typical acid solution, that is not concentrated acid, this first reaction would go to completion leaving very little or none of the original H_2SO_4 because it is a strong acid. But, due to the limited water, only a small amount of it can dissociate. In dilute solutions, the HSO_4^{-1} would also dissociate nearly completely because it is also very strong. This then would make SO_4^{-2} of higher concentration than the undissociated acid. Obviously, a very difficult question as few of us got it correct - yet, it is based on simple concepts.

This is a camouflage/distraction question **(SB A.1.3)** as it is really dealing with acid-base equilibria **(CHM 6.1, 6.2)** understanding the relative strengths of acids and bases.

This is also three out of four **(SB A.2.8)** type question. There are two sets of three out of four which are A, B and D (all contain sulfate) and A, C and D (all are charged). Combining these, the possible options are A and D. You can either guess from either of the three out of fours or from the combination. Either guess will result in the possible correct option at greater than the 30% guess rate that the general student body had.

Q48 — Pre-Study Suggestions

Review the following if needed:
1) Oxidation Reduction Reactions **CHM 10.1**
2) Half Reactions **CHM 10.1**
3) Galvanic Cells **CHM 10.2**
4) Anode **CHM 10.1**
5) Cathode **CHM 10.1**
6) Internally Inconsistent **SB A.2.5**
7) Dichotomy of Options **SB A.2.3**
8) Solve the problem.

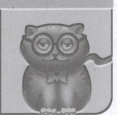

Solution Discussion

The first step is to determine what the starting reactants are. The reactants are Zn (s) and H^+(aq) from HCl. Then knowing this, you can determine the possible half-reactions and if they will occur or not. The half-reactions must be consistent with your starting reactants.

The two reductions, this is the standard method of writing, half reactions (**CHM 10.1**) are:

$$Zn^{+2} (aq) + 2e^- \rightarrow Zn(s) \quad E^o = -0.763 \text{ V}$$

$$2H^+ (aq) + 2e^- \rightarrow H_2(g) \quad E^o = 0.0 \text{ V}.$$

The Cl⁻ does not change and is ignored in the half reactions. This will be a galvanic cell (**CHM 10.2**) because the voltage (**PHY 9.1.4**) will be created as a result of a chemical reaction. A cell will only operate if the cell potential is positive. Then the reaction must be written as follows (which is consistent with the starting reactants):

$$Zn(s) \rightarrow Zn^{+2} (aq) + 2e^- \quad E^o = +0.763 \text{ V}$$

$$2H^+ (aq) + 2e^- \rightarrow H_2(g) \quad E^o = 0.0 \text{ V}.$$

Since the electrons will now cancel out, the half reactions may be added to give the galvanic cell:

$$2H^+(aq) + Zn(s) \rightarrow Zn^{+2}(aq) + H_2(g)$$

$$E^o = +0.763 \text{ V}$$

This reaction will proceed as written because the potential (voltage) is positive. The Cl⁻, which is a spectator ion (not involved directly in the oxidation reduction (**CHM 10.1**) may now be added back:

$$2HCl(aq) + Zn(s) \rightarrow ZnCl_2(aq) + H_2(g)$$

$$E^o = +0.763V.$$

The oxidation half reaction is the:

$$Zn \rightarrow Zn^{+2} + 2e^-$$ and this is the anode. (**CHM 10.1**)

The reduction half reaction is the:

$$2H^+ + 2e^- \rightarrow H_2$$ and this is the cathode. (**CHM 10.1**)

If the potential (voltage) (**PHY 9.1.4**) for the

reaction would have been negative, then the half reactions would have to be reversed to have a spontaneous reaction. Remember, you do not multiply the voltage, as you do for thermodynamic terms **(CHM 7.2)**, when you multiply the equations.

Option A is incorrect. This should have been eliminated because the formula for zinc chloride is incorrect. You are given that the zinc is +2. From the HCl formula, you should be able to determine that the Cl must be -1 since H is +1 in this molecule. This means ZnCl cannot be correct.

Option C is incorrect. This question is not a matter of less reactivity per se. It is a matter of one of the half reactions being the reduction half and the other being the oxidation half so the electron flow may cancel. Then it is a matter of the potential of the cell being positive and not negative. Again, if the cell potential, the sum of the two half reactions, is negative, the

half reactions must be reversed to get a positive potential and a spontaneous reaction. You could compare relative reactivity's for a reduction half reaction or for an oxidation half reaction, but it makes little sense to compare oxidation vs. reduction. So, for Zn to react, it must undergo oxidation **(CHM 10.1)** which it does in this reaction. For H_2 to react, it must undergo an oxidation as well, which it does not do in this reaction. Since both options are oxidation, you can then compare reactivities by comparing the oxidation potentials **(CHM 10.1)**. The oxidation potential for Zn is +0.763 V and for H_2, it would be 0.00 V. The greater, more positive, the potential for the direction of reaction, the greater the reactivity. Since the oxidation potential of Zn is greater than H_2, this means Zn is more reactive than H_2. You could also determine this because H_2 is the product in the reaction shown above. If H_2 was more reactive than Zn in the oxidation reaction, it would be the reactant and not the product. This option is false **(SB A.1.2)** and incorrect **(SB A.1.2)**.

Option D is incorrect. This is the same reasoning as for option C, except now we must compare the reduction potentials **(CHM 10.1)** because Zn^{+2} will be reduced and H^+ will also be reduced. Now the one with the most positive reduction potential will be the most reactive. The reduction potential, written as a reduction half-cell, for Zn^{+2} is -0.763 V and for H^+ it is 0.00 V. Since $0 > -0.763$, this means H^+ is more reactive than Zn^{+2} in

a reduction half-reaction. Now this statement is true **(SB A.1.2)** but not correct. It is not correct, because a reaction does occur and is not dependent on this fact.

Option B is correct. These products are produced as shown above.

Test Taking Skills Comment

See the discussion above. The only other information you are required to know is the standard potential of the hydrogen gas/ hydrogen ion half reaction which is 0.0V because it is the standard half cell set to 0V. This is a dichotomy question **(SB A.2.3)**. You may be able to determine that 'reactivity' is not the issue here as you are looking for an oxidation half reaction and a reduction

half reaction represented by the molecules listed. This allows you to eliminate options C and D. If the issue was about more reactivity as a reducing agent, or the reduction half reaction, or vice-versa for the oxidation, then it would make sense to compare reactivities. Option A is an example of internal inconsistency **(SB A.2.5)** in that ZnCl is not consistent with the charges given for Zn.

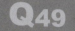
THE SILVER BULLET Real MCATs Explained

Physical Sciences PASSAGE QUESTIONS 3.PS.NPIII

Q49   Pre-Study Suggestions

Review the following if needed:
1) Mechanical Power **PHY 9.1.4**
2) Kinetic Energy (KE or K = mv^2/2) **PHY 5.3**
3) Work (W = Fd or W = Fdcosθ) **PHY 5.1, 9.1.4**
4) Equation Interpretation
5) Internal Inconsistency of Options **SB A.2.5**
6) Solve the problem.

Solution Discussion

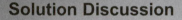

Energy **(PHY 5.2)** may be substituted for work **(PHY 9.1.4)** as they may be interchangeable and both have the units of joules and the power formula **(PHY 9.1.4)** is:

P = energy (work) change / time
  = joules / seconds = J/s.

Another formulation of the power formula using work is:

P = W / t = Fd / t = F (d / t) = Fv
v = d/t = velocity.

The force **(PHY 2.2)** and velocity **(PHY 1.3, 1.4)** would be the averages over the time period.

Work is a scalar **(PHY 1.1)** and power is a scalar.

Option A is incorrect. The final velocity and height cannot be used to determine power by themselves. You must have a work (energy) term and elapsed time. The final velocity could be used to determine the kinetic energy **(PHY 5.3)** contribution if the mass was known. The height could be used to determine the gravitational potential energy **(PHY 5.4)** if the mass and g, gravitational acceleration **(PHY 2.5)**, are known.

Option B is incorrect. The mass would not be needed. The amount of work is needed but again there is no elapsed time given.

determine the work performed. But, again the elapsed time is needed to determine the power.

Option C is incorrect. Force exerted and distance moved under the force could be used to

Option D is correct. Power is defined as the work done in a given time period.

Test Taking Skills Comment

See the discussion above. You must know the definition of power in mechanical terms to solve the problem. There is some internal inconsistency **(SB A.2.5)** of options, but this is only evident if you know what power is - these options are A, B and C and are discussed above.

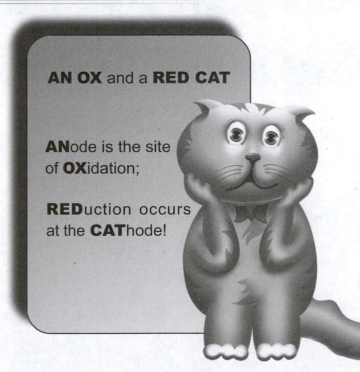

AN OX and a **RED CAT**

ANode is the site of **OX**idation;

REDuction occurs at the **CAT**hode!

Q50 — Pre-Study Suggestions

Review the following if needed:
1) Periodic Table **CHM 2.3**
2) Periodic Trends **CHM 2.3**
3) Atomic Radius **CHM 2.1**
4) Chemical Structures **CHM 2.2**
5) Sigma Bonds **CHM 3.5**
6) Pi Bonds **CHM 3.5**
7) Bond Lengths **CHM 3.1, 3.2**
8) Resonance of Molecules **ORG 1.4, 7.1, 8.1**
9) Camouflage and Distraction **SB A.1.3**
10) Mutually Excluding Options **SB A.2.6**
11) Three Out of Four Options **SB A.1.4**
12) Negative Question **SB A.1.2**
13) Solve the problem.

Solution Discussion

The molecule is nitric acid:

HNO_3.

The line and stick structure of nitric acid is:

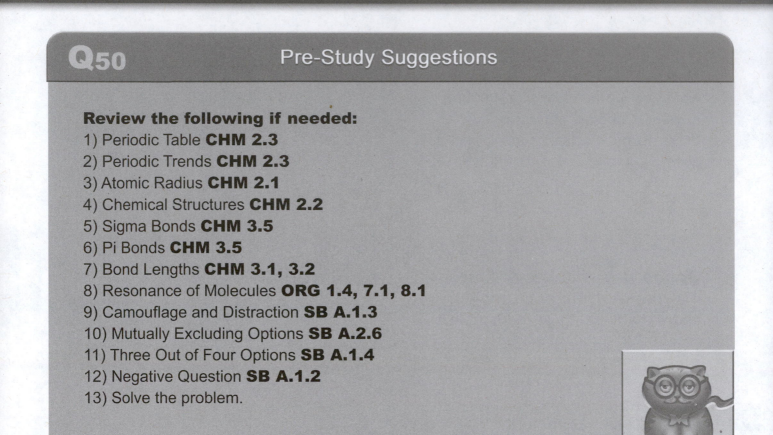

Resonance hybrid of the nitric acid molecule

The bonds of the molecule are labeled as shown below:

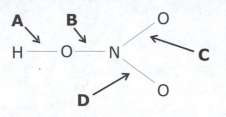

The largest atoms are the O and N with the H being much smaller. Since the O-H bond is between a larger atom and a smaller one and is a single bond, it would be expected to be shorter than the others. Nitrogen and oxygen are both in the second row of the periodic table (**CHM 2.3**) whereas hydrogen is in the first row. The atomic radii (**CHM 2.1**) of the oxygen and nitrogen are expected to be greater than the hydrogen. This means *option A will be incorrect.* All of the other bonds are between nitrogen and oxygen. From the discussion of the resonance hybrids (**ORG 1.4, 7.1, 8.1**), it should be clear that bond B is a single bond (**CHM 3.5**). The bonds C and D are somewhere between a single bond and a double bond (**CHM 3.5**). Since single bonds are longer than double bonds which are longer than triple bonds (**CHM 3.5**), *options C and D are incorrect. Option B is correct.* Notice the resonance hybrid (**ORG 1.4, 7.1, 8.1**) suggests that bonds C and D would be longer than a typical double bond but shorter than a single bond.

Test Taking Skills Comment

This question could be rephrased (**SB A.1.3**) to determining which bonds are double bonds and the effect of resonance on bonds and bond lengths. This is also a mutually excluding question (**SB A.2.6**) as options C and D are identical. If you look carefully at the options C and D bonds, there is really no way to make them different. Since both C and D cannot be the answer, and they are identical, neither can be the answer, they are mutually excluding. This is also a three out of four question (**SB A.1.4**) with options B, C and D being the three and option A being the outlier. Outliers are usually incorrect and should be excluded when you are in the guess mode. Notice that C and D are not a similar pair (**SB A.2.7**) because they are identical.

CHAPTER 1

Q51 — Pre-Study Suggestions

Review the following if needed:
1) Kinetic Energy **PHY 5.3**
2) Conservation of Energy **PHY 5.5**
3) Electronic Transitions **PHY 12.5**
4) Electric Potential **PHY 9.1.5**
5) Ionization Energy **CHM 2.3**
6) Rephrasing of Question **SB A.1.3**
7) Solve the problem.

Solution Discussion

The definition of the electric field potential **(PHY 9.1.5)**, V, is

$$V = \text{potential energy}(U) / \text{charge}(q),$$

then the potential energy **(PHY 9.1.4)** related to a charge would be,

$$U = q\,V.$$

An electron volt is then a measure of energy because it is the same as the formula for U:

electron volt
= 1 electron charge x 1 volt
= energy = coulombs x volt
= coulombs x (joules / coulomb)
= joules.

So, the electron volt, eV, is another unit for energy. Since the charge on an electron is 1.6×10^{-19} C, the eV is equal to,

$$eV = 1.6 \times 10^{-19} \text{ C} \times 1 \text{ V} = 1.6 \times 10^{-19} \text{ J}.$$

This is not needed to solve the problem, but is critical conceptually to show you are dealing with energy.

The photon then has an energy of 15.0 eV and then ionizes the hydrogen atom. The ionization is an electron transition **(PHY 12.5)** in which the electron escapes the atom. Another term for this is the ionization energy **(CHM 2.3)** or ionization potential. This process must obey the Law of Conservation of Energy **(PHY 5.5)**:

energy before = energy after

energy before = the energy of the photon

energy after = the energy to remove the electron + kinetic energy of the electron

then,
energy of the photon = energy to eject the electron + kinetic energy of the electron(K_e).

This is then,

$$15.0 \text{ eV} = 13.6 \text{ eV} + K_e$$
$$K_e = 15.0 - 13.6 = 1.4 \text{ eV}.$$

This means **option A is correct**.

Test Taking Skills Comment

This problem is well disguised and is a camouflage/distraction **(SB A.1.3)** type question. It is a problem of the conservation of energy **(PHY 5.5)** and nothing more. You are given a before and after with energies-when this happens, you have to, at least, consider the possibility that conservation of something can solve the problem. It also stresses tests, your general knowledge in chemistry and physics. Instead of being given the energy in electron volts, a type of camouflage/distraction, the energy could have been given as Joules-would have this made it easier to see through the camouflage It also tested your understanding of atomic structure **(CHM 2.1)** and electron transitions **(PHY 12.5)**. You had to know there is energy required to eject the electron from the atom and that any extra energy results in the kinetic energy **(PHY 5.3)** of

the electron. The energy to eject the electron is found in the potential energy **(PHY 9.1.4)** of the system (nucleus and electron). The structure of the answers is also simple. They are a repetition of the original numbers, their sum and their difference. You had to decide which way to go. The test makers are not going to announce what concepts you need to solve the problem. If they had told you this was a conservation of energy problem, probably 95% or more would have gotten it correct instead of the 55%. Before you leap to an answer, or leap to defeat, try to visualize what is occurring in the context of your knowledge. By remembering that it takes energy to ionize an electron and energy to give it a velocity, kinetic energy, this must have come from somewhere and the only place is the photon.

CHAPTER 1

Q52 Pre-Study Suggestions

Review the following if needed:
1) Nuclear Reactions **PHY 12.4**
2) Radioactive Decay **PHY 12.4**
3) Periodic Table **CHM 2.3**
4) Dichotomy of Options **SB A.2.3**
5) Solve the problem.

Solution Discussion

An electron is symbolized as:

$$_{-1}\beta^0,$$

a positron, or positive electron, is symbolized as,

$$_1\beta^0.$$

The equation for the reaction may be written in terms of the electron or the positron:

"by electron capture"

$$_4Be^7 + {_{-1}\beta^0} \rightarrow {_3?^7}$$

or by,

"a form of β^+ decay"

$$_4Be^7 \rightarrow {_1\beta^0} + {_3?^7}$$

The ? is the unknown element. The results are the same. Looking at the periodic table **(CHM 2.3)** included with the test, the element with the atomic number of 3 is lithium, and this becomes:

$$_4Be^7 + {_{-1}\beta^0} \rightarrow {_3Li^7}$$

or,

$$_4Be^7 \rightarrow {_1\beta^0} + {_3Li^7}$$

The correct option is B.

Test Taking Skills Comment

This is a matter of knowing the information presented. This is a dichotomy type question **(SB A.2.3)**. If you realized the mass number, the top number, would not change, then you would have to eliminate options A and D. If you knew the addition of an electron could only mean the loss of a proton being converted to a neutron, you would know the element would have to change and could not be Be any more. This would eliminate options C and D. For a positron emission **(PHY 12.4)**, you would have a proton being converted to neutron and again a change of element. Remember in nuclear reactions **(PHY 12.4)**, the electrons come or go to the nucleus and not the outer shells or orbits.

A physicist, a biologist and a chemist were going to the ocean for the first time.

The physicist saw the ocean and was fascinated by the waves. He said he wanted to do some research on fluid dynamics and so he walked into the ocean. Unfortunately, he drowned and never returned.

The biologist said he wanted to do research on underwater flora/fauna and so also walked into the ocean. He too, never returned.

The chemist waited for a long time and afterwards, wrote the observation, "The physicist and the biologist are soluble in ocean water".

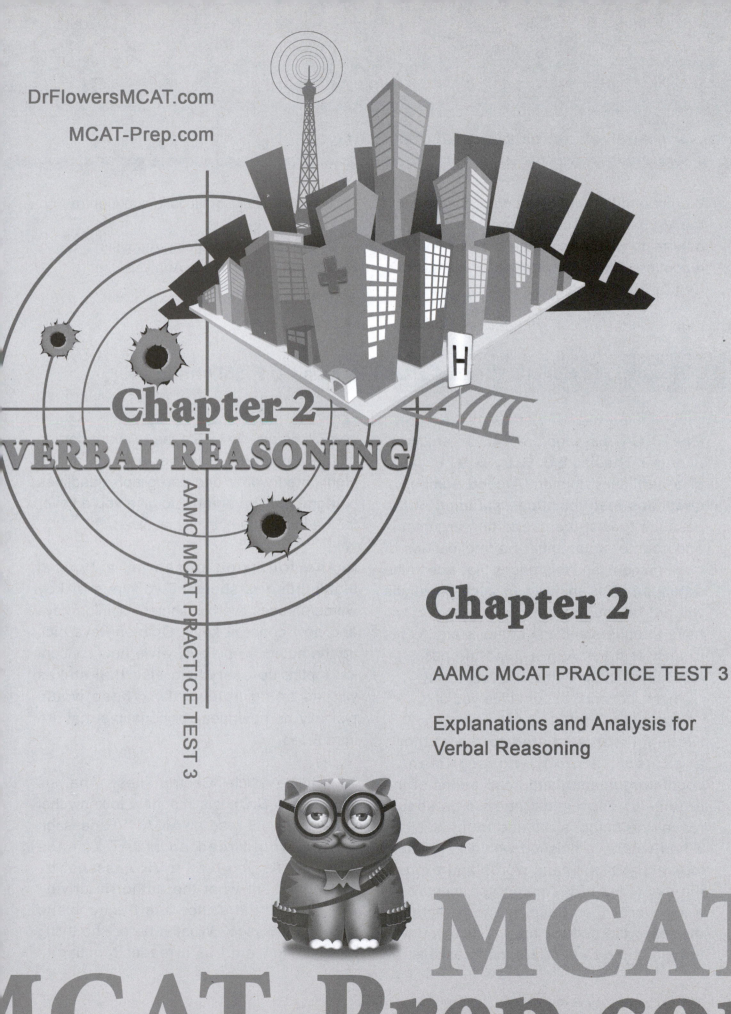

Chapter 2
VERBAL REASONING

Chapter 2

AAMC MCAT PRACTICE TEST 3

Explanations and Analysis for
Verbal Reasoning

MCAT

MCAT-Prep.con

Passage Analysis (use this for all questions)

We present three different ways to approach the Verbal Reasoning subtest. You should determine which works the best for you. We recommend the "Highlighting for Holistic and Central Thesis Analysis":

1) Highlighting for Holistic and Central Thesis Analysis
2) Standard Highlighting Analysis
3) Option Elimination Analysis

A Note on the Holistic (Central Thesis Emphasis) Highlighting

Every MCAT passage presents an argument (Central Thesis; **SB B.8, B.9**) in favor of a particular opinion. A good number of questions test your understanding of the passage thesis, the supporting arguments and counterarguments, the implications of the argument, and inferences that extend the argument. The answers to such questions will not be found in the passage; you will have to understand the author's arguments to answer them. As you read the passage, focus on what the author is trying to say.
* What is he trying to persuade you of?

Highlight words related to the author's argument, supporting arguments, counterarguments, and implications of the argument. The highlighted words should reveal the author's attitude to the subject. When you have finished with a paragraph, look at the highlighted words and express the main idea of the paragraph mentally in a few words (i.e., headline the paragraph), the fewer the better. This will help you with the direct passage reference questions, as

you will be able to locate the relevant portion of the passage easily. Let us look at the highlighted words and paragraph headlines paragraph by paragraph, to give you a flavor for the thought processes involved.

In the following passage, a typical highlighting is shown. Two types of key words/phrases are highlighted: opinion keys and new concept keys. Opinion keys pick up the author's opinions, while new concept keys pick up everything else that strikes you as being noteworthy. These would typically be new ideas or concepts that are introduced.

* From the article "Central Thesis Analysis Part 2" **(SB B.9)**: It is important to know that you should not read an MCAT VR passage as you would read an MCAT science passage. As you read a VR passage, try and figure out what the author is driving at. Why did the author take the trouble to write the passage? What is he or she trying to say? How am I as a reader reacting to

the author's persuasion? Do I find myself in agreement with the writer? Do I violently disagree with the writer? What is the purpose of this sentence or paragraph? (These are questions you do not need to ask when reading a science passage.) Engaging with the passage in this way will help you grasp the contours of the author's argument. (Most MCAT passages present arguments.) Look out for key words such as obviously, clearly, on the contrary, nevertheless, thus,

however, further, but, also, etc. These words are clues to the writer's thought processes. Your goal should be to view the passage as a unified argument, not a bunch of facts. So, do not try and remember details; rather, understand how details contribute to the overall argument, how they relate to a central point. Also, you do not have to understand everything in the passage to understand the passage argument. Try and get the big picture.

Putting It All Together: The Critical Path

We know what you're thinking. You're looking at the mass of theoretical explanations above and saying to yourself: Look, I get just x minutes to work on this passage. You expect me to compress this much thought in a few minutes? You've got to be kidding! I need something that works, something practical.

We understand. Dude, look at it this way. We divide the process of tackling each passage into two tasks: (1) reading the passage and (2) answering the questions.

While reading, you should build a mental outline of the passage as you read, highlighting as many words as are necessary for you to be able to mentally answer the following question after you finish reading a paragraph: What was this paragraph about? We call this the process of headlining

or signposting a paragraph. If you are an experienced reader, highlighting may not be necessary. Do not underestimate your speed of thought. Headlining a passage will become faster with practice. See the passage outline above to see how it's done.

Now for the second task: once you have finished reading, you come up against the questions. This is the moment of truth. You find yourself in the hot seat. Decisions have to be made — now! We describe next how you would typically determine the correct option under examination conditions. We break down the process into discrete steps, mimicking the truncated messages that would travel from neuron to neuron inside your head as you close in on the right option. Therefore, the steps are typically expressed in terse, telegraphic style.

During the exam, you will not have the luxury of sitting back in an armchair and weighing the pros and cons of various choices. If you take 3 minutes to read the passage, you will have just over a minute to answer each question. So, it pays to work fast. Verbal reasoning is not an exact science, so there are many ways of arriving at the correct option. In this section, we will pretend that we are working under test conditions and identify the most efficient route (the critical path) to the answer. So, there will be no detailed explanations; you will find those earlier. Instead, the answers will often be written in telegraphic style, to mimic the workings of the mind under test conditions. One factor is on your side. No question in the VR section of the MCAT requires the application of time-consuming deductive logic or other sophisticated strategies. Usually, one or two options can be discarded at once as inappropriate, and you will use the main idea of the passage and passage information to zero in on the correct option. There will be the occasional hard question that confuses even experienced readers who think about it at leisure, so do not obsess over any question; take a call and move on.

We hold these truths to be self-evident: that all men are created equal; that they are endowed by their Creator with inherent and inalienable rights; that among these are life, liberty, and the pursuit of happiness.

Thomas Jefferson

Highlighting For Holistic and Central Thesis Analysis

Holistic Highlighting

You should attempt to go through the passage in 3 minutes or less highlighting the following (or simply read the passage and try to focus on/remember the following). Remember blue means author's opinion and italic means all other important points. To appreciate the continuity of the passage, you should then highlight your passage (either on the computer or print out on paper) with the following excerpts.

Paragraph 1: "drug problem"; Sentence 2;
Paragraph 2: serious public debate; far more attention; policy option; legalization;
Paragraph 3: important; legalization scenarios; hostile; Sentences 2-4;
Paragraph 4: dramatic increase in drug enforcement efforts; little effect;
Paragraph 5: federal expenditures; tripled; five billion dollars;
Paragraph 6: Of greater concern; diversion of limited resources;
Paragraph 7: connections between drugs and crime; much diminished;
Paragraph 8: hundreds and even thousands of dollars a week; significantly cheaper; decline dramatically;
Paragraph 9: susceptible to corruption; tremendous amounts of money; Sentence 3;
Paragraph 10: that cannot be suppressed;
Paragraph 11: tremendous advantages;

Sentences 2-5;
Paragraph 12: good reason to doubt; two assumptions; not so dangerous; unlikely to prove appealing;
Paragraph 13: repeatedly and vociferously dismissed; openly and objectively;

Headlining or Signposting the Passage

Paragraph 1: The passage is about the drug problem, which is becoming more serious over time.

Paragraph 2: Drug legalization is an option that is not given much attention.

Paragraph 3: Three reasons to legalize drugs are given.

Paragraph 4: Drug enforcement has failed despite tremendous efforts.

Paragraph 5: Federal expenditure on drug enforcement has greatly increased. Note that this paragraph supports the previous paragraph with details.

Paragraph 6: This paragraph describes the resource crunch.

Paragraph 7: The link between crime and drugs would weaken with legalization.

Paragraph 8: Legalization would lower drug prices, which would in turn greatly reduce crime.

Paragraph 9: Police corruption. Drug prohibition is compared with alcohol prohibition, well known to be a colossal failure.

Passage I - Questions 53-57

Paragraph 10: Some police officers also accept the Prohibition analogy.

Paragraph 11: Some of the advantages of drug legalization are given: financial, law and order.

Paragraph 12: The argument that drug legalization would increase drug consumption is countered.

Paragraph 13: Repealing the drug prohibition laws would eliminate or greatly reduce the "drug problem." This is the central thesis of the passage. Note that the central thesis, or main idea, of the passage is usually found in the beginning or end of the passage.

The Central Thesis

"Repealing the drug-prohibition laws would eliminate or greatly reduce the "drug problem."" (Note that a hint regarding the central thesis can be obtained from an unexpected source: the source line of the passage. In this case, The Case for Legalization sums up the central thesis neatly in just a few words. Note also that the central thesis of a passage is often found toward the beginning or end of the passage. In this case, the central thesis is stated in the first line of the last paragraph. Sometimes the central thesis is restated elsewhere in the passage. In our passage, the CT is restated in the first line of the 11th paragraph.)

Paragraph 1
The passage is about the drug problem, which is becoming more serious over time.

Paragraph 2
Drug legalization is an option that is not given much attention.

Paragraph 3
Three reasons to legalize drugs are given.

Paragraph 4
Drug enforcement has failed despite tremendous efforts

Paragraph 5
Federal expenditure on drug enforcement has greatly increased.

Paragraph 6
This paragraph describes the resource crunch.

Paragraph 7
The link between crime and drugs would weaken with legalization.

Central Thesis
Repealing the drug-prohibition laws would eliminate or greatly reduce the " drug problem."

Paragraph 13
First sentence gives the central thesis of the passage.

Paragraph 12
The argument that drug legalization would increase drug consumption is countered.

Paragraph 11
Some of the advantages of drug legalization are given: financial, law and order.

Paragraph 10
Some police officers also accept the Prohibition analogy.

Paragraph 9
Police corruption. Drug prohibition is compared with alcohol prohibition, well known to be a colossal failure.

Paragraph 8
Legalization would lower drug prices, which would in turn greatly reduce crime.

Passage at a Glance

Genre: Sociology/Controversy/Social Policy
Passage difficulty level: Simple.
Abstract/concrete: Concrete
Subject: Drug legalization
Author's attitude to subject: Strongly in favor of drug legalization

Question types: One stand-alone inference, one central thesis related, two direct passage reference, one indirect passage reference.

Standard Passage Highlighting

Passage Highlighting (this is done as if skimming during an actual test and is not meant to be a "perfect" highlighting - learn from the following discussion): *see* Highlighting **(SB B.6, B.7)**.

Paragraph 1-""drug problem"", "war", "government funding", "not going away", "worse"

Paragraph 2- "serious public debate", "given to on policy", "legalization"

Paragraph 3- "three reasons", "Americans remain hostile", "drug-control policies have failed", Sentences 2-3

Paragraph 4- "drug-enforcement efforts", "little effect"

Paragraph 5- "expenditures", "18 percent of total investigative resources"

Paragraph 6- "diversion of limited resources"

Paragraph 7- "drugs and crime ... diminished if drug-prohibition laws were repealed"

Paragraph 8 - Sentence 1, "significantly cheaper", "crimes committed ... decline"

Paragraph 9 -Sentence1, "tremendous amounts of money", "police corruption is more pervasive"

Paragraph 10 - "enforcing the drug ... predators", "regulates an illicit market", Sentence 2

Paragraph 11- "repealing", "advantages", "reduced government expenditures", "new tax revenue", "public treasuries ... net benefit", Sentence 3-4

Paragraph 12 - Sentence 1, "logic of legalization", "most illegal ... dangerous", "unlikely to prove appealing to"

Paragraph 13 - "repealing the drug-prohibition", "eliminate ... "drug problem"", "openly and objectively"

CHAPTER 2

QUESTION 3R.VR.I.53

Question Discussion Using Holistic Approach

This is a stand-alone question, in the sense that it can be answered based on information provided in the question itself. Reference to the passage is not necessary. The fastest way to answer is to latch onto a couple of give-away negative expressions in the stem: "debases" and "alters one's soul." The clear inference is that this authority has a highly negative view of illegal drugs such as cocaine, and is also likely to be a supporter of the War on Drugs.

We can immediately eliminate options A and C on this count alone. How do we decide between options B and D? There is no evidence in the stem for option B, which leaves option D (the right option).

Note: You should understand that there is nothing absolute about the correctness of option D. It just happens to be the best option among those available. For example, suppose option D had been the following sentence: "consider tobacco more dangerous than cocaine." Now option B becomes the only reasonable choice.

Putting it all together: the critical path

Step 1: Understand that authority opposes drug legalization.

Step 2: So eliminate options A and C.

Step 3: Pick option D (clue words in stem: "debases," "alters one's soul"). No evidence for option B.

Question Discussion Using Standard Highlighting (HL) Analysis

There is nothing from the passage needed to answer this question. This is a type of "rephrasing **(SB A.2.2)** in the stem". All of the information you need is found restated in the stem itself. So, there is no need to refer neither to the passage nor to your highlighting. It is valuable to recognize these "rephrasing" types of questions rapidly as you can determine there is nothing in the passage that really help you answer it and you can focus your time on the stem and options **(SB A.1)**.

Question Discussion Using Option Elimination Analysis

Q53 — Pre-Study Suggestions

Review the following if needed:
1) Similar Pair Options **SB A.2.7**
2) Internal Inconsistency of Options **SB A.2.5**
3) Complex Sounding Option(s) **SB A.2.2**

Solution Discussion

Please review the AAMC solution for this problem.

Test Taking Skills Comment

Option A is incorrect. Option A is an Internal Inconsistency of Options **(SB A.2.5)**. Option A is illogical based on the stem. It is inconsistent for an authority to view tobacco and cocaine in a negative way and still want to legalize either one, especially cocaine.

Option B is incorrect. There is some consistency of the intent to abolish sales, but from General Knowledge **(SB A.2.2)** you should know that there are no cocaine sales to be abolished. Also, the authority appears to be more critical of cocaine than of tobacco. It is possible that the authority would want both abolished, but there is not firm enough evidence for this making this a Complex Sounding Option(s) **(SB A.2.2)**.

Option C is incorrect. Options C and D are a reasonable Similar Pair Options **(SB A.2.7)**. Each deals with the concept of 'harm' or 'danger', which are similar concepts. Option C is also an Internal Inconsistency of Options **(SB A.2.5)**; based on the statement highlighted previously, it is not logical that an authority making these statements would not consider tobacco and cocaine to be particularly dangerous.

Option D is correct. This is the Best Option **(SB A.1.2)**.

Notice that there is nothing from the passage required to answer this question.

QUESTION 3R.VR.I.54

Question Discussion Using Holistic Analysis

This question involves knowledge of the CT. Option A is eliminated because mandatory drug treatment is against the liberal spirit of drug legalization. Option D is eliminated because a supporter of drug legalization is not going to commit more resources on prohibition related efforts. That leaves options B and C. The passage author is a supporter of drug legalization and believes that the dangers of drug use are exaggerated. However, he is not a Timothy Leary; he does not promote drug use. Exempting drug trade income from tax is a measure that would promote drug use. Hence, this option can be eliminated.

Option C is selected because distribution of free needles to addicts is in line with the basic premise of drug legalization, that the dangers of drugs are overestimated. A person against drug legalization would oppose to this, arguing that free distribution of needles to addicts would encourage them to consume more drugs, although in a healthier manner.

Putting it all together: the critical path

Step 1: Understand that the author supports drug legalization.

Step 2: So eliminate options A and D.

Step 3: Recognize option B as being a "loony" idea. Pick option C.

Question Discussion Using Standard Highlighting (HL) Analysis

CHAPTER 2

Option A is incorrect. (There are no HL phrases.) This policy would be unlikely because the gestalt of the article was not to discuss options against or for the drug users themselves. Besides, it is Inconsistent **(SB A.2.5)** to "mandate" treatment if drugs have been legalized.

Option B is incorrect. Option B is found rapidly by scanning and noting in paragraph 11, "advantage" and "new tax revenue". This means the author would not "grant tax-exempt status".

Option D is incorrect. This option is in contrast to the passage. Looking at paragraph 2, it should be clear that "intercepting drugs" is not consistent with "legalization".

> ***Option C is correct.*** The policy in option C is consistent with paragraph 8: "crimes committed by drug addicts" and "decline".

This means option C is the Best Option **(SB A.1.2)**. Notice carefully that none of the options were explicitly stated in the passage, but each was a short inference **(SB B.5)** from something presented in the passage. So, you will need to use your HL directly and indirectly to help you answer questions. You will have to become good at doing this to excel on the Verbal Reasoning subtest.

Question Discussion Using Option Elimination Analysis

Q54 — Pre-Study Suggestions

Review the following if needed:
1) Similar Pair Options **SB A.2.7**

Solution Discussion
Please review the AAMC solution for this problem.

Test Taking Skills
Options A and C are Similar Pair Options **(SB A.2.7)**. Both deal with the drug user/addict. Neither B nor D deals with this nor issues related to each other. Since this is the only similar pair present, it is a reasonable set to make a pure guess from.

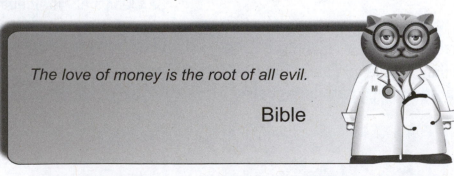

The love of money is the root of all evil.

Bible

QUESTION 3R.VR.I.55

Question Discussion Using Holistic Analysis

This is a direct passage reference question. *See* Paragraph 11 of the passage, which contains the phrase "public treasuries," for the answer. Only I and III are mentioned there. So the right option is option C.

Putting it all together: the critical path

Step 1: Latch onto clues in stem, "public treasuries" and "explicitly presented in the passage," like a shark that has scented blood.

Step 2: Plunge into passage.

Step 3: Sniff out relevant paragraph (Paragraph 11).

Step 4: Only statements I and III mentioned. Pick option C.

Question Discussion Using Standard Highlighting (HL) Analysis

Choice I is readily found in paragraph 11 as "advantages" and "new tax revenue" were HL. You should have known that choice I is right as it is found in all options (A, B, C and D) and you should not have even evaluated it.

Choice II is not directly stated but has allusions to this possibility including paragraphs 5 ("18 percent of their total investigative resources"), 6 ("diversion of limited resources") and 9 ("police corruption is more pervasive") which all suggested that choice II should be true. But, the stem of the question asks for "explicitly presented" as a net benefit, which is only in paragraph 11, and reduced law-enforcement is not explicitly mentioned.

Choice III is found in paragraph 11 as "advantage" and "reduced government expenditures", so it is true. This means choices I and III are true.

Option A, B and D are incorrect.
See previous discussion.

CHAPTER 2

Passage I - Questions 53-57

Option C is correct. *See* previous discussion. So, you must always read the Stem **(SB A.1)** carefully and make sure your answer conforms to it. This is despite options being true or seemingly true as in this question.

Question Discussion Using Option Elimination Analysis

Q55   Pre-Study Suggestions

Review the following if needed:
1) Three Out of Four Options **SB A.2.8**
2) Multiple Choice Options **SB A.1.2**

Solution Discussion
Please review the AAMC solution for this problem.

Test Taking Skills Comment
This is a Multiple Choice Options **(SB A.1.2)** question. For this question, you do not have to waste time with choice I. It must be True **(SB A.1.2)** as it is found in every option. You only have to determine if choice II and III are True or False **(SB A.1.2)**. For these types of questions, it is essential that you are certain about your assessment of each choice (I, II or III) as true or false, so you can eliminate certain options. This is also a soft Three Out of Four Options **(SB A.2.8)** with options B, C and D being similar only because they contain multiple options. This means option A is the outlier. Outliers tend to be Incorrect **(SB A.1.2)**.

QUESTION 3R.VR.I.56

Question Discussion Using Holistic Analysis

This is a direct passage reference question. "The author's belief" referred to in the stem is present somewhere in the passage. Compare the wording of option B ("unlikely to engage in an obviously dangerous activity") with the wording in the penultimate paragraph ("unlikely to prove appealing to many people, precisely because they are so obviously dangerous"). The statement in option B should ring a bell and direct you to this paragraph. Alternatively, you may recall that the main idea of some paragraph dealt with this topic. Once you locate the penultimate paragraph, direct support for option B will be found.

Putting it all together: the critical path

Step 1: Recognize that this is a passage reference question. "The author's belief" must be dealt with somewhere.

Step 2: Scan passage.

Step 3: Locate penultimate paragraph, either by main idea association, or by similarity in option B wording. Pick option B.

Question Discussion Using Standard Highlighting Analysis

Option A is incorrect. See paragraph 3 sentence 1. The author does not relate the hostility to the use of drugs if they were legalized. Yet, you might expect that if this was true, drug use should not rise if they were legalized. So, this option is not definitely eliminated.

Passage I - Questions 53-57

Option C is incorrect. Option C is not specifically discussed and is not an easy Inference **(SB B.5)** from items underlined. This diminishes its possibility especially since option B is such an obvious choice.

Option B is correct. See paragraph 12. This is essentially the gist of option B and the argument used by the author to suggest drug use would not rise.

Option D is incorrect. This is an Internal Inconsistency of Options **(SB A.2.5)**. The Stem **(SB A.1)** explains why legalizing drugs would not increase drug use. Option D states a historical example showing otherwise; this being a direct conflict and negation of the statement trying to be proved.

I have a dream that my four little children will one day live in a nation where they will not be judged by the color of their skin but by the content of their character. I have a dream today.

Martin Luther King, Jr.

Question Discussion Using Option Elimination Analysis

Q56 — Pre-Study Suggestions

Review the following if needed:
1) Three Out of Four Options **SB A.2.8**

Solution Discussion

Please review the AAMC solution for this problem.

Test Taking Skills Comment

The best guess comes from Three Out of Four Options **(SB A.2.8)** analysis. Options A, B and C are a quick assessment for being a three out of four as each has 'Most Americans'. This is a five second evaluation, which is what you want when you are guessing. Option D is the outlier, and outliers tend to be Incorrect **(SB A.1.2)**.

QUESTION 3R.VR.I.57

Question Discussion Using Holistic Analysis

This is an indirect passage reference question. Match "street prices" in the stem with sentences 1 and 2 of paragraph 8 or with the main idea of that paragraph: "Legalization would lower drug prices, which would in turn greatly reduce crime"; clearly making option A the right option. The assumption that prohibition drives prices upward (thus leading users to commit crimes to raise money to buy drugs) is one of the core arguments in favor of drug legalization.

Putting it all together: the critical path

Step 1: Latch onto clue "street prices" in stem.

Step 2: Scan passage and locate paragraph 8 (which deals with street prices).

Step 3: Pick option A.

Summary of Holistic Reasoning for 3CBT Passage I

That's it in a nutshell. You would have got all the questions right if you had only:

• Inferred correctly (Q 53)
• Grasped that the passage author is in favor of drug legalization (Q 54)

• Associated Q 55 with paragraph 11
• Associated Q 56 with paragraph 12
• Associated Q 57 with paragraph 8

Question Discussion Using Standard Highlighting (HL) Analysis

The whole question is found in paragraph 8 as "cocaine and heroin addicts spend" and "significantly cheaper" gives the answer to the question.

answer the question quickly.

Options B, C and D are incorrect. Then options B, C and D are Incorrect **(SB A.1.2)** as they are direct contradictions to this statement. What the HL allowed was the rapid finding of the critical information to

Option A is correct. Option A is a direct paraphrase of the discussion in paragraph 8; more enforcement raises prices. Making the drugs legal = less enforcement = lowers prices.

Summary of Standard Highlighting for 3CBT Passage I

Final comment on HL for this passage: notice that most of the HL was not even used. This emphasizes the need to "skim" and not "read" or "study" and to create means (the HL), to rapidly find the information you need to answer the specific questions. So, some of your HL will be "wasted", but this is ok. This is analogous to much of our screening in public health.

We want tests with high sensitivity which will pick up individuals who do not have the disease, a false positive. What is done then is to do a second test, with high specificity, which can eliminate those with falsely positive tests. This is what you must do with your highlighting. You will select more than you need, but then you use your logic and Inferences **(SB B.5)** to determine what is important for the task, the question, at hand.

> *He who is unable to live in society, or who has no need because he is sufficient for himself, must be either a beast or a god.*
>
> Aristotle

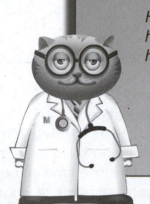

Question Discussion for Option Elimination Analysis

Q57   Pre-Study Suggestions

Concept Review Discussion
1) Three Out of Four Options **SB A.2.8**
2) Similar Pair Options **SB A.2.7**

Solution Discussion
Please review the AAMC solution for this problem.

Test Taking Skills Comment
This is a Three Out of Four Options **(SB A.2.8)** question. Options A, B and C are similar by having an effect on street prices. Option D is the outlier with no relationship present. Outliers tend to be incorrect.

There are also Similar Pair Options **(SB A.2.7)** present. There are two sets. One set is options A and B, which both have 'more strict', and the other set is options A and C, which both have 'higher'. Remember when there is more than one similar pair present, it is best not to use this technique, although in this case, by using both similar pairs, the last option standing is option A which is the correct option.

Highlighting For Holistic and Central Thesis Analysis

Holistic Highlighting

You should attempt to go through the passage in 3 minutes or less, highlighting the following (or simply read the passage and try to focus on/remember the following). Remember blue means author's opinion and italic means all other important points. To appreciate the continuity of the passage, you should then highlight your passage (either on the computer or print out on paper) with the following excerpts.

Paragraph 1: know little; good deal more; imagine

Paragraph 2: wolves as hunters; know where they are going; learn from … ravens; certain wolves … small game; each wolf is a little different; new things

Paragraph 3: their hunting … do not hunt; give gifts; communication … olfactory; pelages; good part … with each other

Paragraph 4: not see him at all

Paragraph 5: powerfulinfluence...imagination; feelings; their fear … curiosity; born killers; isn't true; no healthy … killed anyone

Paragraph 6: perception … of circumstances; only an opinion

Paragraph 7: rigorous; clouds

Paragraph 8: people who loved wolves; people who hated them

Paragraph 9: men do not … create their animals

Headlining or Signposting the Passage

Paragraph 1: Although we know very little about the wolf, it exerts a powerful influence on the human imagination.

Paragraph 2: Examples of wolf lore of Indians from Alaska who have lived in close proximity with wolves since time immemorial.

Paragraph 3: Likeable aspects of wolves; the author likes these animals.

Paragraph 4: How well the wolf can camouflage itself (eerie paragraph).

Paragraph 5: Powerful visceral emotions the wolf arouses in humans.

Paragraphs 6 and 7: The emotional impact of the wolf colors our evaluation of them.

Paragraphs 8 and 9: Describes the research the author undertook, and his conclusion that humans have surrounded the wolf with legends.

The Central Thesis:

"The truth is we know little about the wolf. What we know a good deal more about is what we imagine the wolf to be." (Or, more generally, from the last paragraph: "Men do not discover their gods, they create them. So do they also … create their animals.")

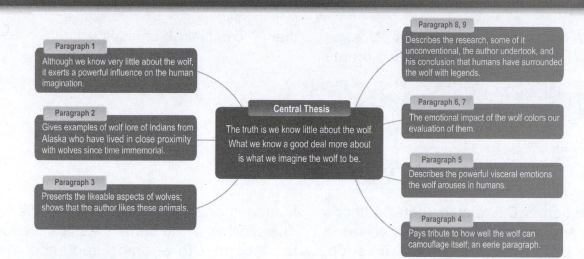

Paragraph 1
Although we know very little about the wolf, it exerts a powerful influence on the human imagination.

Paragraph 2
Gives examples of wolf lore of Indians from Alaska who have lived in close proximity with wolves since time immemorial.

Paragraph 3
Presents the likeable aspects of wolves; shows that the author likes these animals.

Central Thesis
The truth is we know little about the wolf. What we know a good deal more about is what we imagine the wolf to be.

Paragraph 8, 9
Describes the research, some of it unconventional, the author undertook, and his conclusion that humans have surrounded the wolf with legends.

Paragraph 6, 7
The emotional impact of the wolf colors our evaluation of them.

Paragraph 5
Describes the powerful visceral emotions the wolf arouses in humans.

Paragraph 4
Pays tribute to how well the wolf can camouflage itself; an eerie paragraph.

Passage at a Glance

Genre: Symbolism/Folklore/Mythology/Natural History

Passage difficulty level: Moderate

Abstract/concrete: Abstract to some extent because of the symbolism that is the passage theme

Subject: The wolf, especially as a potent symbol in human imagination

Author's attitude to subject: Favorable; author admires and respects the wolf

Question types: One stand-alone inference, two central thesis related, two direct passage reference. (However, the CT plays a role in all questions.)

Standard Passage Highlighting

Passage Highlighting (this is done as if skimming during an actual test and is not meant to be a "perfect" highlighting- learn from the following discussion): *see* Highlighting **(SB B.6, B.7)**.

Paragraph 1: "know little about the wolf", "what we imagine"

Paragraph 2: "Nunamiut Eskimo", "Brooks Range", "hunters", "caribou", "ravens","pack specialize", "each wolf is a little different", "big males … the killing", "Maybe. Sometimes"

Paragraph 3: Sentences 1-3, "pelages", "with their young", "winging … Frisbee"

Paragraph 4: "not see him at all", "Eskimos to smile"

Paragraph 5: Sentences 1, 4-5, "stare", "Bella Coola Indians", "eyes of the wolf", "that stare",

Paragraph 6: "perception … opinion"

Paragraph 7: "rigor of clouds"

Paragraph 8: Sentence 1, 3-6, "captive wolves in Barrow", "people who loved … hated them"

Paragraph 9: "notes ... encounters", "Joseph Campbell", "Primitive Mythology ... create them", "create their animals"

QUESTION 3R.VR.II.58

Question Discussion Using Holistic Approach

This question is CT related (note "author's point" in the stem), but it also involves a passage reference. It's a hard question, because at first glance no option can be dismissed. Upon reflection, option C can be eliminated because the passage does not talk about reverence for the wolf. Option D is tempting, but it is too superficial. Besides, it is not the author's point that wolves and humans resemble each other.

However, options A and B both match the CT, and the focus should be on eliminating one of them. This can only be accomplished by reading the fifth paragraph of the passage, upon which we can eliminate option A, because the legend itself is the product of human imagination stimulated by the wolf. The clincher is the sentence that introduces the legend; the opening sentence of the fifth paragraph, which contains the phrase "powerful influence on human imagination."

Putting it all together: the critical path
- Eliminate option C (no mention of "reverence" in passage)
- Options A & B match CT
- Choose option B because "legend" matches "fanciful"; sentence introducing
- legend in passage mentions "powerful influence on human imagination"
- If totally at sea, take a chance and match "legend" and "fanciful"

Question Discussion Using Standard Highlighting (HL) Analysis

Option A is incorrect. It is found by noting in paragraph 1 "know little about the wolf". But, this has nothing to do with the "Bella Coola" which is found HL in paragraph 5 as "Bella Coola Indians".

Option C is incorrect. Option C is not found directly by the HL. It is a gestalt that wolves were revered, but again, this is not what is found in paragraph 5 which is the specific location of the Bella Coola reference.

Option D is incorrect. Though paragraphs 2-3 suggest some similarities, they are not related to the Bella Coola example. Option D is found in paragraph 5 ("human only the eyes of the wolf"). This does not "resemble humans in certain ways," this is only one aspect and specifically states that animals were not changed into men.

Option B is correct. Option B is found in paragraph 5 with "powerful influence on the human

imagination" and "Bella Coola Indians" where "human imagination" is just a rephrase or paraphrase of "fanciful thinking".

Notice again that many of the options have references within the passage, but note:

1) You often have to make a one or two step leap from what is exactly stated to get to the answer. E.g. "fanciful thinking" = "human imagination";
2) There will be options which have true statements but are not correct such as option A. This was a difficult question as only 60% of students got it correct. These are the types you have to get correct to separate yourself from the crowd.

Question Discussion Using Option Elimination Analysis

Q58   Pre-Study Suggestions

Review the following if needed:
1) Three Out of Four Options **SB A.2.8**

Solution Discussion
Please review the AAMC solution for this problem.

Test Taking Skills Comment
Options A, B and C are similar and are a Three Out of Four Options **(SB A.2.8).** They each deal with thoughts/thinking related to the wolf. Option D is an outlier which deals only with 'resemble' between humans and wolves. Outliers tend to be incorrect. Make your guess from A, B or C.

QUESTION 3R.VR.II.59

Question Discussion Using Holistic Approach

In a way, this is a direct passage reference type of question, but knowledge of the CT helps. If you know the meaning of "rigorous," you will know that the choice is between options B and C. Now, the main idea of the passage is that we have very little concrete knowledge about the wolf. "Precise" matches "concrete" here, and is the right option.

You can refer to the passage if you like; you will see words like "perception" and "opinion" in the sentences leading up to the phrase "To be rigorous about wolves." "Rigorous," which denotes objectivity, contrasts sharply with "perception" and "opinion," which denote subjectivity; it is in this sense that the word is used, not in the sense of harsh climate.

Putting it all together: the critical path
• Eliminate options A and D
• Locate "rigorous" in passage
• Eliminate "harsh" (option B)
• Rigorous knowledge = precise or definite knowledge.

Question Discussion Using Standard Highlighting (HL) Analysis

This is found in paragraph 7 from "rigor of clouds". Even though "rigorous" was not HL, though it could have been as a word which will require definition. The context is then one of understanding the wolf and being specific, accurate and precise.

Options A, B and D are incorrect. *See* previous discussion.

Option C is correct. You will have to determine the meaning in context. But, everything you need is found in connection with the HL phrase. This is another example of a one step mental action to get to the answer.

Question Discussion Using Option Elimination Analysis

Q59 — Pre-Study Suggestions

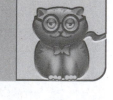

Review the following if needed:
1) Three Out of Four Options **SB A.2.8**

Solution Discussion
Please review the AAMC solution for this problem.

Test Taking Skills Comment
Options A, B and D are similar in terms of being critical/emotional in some manner and are a Three Out of Four Options (SB A.2.8). Option C is the outlier which deals with a non-emotional feature. Outliers tend to be incorrect. You would guess A, B or D but would be incorrect in this question. Remember, guessing is guessing and will be wrong sometimes. But, overall, the techniques lead to greater than the 25% random guess rate of being correct.

QUESTION 3R.VR.II.60

Question Discussion Using Holistic Approach

This is a stand-alone inference question that involves the CT. Note that the CT is mentioned in the stem! The question could have been made harder by asking which of the following would most weaken the author's central thesis.

Option A is incorrect. This states that wolves resemble primates in their playful nature. This weakens the CT, because it represents definite knowledge about the wolf, but keep this option on hold.

Option B is incorrect. This statement strengthens the CT, because folklore is allied with imagination. We are looking for a statement that weakens the CT.

Option C is incorrect. To attribute a behavior to instinct is not an explanation of that behavior. For example, we know that some animals can anticipate earthquakes. Labeling this capability an instinct does nothing to explain it; thus does not weaken the CT.

Option D is correct. If true, this development would kill all the mystery regarding wolves, because even the last vestiges of folklore would have been explained. Thus, this statement would seriously weaken the CT, much more than the statement of option A.

Putting it all together: the critical path

Option D should hit you between the eyes; scientists have a wealth of knowledge that contradicts "wolf is less known".

Question Discussion Using Standard Highlighting (HL) Analysis

Option A is incorrect. Option A is found in paragraph 3 as "winging a piece of caribou". The example "playing with each other" demonstrates this belief. So, without this observation, which weakens that "the wolf is less known than created by us", he would be creating a belief without basis.

Option C is incorrect. Option C is not found anywhere in the passage, as "instinctive" was not discussed. So, this would not weaken the contention.

Option B is incorrect. Option B is found in paragraph 2 as "Nunamiut Eskimo". This actually strengthens the "author's contention that the wolf is less known than created by us" because there is no proof or evidence of the beliefs.

Option D is correct. Option D is found in paragraphs 2 ("Nunamiut Eskimo"), 4 ("Eskimos to smile"), and in other locations. But the key here is that "Scientists" and "wealth of knowledge" means the beliefs of the natives have been independently confirmed by "scientific observation". So, this would mean more is known as facts than created by belief.

CHAPTER 2

Question Discussion Using Option Elimination Analysis

Q60 — Pre-Study Suggestions

Review the following if needed:
1) Guess Question **SB A.2.4**

Solution Discussion
Please review the AAMC solution for this problem.

Test Taking Skills Comment
This is a Guess Question **(SB A.2.4)**. Looking at the other questions in this section, you see they have a shorter Stem **(SB A.1)**. They also have shorter Options **(SB A.1.2)**. Additionally, the question is a Negative Question **(SB A.1.2)**. These factors combine to make this question more difficult and time consuming. You should save it for the end of the test. Otherwise, you simply guess your Lucky Letter of the Day **(SB B.2.3)** and move on.

This question is made easier because the passage is not necessary. You can find all the info/data you need in the stem and options. It is a matter of applying your logic and analysis to the information given.

The only way to make sure people you agree with can speak is to support the rights of people you don't agree with.

Eleanor Holmes Norton

QUESTION 3R.VR.II.61

Question Discussion Using Holistic Approach

This is a passage reference question, but involves CT. First, note that options C and D can be respectively eliminated because the author obviously respects wolves (so "contempt" is a red flag) and because it contradicts what the passage says (that we know little about the wolf). On referring to the passage, we see that option B is right; wolves have been known to kill people (*see* end of fifth paragraph).

Putting it all together: the critical path

Remember the passage states that wolves kill (so choose between options B and C) - "contempt" is a good reason for eliminating option C (author respects wolves).

Question Discussion Using Standard Highlighting (HL) Analysis

Option A is incorrect. Paragraph 5 ("ever killed … isn't true") contradicts option A.

Option D is incorrect. Option D is found in paragraph 1 as "know little about the wolf" and would make this a false option.

Option C is incorrect. It is found in paragraph 5 as "Wolf-haters" and "born killers … isn't true" would suggest this is not a statement the author would make.

Option B is correct. It is found in paragraph 5. So, the only option left is B as the correct option. This is the type of question which forces you to evaluate each option, since each option has a specific reference in the passage. If you do not have effective HL to locate them, you would spend

an inordinate amount of time and frustration trying to determine the answer.

Question Discussion Using Option Elimination Analysis

Q61   Pre-Study Suggestions

Review the following if needed:
1) Three Out of Four Options **SB A.2.8**
2) Similar Pair Options **SB A.2.7**
3) Three or More Steps Analysis **SB A.1.4**

Solution Discussion
Please review the AAMC solution for this problem.

Test Taking Skills Comment
This is a Three Out of Four Options **(SB A.2.8)** question. Options A, B and C all deal with some type of 'harm'/'danger' by wolves. Option D is an outlier and outliers tend to be incorrect. This is also a Similar Pair Options **(SB A.2.7)** question, but there are too many similar pairs present to make a reasonable guess: options A and D ('love' and 'confidence') and options B and C ('caution' and 'contempt'; 'kill humans' and 'dangerous'). It is better not to use this

technique when so many similar pairs are present, unless one of three conditions is met:

1) you have Basic Knowledge (study, passage, general knowledge) **(SB A.2.2)** which supports one pair over another;

2) a similar pair is the mirror image pair; and,

3) the similar pair is part of the Three Out of Four **(SB A.2.8)**. If you push it, because of the statement about 'killed' in paragraph 5, you could make a reasonable argument for A and B as the Similar Pair Options **(SB A.2.7)** to choose.

This is also a Three or More Steps Analysis **(SB A.1.4)** which makes it more difficult than usual because you have to:

1) determine which of the intro words/ emotions is true;

2) conclude if the reason given after the

emotion is consistent with the emotion;

3) determine if the option is True or False **(SB A.1.2)**; and finally,

4) determine if the option is Correct or Incorrect **(SB A.1.2)**.

QUESTION 3R.VR.II.62

Question Discussion Using Holistic Approach

This question is CT related. First, you have to see that the encyclopedia author has a low opinion of wolves ("lack courage and loyalty") and eliminate option D. Option B is the next to go because people do not see themselves as "rapacious" and lacking "courage and loyalty." That leaves options A and C. It becomes clear that though wolves are "excellent hunters," the encyclopedia excerpt does not have anything to say about it! This is a classic distractor: throw in something

that is true but irrelevant. That leaves option C, which is just a restatement of the CT.

Putting it all together: the critical path
• Eliminate option B (people do not view themselves unfavorably);
• Eliminate option D (author's opinion about wolves is favorable); and,
• Eliminate option A (true, but not mentioned in encyclopedia excerpt).

Question Discussion Using Standard Highlighting (HL) Analysis

For this question, you need a gestalt for the paragraph. No specific HL would be helpful other than creating a general feeling for the

passage and the central thesis. This is found in paragraph 1 as "know little about the wolf" and "what we imagine".

Option A is incorrect. Option A would require the HL as shown for paragraph 3.

Option D is incorrect. Option D would be found in the gestalt of the paragraph.

Option B is incorrect. Option B would be found in paragraph 5.

Option C is correct. Option C is the Correct **(SB A.1.2)** option.

Question Discussion Using Option Elimination Analysis

Q62 Pre-Study Suggestions

Review the following if needed:
1) Three Out of Four Options **SB A.2.8**
2) Internal Inconsistency of Options **SB A.2.5**
3) Similar Pair Options **SB A.2.7**

Solution Discussion
Please review the AAMC solution for this problem.

Test Taking Skills Comment
This is a Three Out of Four Options **(SB A.2.8)** question with options B, C and D being similar as they deal with general approach/opinions about wolves. Option A is an outlier being a very specific opinion. Outliers tend to be incorrect.

Option A is incorrect. There is an Internal Inconsistency of Options **(SB A.2.5)**: option A has no basis in the statement of the Stem **(SB A.1)** (there is no logical way to assess that wolves are 'excellent hunters' from 'rapacious, flesh-eating'). This is a type of Complex Sounding Option(s) **(SB A.2.2)**.

Option B is incorrect. Also, option B is inconsistent: humans would believe they possess 'courage and loyalty' like the dog which is stated not to be wolf-like.

Option D is incorrect. *See* the following discussion.

There is a reasonable Similar Pair Options **(SB A.2.7)** present in options B and C. Both relate to how people frame their thoughts about wolves, whereas options A and D do not; one being about hunters and the other about only the author's opinion. So, a reasonable guess would first be from B, C or D using three out of four. With more analysis, a guess could come from B or C using similar pairs.

Option C is correct. Finally, using internal inconsistency, option B could be eliminated and you are left with option C as your guess. Notice, this guess depends on your analysis of the stem and options only and does not require you to read the passage.

CHAPTER 2

Highlighting For Holistic and Central Thesis Analysis

CBT3 Passage III Holistic Highlighting
Paragraph 1: Sentence 1-2, 4; other social … that ruled over them

Paragraph 2: Sentence 1; measure … ambition; difficulties involved; at one level … accurate; visual means … using; in any … way

Paragraph 3: Sentences 1-3; Unconscious; surprisingly unchanged; experience … itself; painting about … abstract art

Paragraph 4: potential freedom … not used; conventions … being dismantled

Paragraph 5: Whole paragraph

Headlining or Signposting the Passage
Paragraph 1: The professional training that was imparted to painters focused on the needs of the ruling classes.

Paragraph 2: Painters of the 19th century tried to extend their training to express the experiences of other classes, but this proved to be difficult to achieve. A painting by Ford Maddox Ford is discussed as an example.

Paragraph 3: In the 20th century, the old tradition stopped, but the experience that painters drew remained the same (the only exception being the introduction of the Unconscious).

Paragraph 4: There was lack of true liberation because the training was still rooted in the old tradition.

Paragraph 5: This limitation led modern art to suffer from the same original defect: a constriction of vision due to a narrow range of subjects and an unjustified claim of universality.

Central Thesis:
It's more or less laid out in black and white in the last paragraph (which is, together with the first paragraph, a very good place to look for the CT). Thus, the extreme of abstract art demonstrates, as an epilogue, the original uncertainty of professional art: an art in reality concerned with a selective, very reduced area of experience, which nevertheless claims to be universal. In plain language: art has been limited to narrow areas of experience over the centuries, because methods used to train artists have not been able to escape the influence of tradition.

Paragraph 5
As a result of this limitation, modern art still suffered from the same original defect: a constriction of vision due to a narrow range of subjects, accompanied by an unjustified claim of universality.

Paragraph 1
The professional training that was imparted to painters focused on the needs of the ruling classes.

Central Thesis
Art has been limited to narrow areas of experience over the centuries, because the methods used to train artists have not been able to escape the influence of tradition.

Paragraph 2
During the 19th century, painters tried to extend their training to express the experiences of other classes, but this proved to be difficult to achieve. A painting by Ford Maddox Ford is discussed as an example.

Paragraph 4
One reason for this lack of true liberation was that their training was still rooted in the old tradition.

Paragraph 3
In the 20th century the old tradition was finally dismantled, but the areas of experience painters drew from remained surprisingly limited (the only exception being the introduction of the Unconscious).

Passage at a Glance

Genre: A mix of literary criticism and sociology.

Passage difficulty level: Moderate (requires close, concentrated reading because of the abstruse subject).

Abstract/concrete: Surprisingly accessible in spite of the recondite nature of the subject. The theme is clear and logically developed.

Subject: How the professional training of artists stagnated over the centuries, denying painters the opportunity to open themselves to new areas of experience.

Author's attitude to subject: Sharply critical of the training process of artists.

Question types: One inference, three central thesis related, one passage reference.

Standard Passage Highlighting

Passage Highlighting (this is done as if skimming during an actual test and is not meant to be a "perfect" highlighting- learn from the following discussion): *see* Highlighting **(SB B.6, B.7)**

Paragraph 1: Sentence 1, 4, "artist's training", "a professional," "conventional skills","other social classes", "remote", "mere social … accoutrement","revolt … destroyed"

Paragraph 2: "19th century", "extend … other

classes", "pedestrian example", Sentences 4, 7, 9, "ambivalent"

Paragraph 3: Sentences 1-2, "Unconscious", "serious … narrow experience", "abstract art"

Paragraph 4: "potential freedom gained", Sentences 2-3

Paragraph 5: "extreme of abstract art", "original … art", "reduced area … universal"

QUESTION 3R.VR.III.63

Question Discussion Using Holistic Approach

This question revolves around the CT, as is clear from the language of the stem ("main argument of the passage"). All the options have echoes in the passage, but which option touches the core? The word 'limit' in option C gives the game away. The passage is about how poor training has limited artists.

Sometimes, one word is all it takes.

Putting it all together: the critical path

Recognize that the CT has to be identified and pick out Option C as closely matching the CT.

Question Discussion Using Standard Highlighting (HL) Analysis

Option A is incorrect. Option A is a true statement described in the first sentence of paragraph 1; however this is not the CT.

Option B is incorrect. Option B is found in paragraph 1 as "conventional skills", "corresponded ... social experience", "class ... serving". So, this is a True **(SB A.1.2)** statement but is it the central thesis?

Option D is incorrect. Option D is found in paragraph 3 as "crisis provoked", "extend ... of experience" suggests this is a true statement.

So, options B, C and D all appear true, but which is the Best Option **(SB A.1.2)**? The HL doesn't totally help get the final answer, but it did quickly get you to the locations where the issues were presented. From this point it depends on your knowledge, inferences and analysis.

Option C is correct. Option C is found partially in paragraph 1 as noted in option B but also in paragraph 2 as "extend ... tradition", "experience of other classes" would suggest that the subjects and training were connected but that the training was expanded.

Question Discussion Using Option Elimination Analysis

Q63   Pre-Study Suggestions

Review the following if needed:
1) Three Out of Four Options **SB A.2.8**

Solution Discussion
Please review the AAMC solution for this problem.

Test Taking Skills Comment
Options A, B and D are all similar in dealing with the 'ruling classes' in some manner and are the Three Out of Four Options (SB A.2.8). Option C is the outlier as it does not specifically deal with the 'ruling classes'. Usually outliers are incorrect. It is not in this question. Remember these are guesses and will be occasionally wrong. The goal is to overall increase your chance of guessing correctly which will occur using these techniques.

QUESTION 3R.VR.III.64

Question Discussion Using Holistic Approach

This is a direct passage reference question. Note that option D is ridiculous because the unconscious is a new concept, and hence is far removed from tradition. Also, option A looks plausible but can be ruled out because the author has an unfavorable opinion of tradition, and the option presents an exalted opinion of it. Yes, "preserve eternal artistic truths" does occur in the passage in the context of tradition, but from the point of view of the artist-apprentice. The wording of the stem ("in the context of the passage") makes it clear that the author's point of view is of interest.

The wording "mythological or symbolic" of option C requires attention because it occurs in the text. The author's point is that the artist was unable to depict manual work honestly because realism revealed ugly truths about labor that society was not ready to acknowledge or handle and hence imparted a religious color to the painting. In any case, remarks about a specific painting cannot be generalized as representing tradition as a whole. Hence, option C should be rejected.

The opening sentence of the second paragraph links extension of tradition to portraying the experiences of other classes. So, the existing tradition is related to the needs of the ruling elite option B. You should also note that tradition and convention, although not quite synonyms, are closely related.

I would classify this as a difficult question because all four options have wording from the passage, and to distinguish between them is not a trivial task (except that option D can be discarded at once).

Putting it all together: the critical path
This has to be done the hard way. *See* the previous explanation for details. However, the closeness in meaning between tradition and convention makes option B stand out, which you pick if you have to guess.

Question Discussion Using Standard Highlighting (HL) Analysis

Option A is incorrect. Option A is found in the HL in the discussed in option C and would be a close second choice but the tradition is implied as more the process of training than what results (preserving eternal truths).

Option D is incorrect. Option D is found in paragraph 3 as "Unconscious" as something introduced and not as the tradition itself.

Option C is incorrect. Option C is found in the HL in paragraph 2 as "mythological or symbolic" and this is in the context of an example of the extension of the tradition and not as what it is.

Option B is correct. References to "tradition" are found in paragraph 2 as "extend ... tradition", "experience ... classes". In paragraph 3, tradition is also found and was not HL as "The tradition ... dismantled". Also, in paragraph 4, "dismantling ... tradition" is found.

Question Discussion Using Option Elimination Analysis

Q64 Pre-Study Suggestions

Review the following if needed:
1) Three Out of Four Options **SB A.2.8**

CHAPTER 2

Solution Discussion
Please review the AAMC solution for this problem.

Test Taking Skills Comment
This is a Three Out of Four Options (SB A.2.8) question. Options A, B and D all relate to 'artistic'. Option C does not relate to 'artistic' and is the outlier. Outliers tend to be incorrect. You would make your guess from A, B or D.

QUESTION 3R.VR.III.65

Question Discussion Using Holistic Approach

This is a CT related question. From the central thesis, you should be able to immediately pick out option A. The word that gives it away is transcends, the opposite of the give-away word in option C (reflects) of the first question. A detailed analysis of all the options is unnecessary.

Putting it all together: the critical path
Option A should hit you between the eyes. From the CT, it is clear that the author feels art should break out of the shackles imposed by tradition.

Question Discussion Using Standard Highlighting (HL) Analysis

Option B is incorrect. It is found in paragraph 1 as "recording ... truths". The context of this is specific to the training for the ruling classes and the preservation of their conventions. This is not what the author meant to portray as art.

Option C is incorrect. It is found in paragraph 1 as "social manners", "revolt, ... destroyed", and in paragraph 2 as "extend ... tradition" and in other paragraphs. The author is clear that no "social manner" is art.

Option D is incorrect. Option D is found in paragraph 2 as "religious scene" and there is minimal other discussion of religion as critical to art.

Option A is correct. Option A is found in many locations as paragraph 1, "mere social convention", and in paragraph 4 as "academies … dismantled". These, and the associated phrase not HL, suggest that the issue of conventions were central to what the author is discussing in terms of art.

We live in a moment of history where change is so speeded up that we begin to see the present only when it is already disappearing.

R. D. Laing

CHAPTER 2

Question Discussion Using Option Elimination Analysis

Q65   Pre-Study Suggestions

Review the following if needed:
1) None

Solution Discussion
Please review the AAMC solution for this problem.

Test Taking Skills Comment
No specific techniques for this question.

Passage III - Questions 63-67

QUESTION 3R.VR.III.66

Question Discussion Using Holistic Approach

This is an inference type question. The question is not explicitly answered anywhere in the passage. Option A is suspicious because of the mention of "historical phenomenon." Why should artists be interested in history? There is no mention in the passage about artists displaying such an interest.

Option B can be eliminated because the passage mentions that some artists did try and reflect the experiences of other classes in their work. That leaves options C and D. The aspiration mentioned in option C is a normal aspiration, so it's not easy to decide. Since the passage has social inequality as an underlying subtext, option D is the better choice. Patronage often comes with strings attached.

Putting it all together: the critical path
Rule out options A and B, after which you pick the most sociological sounding option.

Question Discussion Using Standard Highlighting (HL) Analysis

There is really nothing in terms of HL to answer this question. This takes logic. Everyone has to pay the rent, buy clothes and food. The poor did not provide this, the ruling classes did. So, option D is the most logical of the set.

typical Complex Sounding Option **(SB A.2.2)**.

Option A is incorrect. This option requires a lot of assumptions. How would you know of an interest "in the narrowness and isolation", as a "historical phenomenon"? This is a

Option B is incorrect. Based on the HL of paragraph 2 artists did "extend the professional tradition" to other classes but faced struggle.

Option C is incorrect. Option C is certainly possible and logical and may be a reasonable guess if there is nothing better.

reason-basic support. In these types of questions and options, don't go for complexity ... keep it simple. The question states "According to the passage", but we are not sure what specific info was provided in the passage to legitimately answer this question ... refer to the AAMC Solution for this problem.

Option D is correct. But option D is the most simple and logical

Question Discussion Using Option Elimination Analysis

Q66 — Pre-Study Suggestions

Review the following if needed:
1) None

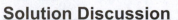

Solution Discussion
Please review the AAMC solution for this problem.

Test Taking Skills Comment
No specific techniques for this question.

CHAPTER 2

QUESTION 3R.VR.III.67

Question Discussion Using Holistic Approach

This is a CT-related question. (One could argue that this is an inference type question, the inference being the significance of the Maddox painting, but the inference agrees so closely to the CT that the distinction is academic.) The giveaway word here is 'expands', which plays the same role that 'transcends' plays in option A of Q 65. A detailed analysis of all the options is unnecessary.

Putting it all together: the critical path

Pick the option that matches the CT, namely option A.

Question Discussion Using Standard Highlighting (HL) Analysis

Option B is incorrect. Option B is False **(SB A.1.2)** because the example does not specifically talk of "abstract art". Paragraph 3 deals more specifically with this subject.

the example. There are further discussions related to this in paragraphs 3, 4 and 5 and the HL done.

Option C is incorrect. Option C is not specifically discussed in paragraph 2 in reference to

Option D is incorrect. Option D is found in paragraph 1 as "complicated, various and should not be simplified". While this is True

(SB A.1.2), it has nothing to do with the "Ford Madox Brown's" of paragraph 2.

Option A is correct. Option A is found in paragraph 2 as "pedestrian example" and "Ford Madox

Brown's" directs you rapidly to the correct location for the answer. Then as you read quickly, you find "pedestrian … difficulties involved". This is the answer, so this is the Correct **(SB A.1.2)** option. This is nearly a direct restatement of the stem.

Question Discussion Using Option Elimination Analysis

Q67 — Pre-Study Suggestions

Review the following if needed:
1) Similar Pair Options **SB A.2.7**

Solution Discussion
Please review the AAMC solution for this problem.

Test Taking Skills Comment
There is a reasonable Similar Pair Options **(SB A.2.7)** present. Options A and C both deal with similar concepts regarding 'expanding'. Neither options B nor D deal with this. There are no other reasonable similar pairs present. So, a reasonable guess would be A or C.

Passage IV - Questions 68-74

Highlighting For Holistic and Central Thesis Analysis

CBT3 Passage IV Holistic Highlighting

Paragraph 1: Sentence 1; coalesced ... gravity; dense, metallic ... top; earth's internal heat; cooling slowly ever since; tens of ... years

Paragraph 2: heat generated ... elements; forty-two terawatts; a thousandth; Sentence 4

Paragraph 3: 4,000 miles across; completely ... solid; Sentence 3

Paragraph 4: Sentences 1, 7, 8; by-product ... currents; magnetized ... years

Paragraph 5: dynamo; converts ... electric current

Headlining or Signposting the Passage

Paragraph 1: The structure of the earth (mantle and core) and the heat stored in it as well as its loss are explained in terms of the events that accompanied the planet's formation.

Paragraph 2: The sources and amounts of heat originating from the earth and the phenomena caused by discharge of the heat are described.

Paragraph 3: The structure of the core is described; the inner third of the core is solid despite its higher temperature, because it is under greater pressure.

Paragraph 4: The dynamo theory is used to infer that the core is cooling, the evidence being the earth's magnetic field.

Paragraph 5: The dynamo theory is explained.

Central Thesis:

The earth's core has been cooling continuously for a long time. The energy thus released sets up fluid movements in the outer core, resulting in an electric current that sets up the earth's magnetic field.

CHAPTER 2

Paragraph 1
The structure of the earth (mantle and core) and the heat stored in it as well as its loss are explained in terms of the events that accompanied the planet's formation.

Paragraph 2
The sources of heat originating from the earth and its amount, and the phenomena caused by discharge of the heat are described.

Central Thesis
The earth's core has been cooling continuously for a long time. The energy thus released sets up fluid movements in the outer core, resulting in an electric current that sets up the earth's magnetic field.

Paragraph 5
The dynamo theory is explained.

Paragraph 4
The dynamo theory is used to infer that the core is cooling, the evidence being the earth's magnetic field.

Paragraph 3
The structure of the core is described; the inner third of the core is solid despite its higher temperature, because it is under greater pressure.

Passage at a Glance

Genre: Hard science (descriptions and explanations of processes).

Passage difficulty level: Moderate (requires close, concentrated reading because of the hard science element).

Abstract/concrete: Concrete.

Subject: Causes and implications of heat trapped beneath the earth's surface.

Author's attitude to subject: Supports the dynamo theory.

Questions' difficulty level: Easy (of seven questions, no fewer than five are direct passage reference type).

Question types: Five passage reference, one inference, one CT related.

Putting It All Together: The Critical Path

Out of 7 questions, no fewer than 5 were direct passage reference questions. What is more, there were no confounding options or red herrings: the choice in each case is straightforward, so that no time need be wasted in considering other options. All you need to do is recognize that a question involves a direct passage reference, through your intense, concentrated reading of the passage and highlighting. Even the CT related and inference questions were relatively simple.

Therefore, the critical path for this passage is identical to the earlier discussion of questions.

General Comments:

It would seem to be a good idea to highlight important facts, including numbers, in passages about scientific processes, to exploit any direct passage reference questions that may be asked.

Note that the passage is a straightforward presentation of the dynamo theory. No criticisms of the theory are offered, nor are alternative theories discussed, which explains why the questions were so simple. Also note that though the passages in general become progressively more difficult, exceptions, such as this passage, are common.

Standard Passage Highlighting

Passage Highlighting (this is done as if skimming during an actual test and is not meant to be a "perfect" highlighting-learn from the following discussion): see Highlighting **(SB B.6, B.7)**.

Paragraph 1: "memory ... 4.5 billion", "disk ... energy", Sentence 3-4, "cooling slowly ever since"

Paragraph 2: Sentences 1-2, 5, "thousandth ... quantity", "Most ... mantle"

Paragraph 3: Sentences 1-3

Paragraph 4: Sentences 1, 4, 7, 8, "by-product ... currents", "bar magnet", "magnetized rocks ... billion years"

Paragraph 5: Sentences 1, "laws ... current", "force ... conductor", "working ... outer core"

QUESTION 3R.VR.IV.68

Question Discussion Using Holistic Approach

This is a CT-related question. From our central thesis above, we see that it is the internal heat of the earth that is responsible for fluid movements, and not the other way around. So, option A is the right option. In fact, the primordial processes described in the remaining options, namely, gravitational forces, decay of radioactive elements, and separation of lighter from heavier materials, are described in the first paragraph as being responsible for the earth's "internal heat."

Putting it all together: the critical path
See general discussion on previous critical path.

Question Discussion Using Standard Highlighting (HL) Analysis

Option B is incorrect. Option B is found in paragraph 1 as "gravitational energy". And, then reading the sentences around this, you note "gravitational energy was released to melt". This is clearly the generation of heat.

Option C is incorrect. Option C is found in paragraph 2 as "casts off the heat generated by the decay of radioactive". This is a true statement and is wrong.

Option D is incorrect. Option D is found in paragraph 1 as "heavier materials ... energy" HL. This option is a true option and cannot be correct.

Option A is correct. In paragraph 4, "fluid motions", "motions ... the core", refer to the generation of the magnetic field and not the heat generation. So, this is false. Since the question is a Negative Question **(SB A.1.2)**, this is probably the answer.

CHAPTER 2

Question Discussion Using Option Elimination Analysis

Q68   Pre-Study Suggestions

Review the following if needed:
1) Similar Pair Options **SB A.2.7**
2) Negative Question **SB A.1.2**

Solution Discussion

Please review the AAMC solution for this problem.

Test Taking Skills Comment

Options B and D are a Similar Pair Options **(SB A.2.7)** with 'primordial'. Since, this is the only reasonable similar pair, this would normally be a good guess. But, this is a Negative Question **(SB A.1.2)** and you have to be very careful. With negative questions, often the opposite options may be the best options to guess from; this means the best guess may be from A and C. The take home message is to be very careful when a question is a negative question; you may have to guess the reverse of what you would ordinarily guess.

QUESTION 3R.VR.IV.69

Question Discussion Using Holistic Approach

This is a direct passage reference question. It is mentioned in the second paragraph that the heat released by the earth is 42 terawatts, which is one thousandth of the energy provided by the sun. **Option C is correct.**

Putting it all together: the critical path

See general discussion on critical path for this passage.

Question Discussion Using Standard Highlighting (HL) Analysis

The HL information is found in paragraph 2 as "All told, about forty-two terawatts (forty-two trillion watts) continuously escapes from the earth's surface. That is only about a thousandth of the heat provided by the sun."

Since the question is asking about the sun, its heat must be 1000 times that of the earth or:

1000 x 42 terawatts = 42,000 terawatts.
This means option C is correct.

Question Discussion Using Option Elimination Analysis

Q69   Pre-Study Suggestions

Review the following if needed:
1) Three Out of Four Options **SB A.2.8**
2) Internal Inconsistency of Options **SB A.2.5**

Solution Discussion
Please review the AAMC solution for this problem.

Test Taking Skills Comment
This is a Three Out of Four Options **(SB A.2.8)** question. Options A, B and C do not have 'trillion' after the number. Option D does have 'trillion' and is the outlier. Outliers tend to be incorrect. Option A is also an Internal Inconsistency of Options **(SB A.2.5)** which cannot be correct. In paragraph 2 of the passage, the heat of the earth is stated to be 42 terawatts. Since the sun is noted to be hotter, this cannot possibly be the answer.

So, using the three out of four, the possible guesses are options A, B and C. Since option A should be eliminated, this leaves options B and C as the guess options.

QUESTION 3R.VR.IV.70

Question Discussion Using Holistic Approach

This is another direct passage reference question. It is stated in the third paragraph that the inner 1/3 of the core is solid. This implies that the remaining 2/3 of the core is liquid. Option C is the right option.

<u>Putting it all together: the critical path</u>
See the general discussion for the passage.

Question Discussion Using Standard Highlighting (HL) Analysis

The HL information is found in paragraph 3.

Option A is incorrect. Option A would be incorrect, because this description does not discuss "radioactivity".

Option B is incorrect. Option B is incorrect because it states the core is "molten" and "solid" but no mention of "gaseous".

Option D is incorrect. Option D is tricky but incorrect. "Solid" is identified as part of the core, but the "magnetic" is not specifically identified with the core but with the Earth in general as found in paragraph 4 as "earth's magnetic field" and "clearest evidence that the core is cooling". This paragraph goes on to discuss the role of the core in generating the magnetic field and not the core being magnetic.

Option C is correct. Option C is correct because the HL clearly identifies it is made of metals and also contains fluid ("molten").

This is rated as a very difficult question as only 50% of students got it correct. But, the accurate HL rapidly demonstrated the correct option. Notice again, you have to first read and understand the HL and related text first. Then you may need to make some limited and very precise inferences. In this question, "magnetism" is certainly discussed along with the "core", but the magnetic field is not in the core. The magnetic field belongs to the earth but the core helps generate it.

Question Discussion Using Option Elimination Analysis

Q70 — Pre-Study Suggestions

Review the following if needed:
1) Similar Pair Options **SB A.2.7**

Solution Discussion
Please review the AAMC solution for this problem.

Test Taking Skills Comment
This is a potential Similar Pair Options **(SB A.2.7)** question. Options A and D both have 'solid', and options B and D both have 'magnetic'. Since there is more than one similar pair present, neither should be used as a pure guess. In this question, the passage knowledge would suggest that neither is correct because it is neither mostly solid nor mostly magnetic.

QUESTION 3R.VR.IV.71

Question Discussion Using Holistic Approach

This is also a direct passage reference question. The penultimate paragraph states that "magnetized rocks" show that the earth has had a magnetic field for at least three billion years. Option B is the correct option.

Putting it all together: the critical path
See the general discussion for this passage.

Question Discussion Using Standard Highlighting (HL) Analysis

Option A is incorrect. Option A is found by HL found in paragraph 2 as "geological activity" is mentioned. However, the passage is about the motions and heat accounting for the geological activity and has nothing to do with the magnetic field of the earth.

Option C is incorrect. Option C is found in paragraph 5 as "conductive material through a magnetic field" is the primary reference to conduction, but there is no mention of "conductive rocks".

Option D is incorrect. Option D is found by "electric generator" and "conductive material through magnetic field" in paragraph 5. In this area, you also find "converts mechanical energy into electric current", but there is no statement about rocks doing this conversion.

Option B is correct. Option B is found in sentence 6 of paragraph 4 where the answer to the question is explicitly stated.

Question Discussion Using Option Elimination Analysis

Q71 — Pre-Study Suggestions

Review the following if needed:
1) Three Out of Four Options **SB A.2.8**

Solution Discussion
Please review the AAMC solution for this problem.

Test Taking Skills Comment
This is a Three Out of Four Options (SB A.2.8) question. Options B, C and D all contain references to 'rocks'. Option A is the outlier with no reference to rocks. Outliers tend to be incorrect.

> Men prize the thing ungained, more than it is.
>
> Shakespeare

QUESTION 3R.VR.IV.72

Question Discussion Using Holistic Approach

This is also a direct passage reference question. The fourth paragraph states that only the dynamo theory can account for the persistence of the earth's magnetic field and it's propensity for reversing itself. **Option A** *is correct*.

Putting it all together: the critical path
See the general discussion for this passage.

Question Discussion Using Standard Highlighting (HL) Analysis

The "dynamo theory" is found by HL in paragraph 4 as "only theory", "dynamo theory", "fluid motions", and "motions ... core". Sentence 7 is nearly identical phrasing to option A which must be Correct **(SB A.1.2)**. Given this nearly exactness of option A and the finding in passage via the HL clue, there is really little need to look further. Only 65% of students got this question correct. Yet, with the proper HL, the answer literally jumps out of the passage.

Question Discussion Using Option Elimination Analysis

Q72   Pre-Study Suggestions

Review the following if needed:
1) Similar Pair Options **SB A.2.7**

Solution Discussion
Please review the AAMC solution for this problem.

Test Taking Skills Comment
This is a Similar Pair Options **(SB A.2.7)** question with two similar pair sets. One set is options A and B with reference to 'magnetic field'. The other set is options C and D with reference to 'core'. Usually, it is best to ignore the pairs when two or more are present. But one of several exceptions is when Basic Knowledge (study, passage, general knowledge) **(SB A.2.2)** can be used. This question allows the use of passage knowledge as found in paragraph 4. The dynamo theory refers to magnetism/effects as discussed in that paragraph. So, it is reasonable to select the similar pair set with options A and B as your guess.

QUESTION 3R.VR.IV.73

Question Discussion Using Holistic Approach

This is again another direct passage reference question. The fourth paragraph states that the earth's magnetism, like any other, is the product of electric currents. The correct choice is option D. Note that option A (fluid movements) is an attractive candidate. Read our CT now to confirm this. However, the stem refers to magnetic fields in general; there is no mention of the earth's magnetic field in particular, so what is sought is a fundamental principle applicable to all magnetic fields.

Putting it all together: the critical path
See the general discussion for the passage.

Question Discussion Using Standard Highlighting (HL) Analysis

Option A is incorrect. Option A is found in paragraph 4 with the "fluid motions". This is fully associated with the following: "magnetic field results from fluid motions in the outer core". So, this is a True **(SB A.1.2)** statement and appears to be the answer.

Option C is incorrect. Option C is not found in the HL done. As noted previously, it may not have been unreasonable to HL "converts mechanical energy into electric current" as found in paragraph 5. This would have pointed you to this paragraph, but this does not state the magnetic field is due to "mechanical energy".

Option B is incorrect. Option B has no specific HL because there is no mentioning of earth rotation. You would have to be confident that you would have HL this phrase, or you have to go back through the passage searching for it, which you will not find, or believe other options are more credible.

Option D is correct. Option D is found in paragraph 4 as "by-product of electrical currents". Then reading the surrounding sentences, you find that "The earth's magnetic field ... is a by-product of electric currents." So, it is the electric current which is critical. Fluid motion, without electric current or flow, would NOT produce a magnetic field.

Question Discussion Using Option Elimination Analysis

Q73   Pre-Study Suggestions

Review the following if needed:
1) Three Out of Four Options **SB A.2.8**

Solution Discussion

Please review the AAMC solution for this problem.

Test Taking Skills Comment

Options A, B and D are similar in that all relate to motion or movement. Option D is the outlier without a clear motion component. Outliers tend to be incorrect. This is Three Out of Four Options (**SB A.2.8**) question.

QUESTION 3R.VR.IV.74

Question Discussion Using Holistic Approach

This is an inference type question. Looking at the options, we eliminate the last two options on sight, and retain just the first two for consideration. This is because the first two options have one important element in common with the topic discussed in the passage, namely an understanding of past events, and relating them to the present. From the first two options, we eliminate the first because of the motive: "source of artistic inspiration." The motive in the second option, "to develop theories," corresponds closely to the purpose of our passage, which is also to develop theories. Option B is the right option.

Putting it all together: the critical path

See the general discussion for the passage.

Question Discussion Using Standard Highlighting (HL) Analysis

This does not require information from the passage. The key info is Restated (**SB B.7.7**) in the Stem (**SB A.1**). You have to use your logic and Inferences (**SB B.5**) to arrive at the answer. The key here is that you have knowledge from different subjects combined to yield the theory; the Correct (**SB A.1.2**) option must do the same.

Passage IV - Questions 68-74

Option A is incorrect.
Option A deals only with one subject: art.

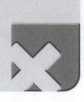

Option D is incorrect.
Option D deals only with one subject: anesthetic effects.

Option C is incorrect.
Option C deals only with one subject: problem solving.

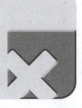

Option B is correct. Option B deals with different subjects in order to come up with a theory. This is entirely similar to the stem's statement.

Question Discussion Using Option Elimination Analysis

Q74 Pre-Study Suggestions

Review the following if needed:
1) Three Out of Four Options **SB A.2.8**

Solution Discussion
Please review the AAMC solution for this problem.

Test Taking Skills Comment
This is a Three Out of Four Options **(SB A.2.8)** question. Options A, B and C each have two or more specific disciplines/areas that are combined to result in the final area of study/research. Option D is an outlier only having 'anesthetics'. Outliers tend to be incorrect.

This is also a question that does not require the passage to answer it. This must be recognized from the manner the stem and options are presented. By recognizing this quickly, you can save valuable time by NOT referring back to the passage.

Highlighting For Holistic and Central Thesis Analysis

CBT3 Passage V Holistic Highlighting

Paragraph 1: not the "dream factory"; reality factory; Sentences 2-4; originality … box; numbing effect; confuse; addicted; Frustration; catharsis … response; staying passive; "stay tuned"

Paragraph 2: recycler and mixer of a confluence of concepts;

Paragraph 3: Television, in fact … already; regularity; how they … credibility; guarantee of quality; human behavior at large

Paragraph 4: Sentence 1; writes our scripts; gives … language; docked … obsessions

Headlining or Signposting the Passage

Paragraph 1: A wholly negative picture of the influence of television is offered, as is evident from this long list of loaded words/phrases: lack of articulacy, grammar, structured argument, oratorical exposition, originality, numbing, confusing, passive, addicted, frustration.

Paragraph 2: Television has no specific vocabulary; instead, it has characters.

Paragraph 3: Television imitates reality with frightening success, and has become the standard by which reality itself is measured.

Paragraph 4: Television, on account of its need to attract and retain audiences, presents a distorted picture of reality.

Central Thesis:

Television began by reflecting life, but has now burst its bonds to become the standard by which life is judged. This is a dangerous development, because television presents a distorted picture of life.

Paragraph 1

A wholly negative picture of the influence of television is offered, as is evident from this long list of loaded words/phrases: lack of articulacy, grammar, structured argument, oratorical exposition, or originality; numbing; confusing; passive; addicted; frustration.

Paragraph 2

Television has no specific vocabulary; instead, it has characters.

Central Thesis

Television began by reflecting life, but has now burst its bonds to become the standard by which life itself is judged. This is a dangerous development, because television presents a distorted picture of life.

Paragraph 4

Television, on account of its need to attract and retain audiences, presents a distorted picture of reality.

Paragraph 3

Television imitates reality with frightening success, and has become the standard by which reality itself is measured..,

Passage V - Questions 75-79

Passage at a Glance

Genre: Sociology/psychology

Passage difficulty level: Moderate (requires close, concentrated reading because of the hard science element).

Abstract/concrete: Abstract
Subject: How television affects people and society

Author's attitude to subject: Highly critical of television

Questions' difficulty level: Moderate to difficult (The options are replete with red herrings).

Question types
• One central thesis related,
• One inference type,
• Four passage reference questions.

Standard Passage Highlighting

Paragraph 1.1: (Sentences 1-7)"not the "dream factory"", "dour sociologists", "reality factory", "immediacy … oratorical", Sentences 4, 7, ""Series"", ""characters"… we love", "originality … box"

Paragraph 1.2: Sentences 8-11)""information" … up-to-date", "segmentation … something", Sentence 9, "staying passive", ""stay tuned … commandment"

Paragraph 2: Sentence 1, "cannot be isolated", "voracious … confluence", ""basic television" … vocabulary", "cadges … dictionary"

Paragraph 3: "more authentic", "drama … quotidian", "regularity … calibrated",""Time for Kojak"", "realistic programs … credibility", "guarantee ofquality"

Paragraph 4: "Mass communication", "lacks … articulation", ""good program"", "verisimilitudinous … switch off"

QUESTION 3R.VR.V.75

Question Discussion Using Holistic Approach

This is a direct passage reference question. The question asks for you to look directly into the passage in order to find the correct answer. The keywords "stay passive," "emotional catharsis," "leave the viewing chair," and "confuse" all ring bells since they are all found in the passage. Search the passage for each of the key words and make sure they are coherent with the general idea (What is the main goal of the newscasters?) The main idea here is that the newscasters want the viewers to be updated with what is happening in the world and therefore need the viewers to "stay tuned".

Putting it all together: the critical path

Main idea questions can usually be answered easily if the central thesis is grasped. In this case, we know the newscasters attempt to "keep us fully up-to-date with the world", however the result of this is that they "confuse us" and doing so has the goal to make the viewers "stay tuned" or "passive"

Question Discussion Using Standard Highlighting (HL) Analysis

CHAPTER 2

Option B is incorrect. Option B is found in paragraph 1.2 as ""news" and "catharsis does not follow"; the option is False **(SB A.1.2)** and Incorrect **(SB A.1.2)**.

Option C is incorrect. Option C is contradicted by paragraph 1.2 as ""news"", "staying passive" and ""stay tuned"... commandment" and is therefore False **(SB A.1.2)**. Reading in this location, you also find "if we are moved to leave the viewing chair we may miss the next program". This means they want to stay in the "viewing chair" and not move.

Option D is incorrect. Option D is found in paragraph 1.2 as ""news" and "segmentation and "personalization"". Reading in this area, you find "confuse us with their discontinuous gush". As explained previously, the newscasters do not attempt to confuse their viewers; they attempt to feed them as much information as possible and therefore do so in a segmented way in order to keep the viewers "tuned" and "passive".

Option A is correct. Option A is found in the last sentence of paragraph 1.2 and as "the reward ... staying passive". The final goal of the newscasters is to keep the viewers passive so that they could "stay tuned".

Only 60 percent of students got this question correct. Yet, with the HL, the answer nearly pops out at you.

Question Discussion Using Option Elimination Analysis

Q75 — Pre-Study Suggestions

Review the following if needed:
1) Three Out of Four Options **SB A.2.8**

Solution Discussion
Please review the AAMC solution for this problem.

Test Taking Skills Comment
There is a Three Out of Four Options **(SB A.2.8)** present with options A, B and D being similar in dealing with an emotion of some type. Option C is the outlier and outliers tend to be incorrect. This is a Negative Question **(SB A.1.2)** and it means you must be careful when applying the technique.

QUESTION 3R.VR.V.76

Question Discussion Using Holistic Approach

This is a direct passage reference question. Note how the keywords 'convincing', 'articulating', 'passive', and 'passionate' are confusing because each of them occurs in the passage. However, according to the passage, "inarticulacy" is a quality valued in television; option B can be eliminated.

Options C and D are opposites. The phrase "amateurish or embarrassing passions" makes option C fall. Option A is also a reasonable choice as the passage states that television is more true to life than life itself.

Since the stem is about an argument between two people, we feel "passion" is closer to that context, and pick option D. The tie can also be broken by looking at how 'convince' is used in the text: "Television convinces us by immediacy and by repetition", which argues in favor of filming a real-life argument.

Note: The AAMC Solution makes the point that television is more true to life than life itself because of the use of natural language, not because of professional acting skills. This kind of hair-splitting argument is not completely convincing because the passage states that television teaches viewers how to "behave." The scope of the passage is not restricted to the language dimension alone, as befits a visual medium like television.

Putting it all together: the critical path

You have to recall the sentence in the passage that states "embarrassing passions … to switch off" and connect it to option D.

Question Discussion Using Standard Highlighting (HL) Analysis

Option A is incorrect. Option A is found in paragraph 4 as "more authentic", "clock … calibrated" and "realistic … behave". This suggests the actors can be realistic, but it doesn't specifically compare reality and television fantasy in terms of the actors and real people. This is a borderline response and you want to look for a better Option **(SB A.1.2)**.

does suggest the actors can express emotions.

Option C is incorrect. Option C is found in paragraph 2 with "staying passive" but this refers to the audience.

Option B is incorrect. Option B is found in paragraph 1.1 as "articulacy… sincerity," and in paragraph 1.2 as "emotional responses". Reading in these areas

Option D is correct. Option D is found in paragraph 5 as "good program" and "verisimilitudinous … obsessions". This most clearly

Passage V - Questions 75-79

states what actors do as compared to nonactors and the real people: they don't show "amateurish and embarrassing passions or obsessions" which "might cause our audience to switch off".

This is difficult problem as only 40% of students got it correct.

Question Discussion Using Option Elimination Analysis

Q76 Pre-Study Suggestions

Review the following if needed:
None.

Solution Discussion

Please review the AAMC solution for this problem.

Test Taking Skills Comment

No specific techniques for this question.

And so, my fellow Americans; ask not what your country can do for you - ask what you can do for your country. My fellow citizens of the world: ask not what America will do for you, but what together we can do for the freedom of man.

John F. Kennedy

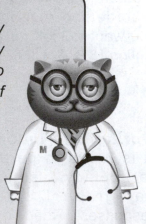

QUESTION 3R.VR.V.77

Question Discussion Using Holistic Approach

This is also a direct passage reference question. Each option statement contains words/phrases from the passage: "originality," "numbing," "truer to life than life," and "immediacy and repetition." This should not confuse you. If you find the place in the first paragraph where familiar characters and loved advertisements are mentioned, you will see that the lack of originality is mentioned in the same context. So the right option is option A.

Putting it all together: the critical path

As in the previous question, you have to link 'familiar characters' and 'loved advertisements' with 'lack of originality" in the passage, and make the connection with option A.

Question Discussion Using Standard Highlighting (HL) Analysis

This refers to a specific claim of evidence by the author. This is found with HL in sentence 6. This is clearly the "overfamiliarity" as found in the Stem **(SB A.1)**. And the author specifically relates it to originality. This is a difficult question; only 35 percent of students got it correct.

Option B is incorrect. Option B is found in paragraph 2 as "numbing effect … news"; it only relates to the news and is not directly tied to the "overfamiliarity" like the "originality" is.

Option C is incorrect. Option C is found in paragraph 1 as "reality factory", "truer to life than life is" and in paragraph 4 as "more authentic", "quotidian" and "Being true to life … life itself." So, this option has passage elements of being True **(SB A.1.2)**, but these comments are not associated with "overfamiliarity".

Note: "Quotidian", from Latin, means daily or routine. In medicine, you may encounter it with "quotidian malaria" which is malaria with daily fevers.

Option D is incorrect. Option D is found in paragraph 1 as "by immediacy and by repetition". But, again, this does not relate to the "overfamiliarity".

Option A is correct. Option A specifically states "little place for originality on television" and this is nearly an exact rephrasing of the information found in the passage.

Question Discussion Using Option Elimination Analysis

Q77 — Pre-Study Suggestions

Review the following if needed:
1) Three Out of Four Options **SB A.2.8**

Solution Discussion
Please review the AAMC solution for this problem.

Test Taking Skills Comment
This is a Three Out of Four Options **(SB A.2.8)** with options A, C and D being related to 'television'. Option B is the outlier not directly noting 'television'. Outliers tend to be incorrect.

QUESTION 3R.VR.V.78

Question Discussion Using Holistic Approach

This is an inference question. The author's contention in the passage is that television is truer to life than life itself because it packages life in a way that viewers find attractive. Thus, "a lack of articulacy" is a desirable trait and "a badge of sincerity"; option C is right.

Putting it all together: the critical path

Inarticulacy and lack of passion are stated in the passage to be hallmarks of good television programming. This connects to option C, in which the television presenter has the opposite characteristics.

Question Discussion Using Standard Highlighting (HL) Analysis

Option A is incorrect. There were no discussions of "critic" in the passage. If you trust your HL, you will not find any "critic" HL and can move on.

resonate with fast-paced. Also, in paragraph 3 "language of television" discusses the lack of any specific language. This is unlikely to be Correct (**SB A.1.2**).

Option B is incorrect. Option B is found in paragraph 1.2 as "information", "news", and "discontinuous gush". These direct you to the correct location and

Option D is incorrect. Option D is found in several locations and especially in paragraph 3 as "voracious ... confluence", "cadges ... parasitism". Cadge means to get by begging. This is a difficult word. It is important to improve your vocabulary as much as possible; study the sections on Vocabulary **(SB B.2.1)** found in Verbal Reasoning. So, option D is consistent with the author and would not challenge information.

Option C is correct. Option C is found in paragraph 1 and 5 as "articulacy" and "verisimilitudinous … obsessions" respectively. This would suggest just the opposite of what the option is stating.

Question Discussion Using Option Elimination Analysis

Q78 — Pre-Study Suggestions

Review the following if needed:
1) Three Out of Four Options **SB A.2.8**
2) Similar Pair Options **SB A.2.7**

Solution Discussion
Please review the AAMC solution for this problem.

Test Taking Skills Comment
This is a Three Out of Four Options **(SB A.2.8)** with options A, C and D directly noting 'television'. Option B is the outlier without a direct link to 'television'. Outliers tend to be incorrect. Options A and D constitute a Similar Pair Options **(SB A.2.7)** as both relate to 'series'. This is a reasonable similar pair as each option is part of the three out of four. So, you can guess from A, C or D based on the three out of four or refine it to the A/D based on the similar pair, but this results in the wrong answer.

QUESTION 3R.VR.V.79

Question Discussion Using Holistic Approach

Again, this is a direct passage reference question. This repeats the same idea as in Q 76. The goal of television programming is to keep the viewer glued to his or her seat, so the right option is option B. Note that option C is ridiculous, because inarticulacy and lack of passion have been identified in the passage as desirable in television. Options A and D sound reasonable but nothing in the passage supports them.

Putting it all together: the critical path
Think "couch potato": option B

Question Discussion Using Standard Highlighting (HL) Analysis

The reference to 'good program' is found in paragraph 5 as "good program", "verisimilitudinous … obsessions".

Option A is incorrect. Paragraph 5 suggests that viewers don't want the full impact of emotions. Also, sentences 9 and 11 of paragraph 2 show that emotion too felt is not wanted.

Option C is incorrect. Option C is the statement as noted in paragraph 5 with "language lacks precise articulation". Additionally, paragraph 2 states it is the lack of articulacy that is wanted. These suggest "passionate and articulate characters" are not wanted.

Option D is incorrect. Option D is found in paragraph 4 as "more authentic" and this section goes on to discuss fantasy may be more real than reality to viewers. Additionally, the excerpt from paragraph 5 suggests real life would not fit with its "amateurish or embarrassing passions or obsessions."

Option B is correct. Option B is found specifically in paragraph 2 as "staying passive" and ""stay tuned" … commandment". This means they don't want viewers to move. This is a True **(SB A.1.2)** statement and a right answer.

Question Discussion Using Option Elimination Analysis

Q79 Pre-Study Suggestions

Review the following if needed:
1) Similar Pair Options **SB A.2.7**

Solution Discussion
Please review the AAMC solution for this problem.

Test Taking Skills Comment
Options A and B are Similar Pair Options **(SB A.2.7)** as both deal with 'viewers'. There are no other significant similar pairs. A good guess would come from A or B.

Highlighting For Holistic and Central Thesis Analysis

CBT3 Passage VI Holistic Highlighting
Paragraph 1: human powers; magical quality;

Sentence 2; "obvious"; new; right; path; li

Paragraph 2: labor... hard; "holy... ceremony"; Sentence 3; essential; human ... own

Paragraph 3: Sentence 1; invisible and intangible; spontaneous ... dignity; esthetic ... spiritual

Paragraph 4: Sentence 1; proper ritual expression; politely ... ceremonially

Paragraph 5: speech ... evoke action; Sentences 2, 5; J. L. Austin; "performative utterance"; "operative" ... instrument

Paragraph 6: not a report; very act of bequeathal itself

Paragraph 7: central lesson; about ceremony; substance ... ceremony; are ... nothing

Headlining or Signposting the Passage

Paragraph 1: Human abilities are in truth extraordinary, and the path to uncovering this magic in the mundane is li.

Paragraph 2: The path of li involves viewing societal conventions as holy ceremonies.

Paragraph 3: The path of li is subtle and based on an acknowledgment of human dignity; its opposite is the ruler who strives to maintain control with a show of force.

Paragraph 4: Demonstrates the power of li to attain physical ends: a polite request to a student enables a book the teacher requires to be in his hands without the teacher himself moving an inch.

Paragraph 5: Words have been traditionally viewed as descriptions of actions, but contemporary linguistic studies show that words often constitute the action (the performative utterance).

Paragraph 6: The wording of wills is given as an example of words constituting action: the words of a will are, in effect, the act of bequeathal.

Paragraph 7: Professor Austin's work (the performative utterance) underscores the central role of ceremony in our everyday lives.

Central Thesis:

Confucius recognized that ceremony lies at the heart of much of everyday life, and the path that he advocated, li, could work wonders by acknowledging this truth.

CHAPTER 2

Passage VI - Questions 80-85

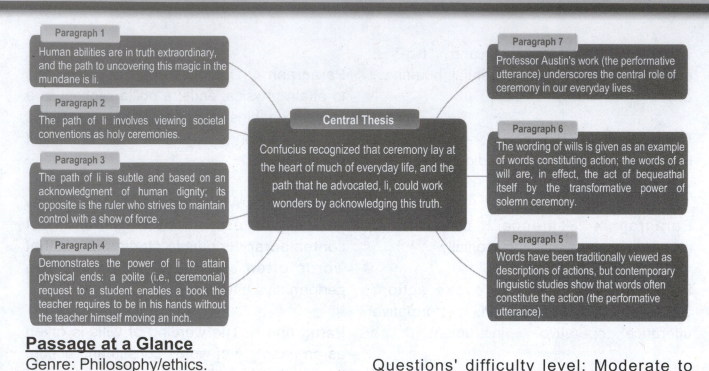

Paragraph 1
Human abilities are in truth extraordinary, and the path to uncovering this magic in the mundane is li.

Paragraph 2
The path of li involves viewing societal conventions as holy ceremonies.

Paragraph 3
The path of li is subtle and based on an acknowledgment of human dignity; its opposite is the ruler who strives to maintain control with a show of force.

Paragraph 4
Demonstrates the power of li to attain physical ends: a polite (i.e., ceremonial) request to a student enables a book the teacher requires to be in his hands without the teacher himself moving an inch.

Central Thesis
Confucius recognized that ceremony lay at the heart of much of everyday life, and the path that he advocated, li, could work wonders by acknowledging this truth.

Paragraph 7
Professor Austin's work (the performative utterance) underscores the central role of ceremony in our everyday lives.

Paragraph 6
The wording of wills is given as an example of words constituting action; the words of a will are, in effect, the act of bequeathal itself by the transformative power of solemn ceremony.

Paragraph 5
Words have been traditionally viewed as descriptions of actions, but contemporary linguistic studies show that words often constitute the action (the performative utterance).

Passage at a Glance

Genre: Philosophy/ethics.

Passage difficulty level: Difficult. This is a slippery passage.

Abstract/concrete: Abstract.

Subject: The Confucian concept li.

Author's attitude to subject: The writer admires Confucius and his philosophy.

Questions' difficulty level: Moderate to difficult (there are many inference questions that test how well the reader has grasped the spirit of the passage).

Question types: One central thesis related, one passage reference, and four inference questions

Standard Passage Highlighting

Passage Highlighting (this is done as if skimming during an actual test and is not meant to be a "perfect" highlighting - learn from the discussion that follows): see Highlighting (**SB B.6, B.7**).

Paragraph 1: "distinctively human powers", "magical quality", "so familiar ... unnoticed", ""obvious" dimension", "new way", "notion of li"

Paragraph 2: "long … learn li", "meaning … ceremony"", "language … medium", "authentic … society", "ability … to li", "will … power"

Paragraph 3: Sentences 1, 3, "force … tangible", "li … dignity",

Paragraph 4: "effortless power of li", "accomplish physical ends", "bring … classroom"

Paragraph 5: Sentence 1, ""linguistic" analysis", "ritual word … action", Sentence 3, ""operative" clause … itself"

Paragraph 6: ""I give … brother"", "bequeathal", "more powerful … force"

Paragraph 7: Sentences 1, 3, "substance … ceremony"

QUESTION 3R.VR.VI.80

Question Discussion Using Holistic Approach

This is a CT-related question. We are asked to pick the main idea of the passage. Option A is misleading. Promises, commitments, etc., are not described as "conventions" but as "ceremonies" (a much more powerful word than convention) in the last line of the passage. Another problem with this option is that a central thesis must be a big idea: where is the bang, the punch, in describing promises, etc., as verbal conventions?

Option B is plausible; the example of the professor in a classroom "teleporting" a book from his office springs to mind. However, the domain of li is not the physical but the spiritual and the aesthetic. This is also underscored by the following wording "teleported book". Turning to option C, the passage does not mention the "honesty" or otherwise of performative utterances at all. This is a red herring. That leaves option D, which also matches our central thesis. The theme of the passage is the power of ceremony.

Putting it all together: the critical path
Main idea questions can usually be answered easily if the central thesis is grasped. Only option D matches the central thesis of the passage.

Question Discussion Using Standard Highlighting (HL) Analysis

Option A is incorrect. Option A is found in sentence 3 of paragraph 7, but this option only gives examples and not the primary or central thesis. Remember the three general themes to monitor in a passage are the central thesis, the secondary contentions or theses, and examples. This was an example.

Option B is incorrect. Option B is found in paragraph 3 and 4 as "ruler ... force", "force of ... tangible", and as "effortless power of li", "accomplish ... ends", "bring ... classroom". This is a True **(SB A.1.2)** statement but these points were made as examples of the power of li and not as the central thesis of the passage.

Option C is incorrect. Option C is found in paragraph 5 as ""performative utterances"", ""operative" ... instrument". This again is True **(SB A.1.2)** but it is not the central thesis.

Option D is correct. Option D is found in paragraph 2 as "long ... learn li", "meaning ... ceremony"", "authentic ... society", and in paragraph 7 as "central ... Austin's", "not so ... ceremony", "substance ... ceremony" and Sentence 3. So, the key is the ceremonial aspects making option D the Best Option **(SB A.1.2)**.

Question Discussion Using Option Elimination Analysis

Q80 — Pre-Study Suggestions

Review the following if needed:
None

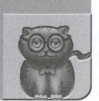

Solution Discussion
Please review the AAMC solution for this problem.

Test Taking Skills Comment
No specific techniques for this question.

QUESTION 3R.VR.VI.81

Question Discussion Using Holistic Approach

This is an inference question. If you have grasped that li has to do with ethics, the "right" way, homing in on the correct option is not difficult. Options B, C and D present motivations that are the opposite of ethical. The right option is option A. Ceremony, the heart of li, upholds the dignity of all participants by the solemnity of the occasion. The third paragraph mentions that li "works through spontaneous coordination rooted in reverent dignity."

Note: To decide between options A and C,

you need to consider the standpoint of the passage. The passage takes a clear moral standpoint. Therefore, the reason preferred by Confucius is likely to be a moral reason, and only option A supplies a moral reason. On the other hand, if the standpoint of the passage were efficiency, option C would be the preferred option.

Putting it all together: the critical path
Pick the most moralistic option, which is option A.

Question Discussion Using Standard Highlighting (HL) Analysis

Option B is incorrect. Option B is found in paragraph 1 as "magical quality". This is again a characteristic of li but not necessarily a reason to endorse its use for something. It is a true option but would be less of a reason to use than "reverent dignity".

Option C is incorrect. Option C is found in paragraph 4 as "effortless power of li", "accomplish physical ends", and a specific example of the use is given. So, this option is true and seems right because a specific example is associated with it.

In this world there are only two tragedies. One is not getting what one wants, and the other is getting it.

Oscar Wilde

Option D is incorrect. Option D is found in paragraph 3 in sentences 1-2 and as "li ... dignity". But, this is not specifically a use but a reason to use.

Option A is correct. Option A is found in paragraph 3 as "spontaneous ... dignity". But, this statement is that this is a characteristic of li which is good but not specifically a reason to use it. Yet, this is a True **(SB A.1.2)** option and must be considered.

The answer by AAMC is option A. We can definitely see how option C could be chosen. You need to read the AAMC solution and then try to sort out the reasoning. We don't fully agree with their reasoning. But, the HL again directed us rapidly to the pertinent areas of the paragraph.

Question Discussion Using Option Elimination Analysis

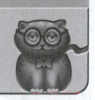

Q81   Pre-Study Suggestions

Review the following if needed:
1) Three Out of Four Options **SB A.2.8**

Solution Discussion
Please review the AAMC solution for this problem.

Test Taking Skills Comment
This is a Three Out of Four Options (**SB**

A.2.8) question. Options B, C and D all involve some action/activity. Option A is the outlier and outliers tend to be incorrect. But, this technique will result in the wrong answer.

CHAPTER 2

QUESTION 3R.VR.VI.82

Question Discussion Using Holistic Approach

This is a passage reference question. The very first line of the passage makes it clear that option A is right. Another way of looking at it is like this: options B, C, and D can be eliminated because of the emphasis on the "supernatural" and the "occult," which are at odds with the central thesis. Note that the "conventions" mentioned in option A are closely allied to "ceremony" mentioned in our central thesis. Therefore, option A is correct.

Putting it all together: the critical path
Options B and C should not be touched with 20-ft barge poles. The red flags in these options are "supernatural" and "occult." Note the source of the passage: Confucius—The Secular as Sacred. The focus is on secular, and not supernatural, aspects of life. So, the choice is between options A and D. It's tempting to pick option D because of the concrete example about the professor using the power of words to have a book brought

to him from his office. Option D is a correct statement, but its focus is too narrow. Why would a great philosopher like Confucius concern himself with moving physical objects? The most philosophical sounding option is option A.

Question Discussion Using Standard Highlighting (HL) Analysis

The word "magical" or its derivations are found by HL in paragraph 1 as "human … powers", "magical quality", "familiar … unnoticed". Paragraph 4's "But there is also magic - the proper ritual expression of my wish will accomplish my wish with no effort on my part" was not HL because it was an example.

entity. This appears to have no basis in the passage.

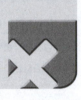

Option B is incorrect. Option B is found in paragraph 2 as "long … learn li", "meaning … ceremony"". But, there is no specific reference to "supernatural phenomena" being harnessed by li. In paragraph 1, what is being harnessed is "distinctively human powers".

Option D is incorrect. Option D is found in paragraph 4 as "effortless power of li", "accomplish physical ends", "bring a book from my office to the classroom". But, this is an example only and is the reason for the use of the word.

Option C is incorrect. Option C is found in paragraph 2 as "long … learn li". It doesn't specifically say it has to be learned from any person or

Option A is correct. The reference to "conventions" is not directly tied to "magic"; it is tied to the "language and imagery" as found is paragraph 2. So, it is True **(SB A.1.2)**, but does not appear to be Correct **(SB A.1.2)**.

Question Discussion Using Option Elimination Analysis

Q82 — Pre-Study Suggestions

Review the following if needed:
1) Three Out of Four Options **SB A.2.8**
2) Similar Pair Options **SB A.2.7**

Solution Discussion
Please review the AAMC solution for this problem.

Test Taking Skills Comment
This is a Three Out of Four Options (**SB A.2.8**) question. Options A, C and D all deal with 'power(s)' of some type. Option B is an outlier and outliers are usually incorrect.

Options B and D are also a Similar Pair Options (**SB A.2.7**) because both deal with the 'supernatural/occult'. But, since this set is not fully part of the three out of four, it should be ignored.

QUESTION 3R.VR.VI.83

Question Discussion Using Holistic Approach

This is an inference question. This is a simple question. Performative utterances have an air of authority, which only II has. I is a request for help, and III is a question.

Therefore, the correct option is option B.

Putting it all together: the critical path
See explanation given earlier.

Question Discussion Using Standard Highlighting (HL) Analysis

This phrase is found in paragraph 5 as ""performative utterances"", ""operative" ... instrument", "execution ... itself". It is further explained in paragraph 6 as ""I give ... brother"", "bequeathal", "more powerful ... force". Looking over these paragraphs, it is reasonably evident that "performative utterance" is an ""operative" clause in a legal instrument". The example of "bequeathal" above shows it is from oneself to another person and is firm and definite.

Choice I ("Please help me") does not fit that pattern and is therefore false. This means options A and C must be Incorrect **(SB A.1.2)**. Your decision now rests on determining the True/False **(SB A.1.2)** status of choices II and III.

Choice II is fairly clearly a "performative utterance" as "I promise to help". This is like a "legal instrument" in that one person has "promised" another to carry out a certain action. This is further found in paragraph 7 as "substance ... ceremony" and in sentence 3. So, a promise would be a "performative utterance".

Question Discussion Using Option Elimination Analysis

Q83   Pre-Study Suggestions

Review the following if needed:
None.

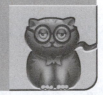

Solution Discussion
Please review the AAMC solution for this problem.

Test Taking Skills Comment
There are no techniques from the Option Elimination Techniques **(SB A.2)**. But, you can eliminate options by using Multiple Choice Options **(SB A.1.2)**.

If you know for sure that any one of the three choices (I, II or III) is True or False **(SB**

A.1.2), then you will be able to eliminate options. E.g. if you knew for sure that choice II is true, then you can eliminate options A and C as only options B/D can be Correct **(SB A.1.2)**.

QUESTION 3R.VR.VI.84

Question Discussion Using Holistic Approach

This is an inference question. Compare this question with Q 81; it's almost a mirror image. Although li is about the right way (the moral way), there is no mention in the passage about the divine or even holy people like prophets. The only reference to holy in the passage is with respect to right actions. (Note the title of the source from which the passage is taken: The Secular as Sacred.) Thus, options B and D can be eliminated.

Option C is psychologically interesting, in that it appeals to common sense. This feeling might be reinforced by the reference to how rulers should conduct themselves in the passage. Please come down to earth. The phrase "refined society" in this option should set off alarm bells if you have absorbed the spirit of the passage, because it smacks of elitism, whereas li is profoundly democratic: recall "familiar and universal." The right option is A, which mirrors option A of Q 81.

Putting it all together: the critical path
Remember "The Secular as Sacred" point mentioned in the main explanation? "Divinely" and "holy persons" are red flags in options B and D. As for option C, I can't see a philosopher kowtowing to refined society, can you? The moralistic option A is right.

CHAPTER 2

Question Discussion Using Standard Highlighting (HL) Analysis

The reference to "holy" is found in paragraph 2 and 3 as ""holy … ceremony"", "authentic … society", "ability … to li", "will … essential" and "li … dignity", "Holy … spiritual".

Option B is incorrect. Option B is not found in the passage as there is no HL related to "divinely sanctioned laws". So, option B is False **(SB A.1.2)**.

Option C is incorrect. Option C is also not found in the passage as there is no reference or HL to "customary in refined society".

Option D is incorrect. Option D is likewise not found in the passage

as there is no HL of "holy persons". Notice that options B, C and D have key phrases or words that would have normally been part of HL if they were present. If you are confident enough, and this will only occur with practice as is suggested in the discussion of highlighting, then you can eliminate options B, C and D as being Complex Sounding Options **(SB A.2.2)**.

Option A is correct. Option A is found in paragraph 3 as shown previously. There is the connection as "reverent dignity" is similar to "expressions of respect". So, this is True **(SB A.1.2)** and a possible answer.

Question Discussion Using Option Elimination Analysis

Q84 — Pre-Study Suggestions

Review the following if needed:
None.

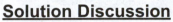

Solution Discussion
Please review the AAMC solution for this problem.

Test Taking Skills Comment
No specific techniques for this question.

QUESTION 3R.VR.VI.85

Question Discussion Using Holistic Approach

This is an inference question. Consider the wording "bind themselves more inescapably" used in the stem. These are strong words! If people rarely try to meet their moral obligations, as stated in option A, obviously a contradiction with the stem arises. This is not the case with the other options. The right option is A.

Putting it all together: the critical path
Option A states that people rarely bind themselves to commitments they have given. That directly contradicts the premise of the stem.

Question Discussion Using Standard Highlighting (HL) Analysis

There is nothing specifically needed from the passage as the key information is Rephrased

(SB B.7.7) and stated in the Stem (SB A.1) of the question. You do not have to use your HL or refer back to the passage for this type of question. The correct option is A. Please refer to the AAMC discussion for this problem. Note that only 30% of students got this correct; it is essentially a Guess Question **(SB A.2.4)**.

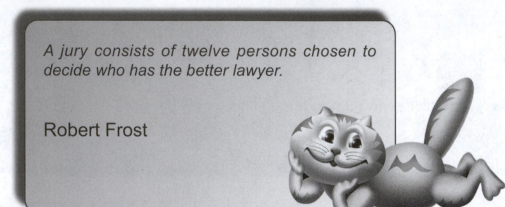

A jury consists of twelve persons chosen to decide who has the better lawyer.

Robert Frost

Question Discussion Using Option Elimination Analysis

Q85 — Pre-Study Suggestions

Review the following if needed:
1) Dichotomy of Options **SB A.2.3**
2) Similar Pair Options **SB A.2.7**

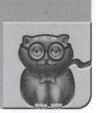

Solution Discussion
Please review the AAMC solution for this problem.

Test Taking Skills Comment
This is a Dichotomy of Options **(SB A.2.3)** question with the dichotomy being 'rarely' versus 'often'. To use a dichotomy, you need to use Basic Knowledge (study, passage, general knowledge) **(SB A.2.2)**, however there is none from the passage or General Knowledge **(SB A.2.2)** which will help you make this choice.

This is also a Similar Pair Options **(SB A.2.7)** with options A and D being similar in dealing with 'obligation/promise' which are similar. There is no other clear similar pair, so your guess from A or D is reasonable.

Highlighting For Holistic and Central Thesis Analysis

CBT3 Passage VII Holistic Highlighting

Paragraph 1: traditionally a religious; always … tendency; familiar flippancy; rationalist movements; later fifth century; further battering; Euripides; profound … forces; shady seducers; discredited … fun; Socrates; whole traditional fabric; "not … believes."

Paragraph 2: Sentence 1; merely symbolic … Providence; allegorical … phenomena; much … favoured; Callimachus and Theocritus; old gods; no longer …concern

Paragraph 3: Euhemerus; great human kings; rationalization of atheism; Strato … all; indifferent; do nothing … Hellenistic life

Paragraph 4: misleading; deviated; classical Olympian cults; impressive … worship; Divine Saviours; Sentence 5

Headlining or Signposting the Passage

Paragraph 1: A strong religious tradition in Greece coexisted with an undercurrent of skepticism.

Paragraph 2: Examples are given showing that this skepticism gained in strength in the early Hellenistic age, which succeeded the period underconsideration in the previous paragraph.

Paragraph 3:More examples are given of writers who cast doubt on traditional religious beliefs.

Paragraph 4: Although the traditional Olympian religious beliefs were weakened, the vacuum was not filled by atheism: instead, their place was taken by deviant cults based on the concept of the divine savior.

Central Thesis:

The Greeks have always been religious, but had slowly begun disassociating themselves from classical Olympian religion and turning instead to a number of deviant cults.

Paragraph 1
A strong religious tradition in Greece coexisted with an undercurrent of skepticism.

Paragraph 2
Examples are given showing that this skepticism gained in strength in the early Hellenistic age, which succeeded the period under consideration in the previous paragraph.

Central Thesis
The Greeks have always been a religious people, but had slowly begun disassociating themselves from classical Olympian religion and turning instead to a number of deviant cults.

Paragraph 4
Although the traditional Olympian religious beliefs were weakened, the vacuum was not filled by atheism: instead, their place was taken by deviant cults based on the concept of the divine savior.

Paragraph 3
More examples are given of writers who cast doubt on traditional religious beliefs.

Passage at a Glance
Genre: Religion/philosophy.

Passage difficulty level: Simple (despite the seriousness of the subject, the ideas are clear and the language is direct. The fudge/obfuscation factor is nil).

Abstract/concrete: Concrete.

Subject: Hellenistic religious tradition: a historical survey.

Author's attitude to subject: Objective (The author examines religion as a social and cultural phenomenon without projecting his biases into the writing).

Questions' difficulty level: Four questions are straightforward. The other three have varying degrees of murkiness.

Question types:
• Three inference
• four passage reference

Standard Passage Highlighting

Paragraph 1: Sentence 1, "gods … Hymns", "rationalistic … century", "divine … battering", "Euripides", "Bacchae", "gods … of fun", "Socrates was questioning", " "not … city believes".

Paragraph 2: "Hellenistic … powers", Sentence 2, "Hellenistic sculptors", "much … forms", "Callimachus and Theocritus", "old gods … belief"

Paragraph 3: "more specific", "Euhemerus … equals", "rationalization of atheism", "Strato of Lampsacus", "did not … gods", Sentence 3, "St Paul", "pagan Hellenism … God""

Paragraph 4: "impression was misleading", "Pagan religion", "Christianity overtook", "deviated … Hellenistic", "no longer … Saviours", "distinct … gifts", "conferment … holiness", "immortality … death", Sentence 6

QUESTION 3R.VR.VII.86

Question Discussion Using Holistic Approach

This is a direct passage reference. Euripides represented the gods both as "psychological forces" and as "shady seducers or discredited figures of fun". Though these representations are negative, the first interpretation is relatively more favorable making option A the right answer. Note that "divine saviours" in option B is a red herring, as divine saviours appear in a much later period.

Putting it all together: the critical path

This is a simple question; see explanation given earlier.

Question Discussion Using Standard Highlighting (HL) Analysis

Option B is incorrect. Option B is found in paragraph 4 as "no longer … Divine Saviors". By a quick review of this location, it should be apparent that it has nothing to do with Euripides.

Option D is incorrect. Option D is found in paragraph 1 as "shady seducers or discredited figures of fun". This was by Euripides, but this is hardly the "most favorable portrayal" because "discredited" precedes "figures of fun".

Option C is incorrect. Option C is found in paragraph 1 but is not HL as "inquisitive … Euripides". So, this was a description of Euripides and not a description of the gods by him.

Option A is correct. The HL is found in paragraph 1 as "Euripides", "Bacchae", and "gods … forces". So, this suggests the Correct option **(SB A.1.2)** is A.

Passage VII - Questions 86-92

Question Discussion Using Option Elimination Analysis

Q86 — Pre-Study Suggestions

Review the following if needed:
1) Three Out of Four Options **SB A.2.8**

Solution Discussion
Please review the AAMC solution for this problem.

Test Taking Skills Comment
This is a Three Out of Four Options **(SB A.2.8)** question. Options B, C and D all represent an entity of some type. Option A does not represent an entity and is the outlier. Outliers tend to be incorrect. The outlier is correct in this question.

QUESTION 3R.VR.VII.87

Question Discussion Using Holistic Approach

This is an inference question. Options A and B are diametrically opposite, and so are options C and D. To answer this question, you have to know that the Olympian gods are the city gods. Thus, it becomes clear that the accusation against Socrates can be justified only if the god Socrates refers to as "my god" is NOT an Olympian figure. Option D is the right option.

OK, confession time now. :-) Honestly, option B is in this reviewer's opinion as objectively

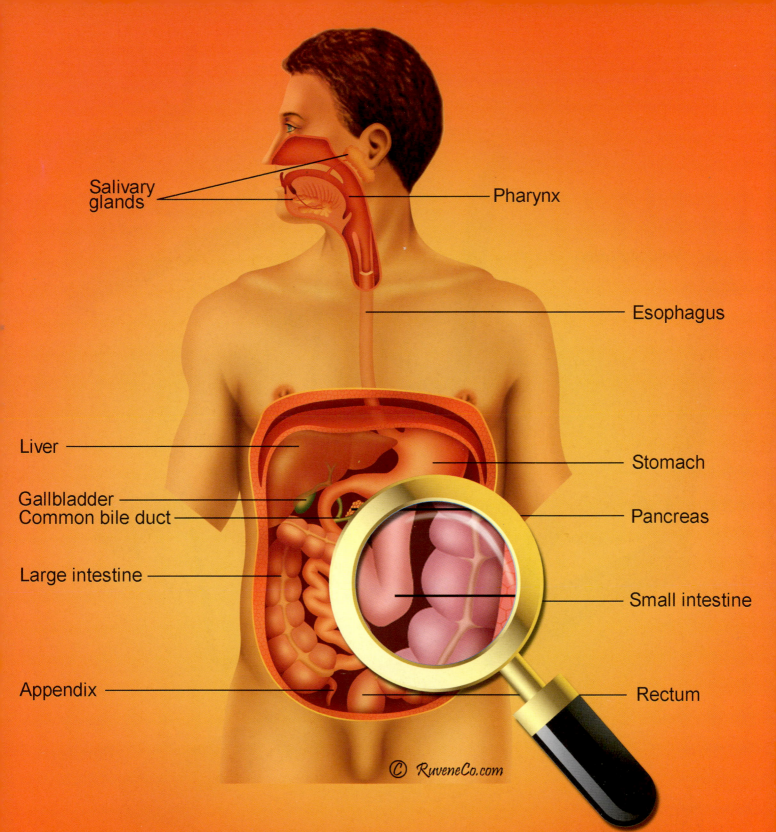

Salivary glands

Pharynx

Esophagus

Liver

Stomach

Gallbladder

Common bile duct

Pancreas

Large intestine

Small intestine

Appendix

Rectum

© RuveneCo.com

Figure IV.A.9.1: Schematic illustration of the major components of the digestive system.

MCAT-Prep.com

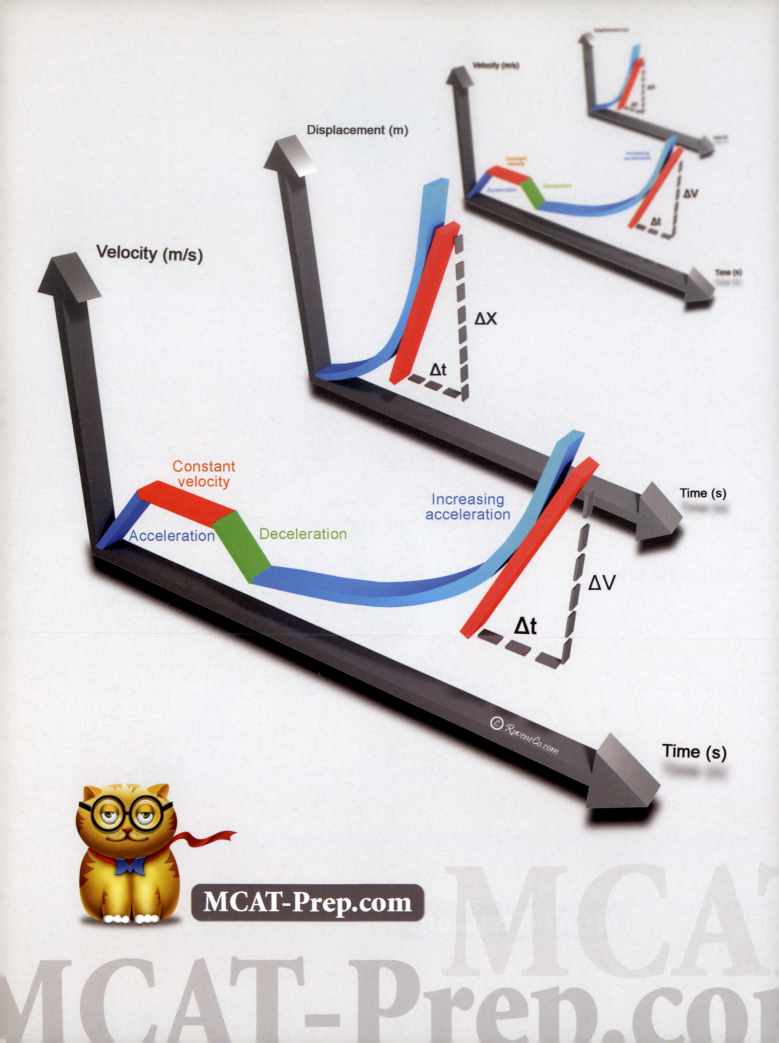

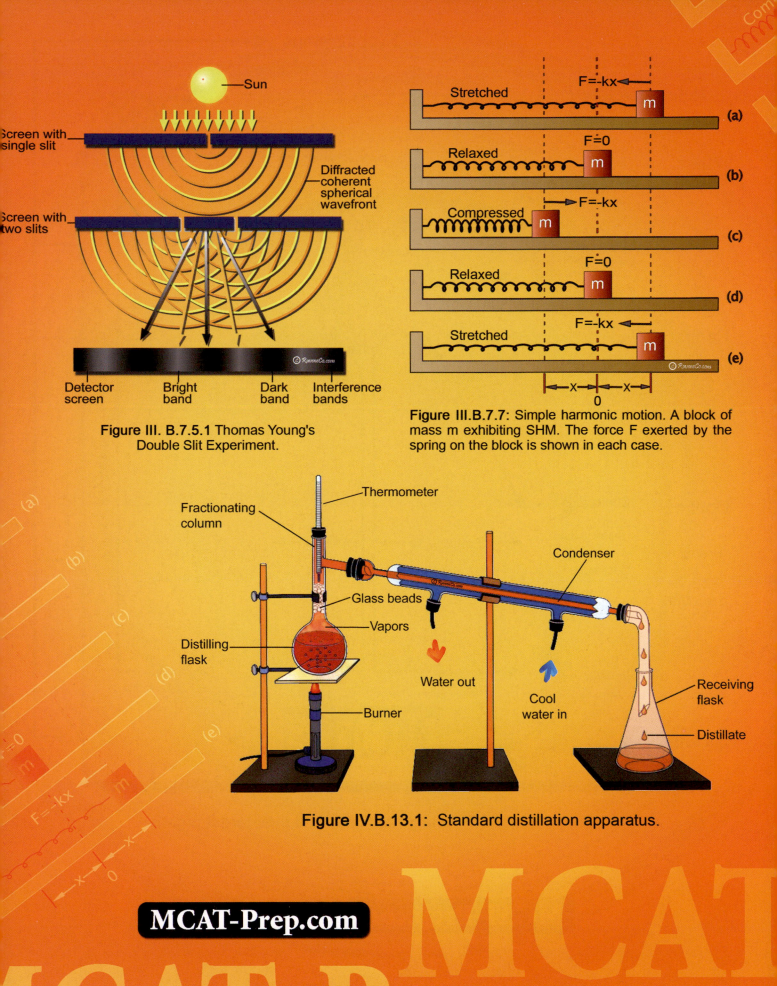

Figure III. B.7.5.1 Thomas Young's Double Slit Experiment.

Figure III.B.7.7: Simple harmonic motion. A block of mass m exhibiting SHM. The force F exerted by the spring on the block is shown in each case.

Figure IV.B.13.1: Standard distillation apparatus.

MCAT-Prep.com

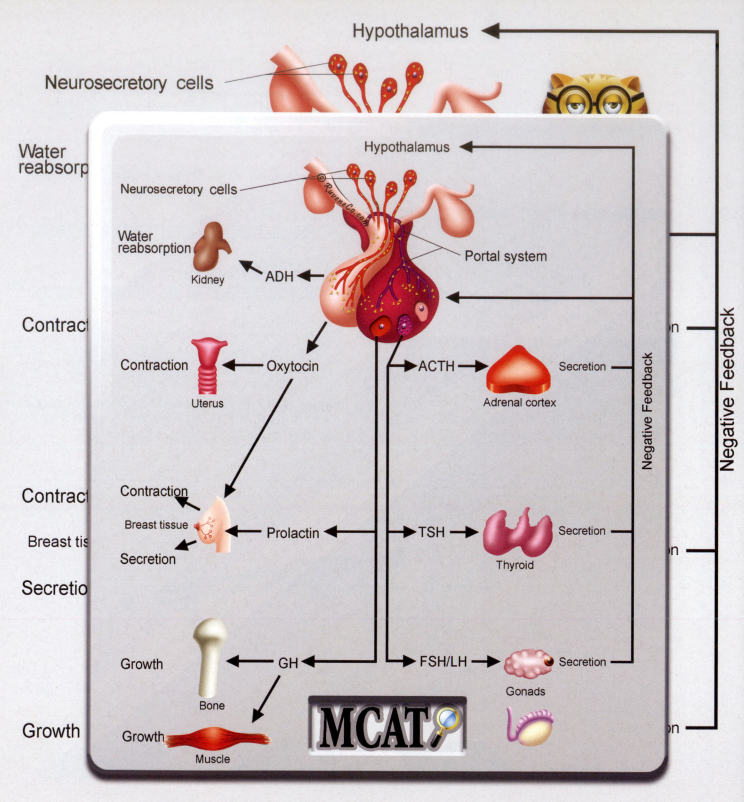

Figure IV.A.6.6: Pituitary hormones and their target organs.

MCAT-Prep.com

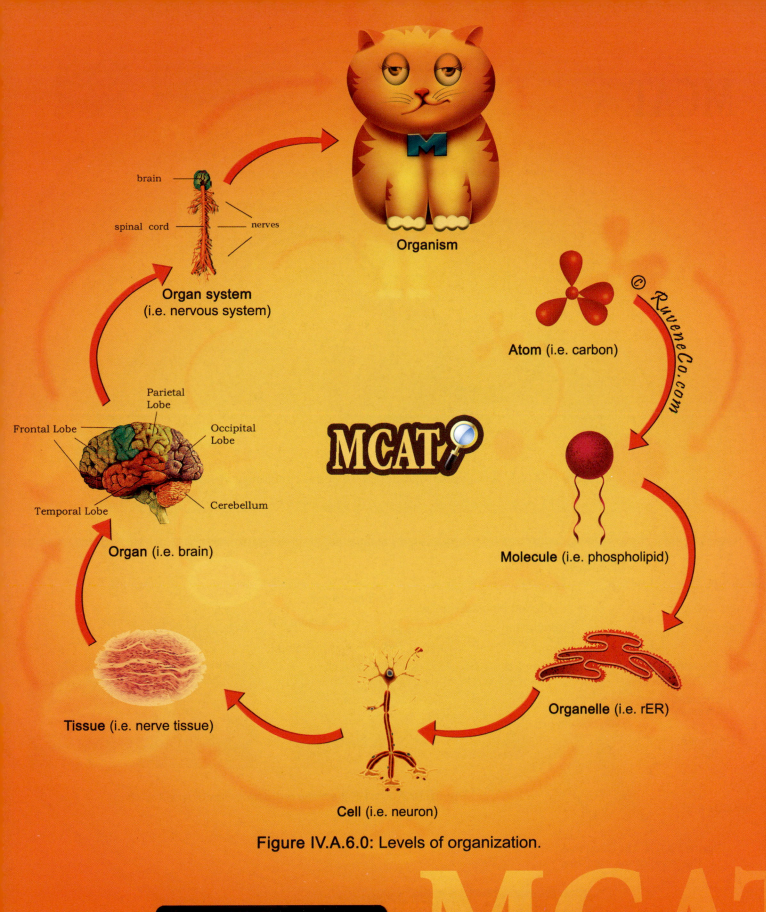

brain

spinal cord — nerves

Organism

Organ system
(i.e. nervous system)

Atom (i.e. carbon)

© *RuveneCo.com*

Parietal
Lobe

Frontal Lobe

Occipital
Lobe

Temporal Lobe

Cerebellum

Organ (i.e. brain)

MCAT

Molecule (i.e. phospholipid)

Tissue (i.e. nerve tissue)

Cell (i.e. neuron)

Organelle (i.e. rER)

Figure IV.A.6.0: Levels of organization.

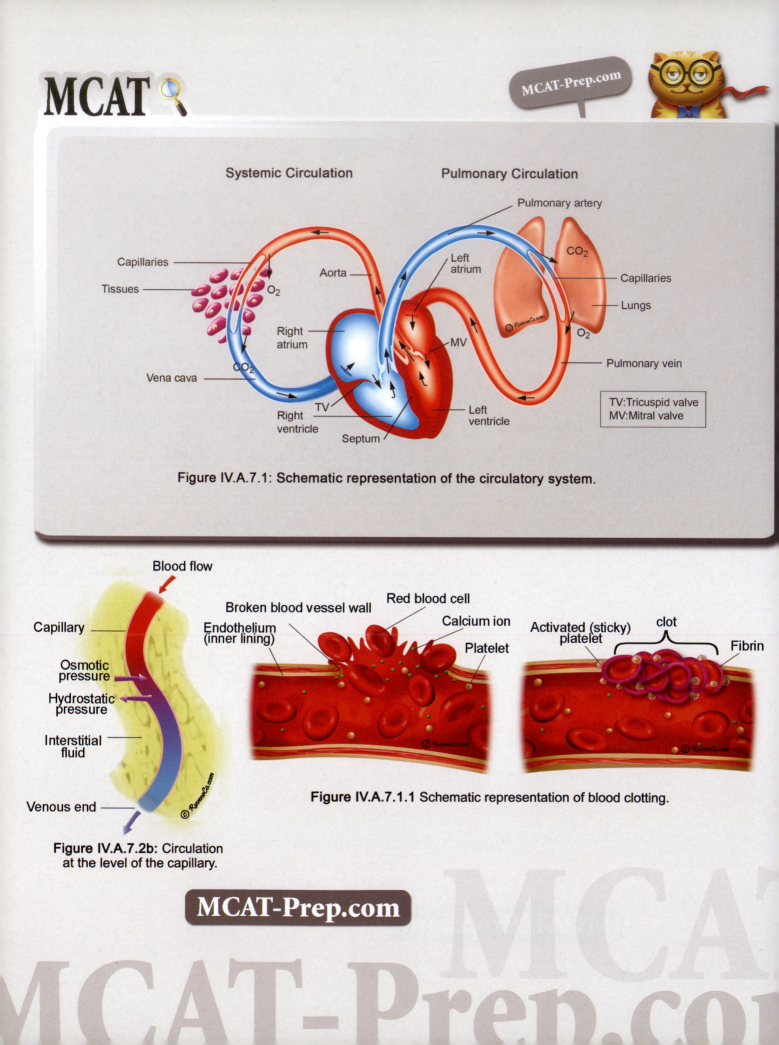

Systemic Circulation

Pulmonary Circulation

Capillaries

Tissues

O_2

Aorta

Right atrium

CO_2

Vena cava

CO_2

TV

Right ventricle

Septum

Pulmonary artery

Left atrium

CO_2

Capillaries

Lungs

O_2

Pulmonary vein

MV

Left ventricle

TV:Tricuspid valve
MV:Mitral valve

Figure IV.A.7.1: Schematic representation of the circulatory system.

Blood flow

Capillary

Osmotic pressure

Hydrostatic pressure

Interstitial fluid

Venous end

Broken blood vessel wall

Red blood cell

Calcium ion

Endothelium (inner lining)

Platelet

Activated (sticky) platelet

clot

Fibrin

Figure IV.A.7.1.1 Schematic representation of blood clotting.

Figure IV.A.7.2b: Circulation at the level of the capillary.

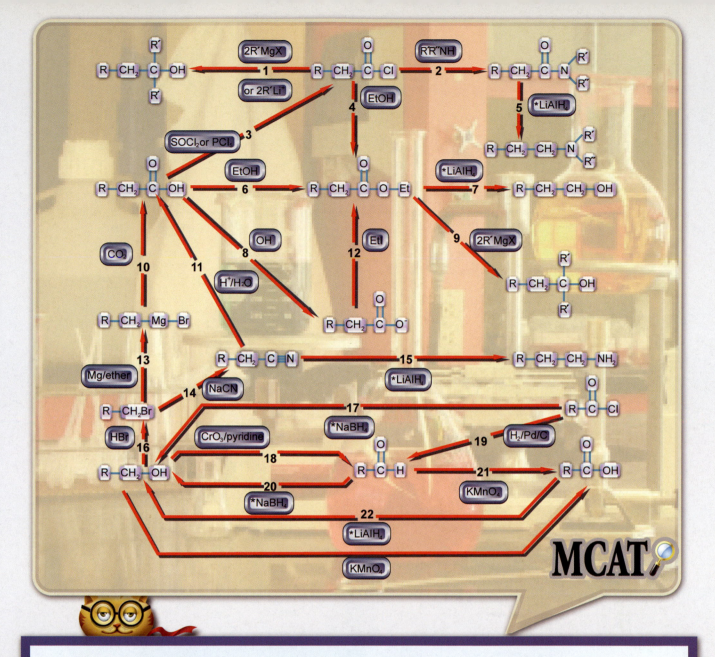

R = alkyl   **Et** = ethyl   **X** = halide

R⁻ MgX⁺ = Grignard reagent   **R⁻ Li⁺** = alkyl lithium

Grignard reagents and alkyl lithiums are special agents since they can create new C—C bonds (*see* **ORG 1.6**).

*Reduction = addition of hydrogen or subtraction of oxygen. Mild reducing agents add fewer hydrogens/subtract fewer oxygens. Strong reducing agents add more hydrogens/subtract more oxygens.

**You must also memorize at least the following IR spectra data for the MCAT: approx. 3300 cm⁻¹ for -OH (alcohol functional group) and approx. 1700 cm⁻¹ for C=O (carbonyl functional group).

Most reactions presented can be derived from basic principles (**i.e. ORG 1.6, 7.1**). In other words, memorization is usually not necessary for MCAT mechanisms as long as you understand the basic rules of organic chemistry.

Cross-referencing to The Gold Standard MCAT text are found below.

1 An acid chloride reacts with a Grignard reagent to produce a tertiary alcohol.
    ORG 1.6, 9.1
2 An acid chloride reacts with a primary or secondary amine to produce an amide.
    ORG 9.3 & 11.2
3 A carboxylic acid reacts with SOCl₂ or PCl₅ to produce an acid chloride.
    ORG 9.1
4 An acid chloride reacts with an alcohol (e.g. ethanol) to produce an ester.
    ORG 9.4

5 An amide reacts with LiAlH₄ to produce an amine.
    ORG 8.2, 9.3
6 A carboxylic acid reacts with an alcohol (e.g. ethanol) to produce an ester.
    ORG 8.2
7 An ester reacts with LiAlH₄ to produce a primary alcohol.
    ORG 8.2, 9.4
8 A carboxylic acid reacts with base to produce a carboxylate anion.
    CHM 6.3 & ORG 8.1
9 An ester reacts with a Grignard reagent to produce a tertiary alcohol.
    ORG 1.6, 8.1.1, 9.4
10 A Grignard reagent reacts with carbon dioxide to produce a carboxylic acid.
    ORG 8.1.1
11 A nitrile reacts with aqueous acid to produce a carboxylic acid.
    ORG 8. 1.1
12 A carboxylate ion reacts with ethyl iodide to produce an ester.
    ORG 8.2
13 An alkyl halide reacts with Mg/ether to produce a Grignard reagent.
14 An alkyl halide reacts with NaCN to produce a nitrile.
    ORG 6.2.3
15 A nitrile reacts with LiAlH₄ to produce an amine.
    ORG 8.2
16 A primary alcohol reacts with HBr to produce an alkyl halide.
17 An acid chloride reacts with NaBH₄ to produce a primary alcohol.
    ORG 8.2, 9.1
18 A primary alcohol reacts with CrO₃/pyridine to produce an aldehyde.
    ORG 6.2.2, 7.2.1
19 A acid chloride reacts with H₂/Pd/C to produce an aldehyde.
    ORG 7.1, 7.2.1, 9.1
20 An aldehyde reacts with NaBH₄ to produce a primary or secondary alcohol.
    ORG 7.1, 8.2
21 An aldehyde reacts with KMnO₄ to produce a carboxylic acid.
    ORG 7.2.1, 8.1.1
22 A carboxylic acid reacts with LiAlH₄ to produce a primary alcohol.
    ORG 8.2

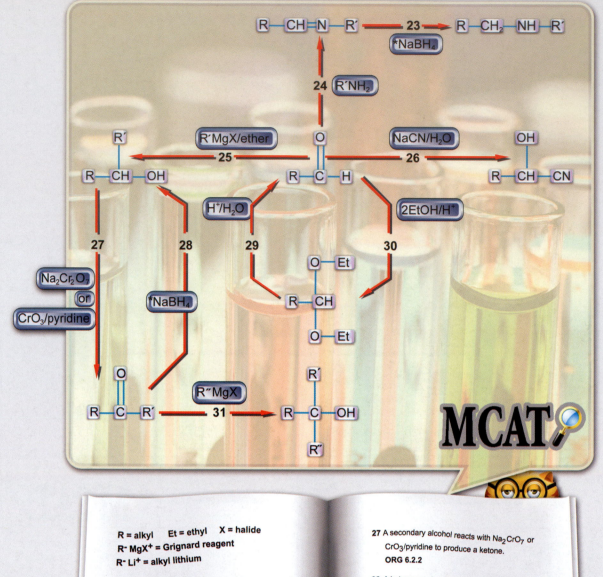

R = alkyl   Et = ethyl   X = halide
R⁻ MgX⁺ = Grignard reagent
R⁻ Li⁺ = alkyl lithium

23 An imine reacts with $NaBH_4$ to produce a secondary amine.
   ORG 7.2.3, 8.2

24 An aldehyde reacts with a primary amine to produce an imine.
   ORG 7.2.3

25 An aldehyde reacts with a Grignard reagent and ether to produce a secondary alcohol.
   ORG 1.6, 7.1

26 An aldehyde reacts with aqueous NaCN.
   ORG 7.1

27 A secondary alcohol reacts with Na_2CrO_7 or CrO_3/pyridine to produce a ketone.
   ORG 6.2.2

28 A ketone reacts with $NaBH_4$ to produce a secondary alcohol.
   ORG 7.2.1

29 An acetal reacts with aqueous acid to produce an aldehyde.
   ORG 7.2.1/2

30 An aldehyde reacts with an alcohol (e.g. ethanol) and acid to produce an acetal. Note that using with less $EtOH/H^+$, a hemiacetal will form.
   ORG 7.2.2

31 A ketone reacts with a Grignard reagent to produce a tertiary alcohol.
   ORG 1.6, 9.1

correct as option D; the latter option smacks of lawyerly hair splitting. When Socrates says "my god," there is a clear implication that his god is different from the god most people worship. However, from a practical point of view, since option D is present, one would have to prefer it to option B.

Putting it all together: the critical path
The choice is between options B and D. With option D, the tester is displaying how subtle his mind is, so we bow to the tester and pick option D.

Question Discussion Using Standard Highlighting (HL) Analysis

Options A, B and C are incorrect. *See* following discussion.

Option D is correct. The key information is Rephrased **(SB B.7.7)** in the Stem **(SB A.1)** and you must then apply logic to arrive at the answer. The HL passage is found, but not needed, in paragraph 1 as "Socrates was questioning", ""not believing in the gods in whom the city believes". So, by reading in this area, it is evident that the prosecutors wanted him to believe in their city gods. So, the statement "I will obey my god rather than you" is vague in that the god is not specified. Specifically, the god has to be the "city god".

CHAPTER 2

Question Discussion Using Option Elimination Analysis

Q87 — Pre-Study Suggestions

Review the following if needed:
1) Three Out of Four Options **SB A.2.8**
2) Similar Pair Options **SB A.2.7**

Solution Discussion

Please review the AAMC solution for this problem.

Test Taking Skills Comment

First, this is a Three Out of Four Options **(SB A.2.8)** question with options B, C and D being similar because of 'support'. Option A is the outlier without 'support' and outliers are generally incorrect.

Second, this is also a Similar Pair Options **(SB A.2.7)** question with options C and D. This is a good similar pair because it is of the mirror image/opposite type. So, your guess would be from C or D. This is also a borderline Guess Question **(SB A.2.4)** because of the length of the Stem **(SB A.1)** and the length of some of the Options **(SB A.1.2)**.

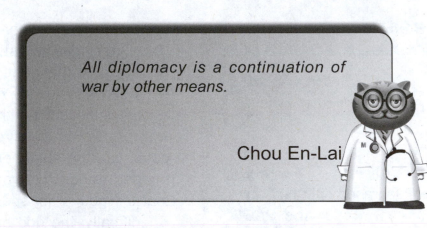

All diplomacy is a continuation of war by other means.

Chou En-Lai

QUESTION 3R.VR.VII.88

Question Discussion Using Holistic Approach

This is an inference question.

Option A is correct. This is a serious contender because of the exact match between "natural phenomena" ("thunder") and "reinterpreted individual deities."

Option B is incorrect. Here Zeus is regarded as the source of thunder and is responsible for the lightning bolts that hit the earth and causing damage. There is nothing symbolic about this interpretation.

Option C is incorrect. This contradicts the passage because thunder (a harbinger of destructive storms) can be interpreted as a vehicle of divine Providence and is attributed to the god Zeus.

Option D is incorrect. The passage does not attribute the "numerous

slighting references" to the Stoics alone but collectively to writers and thinkers of the "early Hellenistic age."

Note: For one thing, the wording "merely allegorical" in the passage is uncomfortably close to "merely symbolic" in option B. There is also a clash between "originated the traditional portrayal" in the stem and "reinterpreted" in option A. However, the stem wording states unambiguously that Zeus is the "source of thunder," and there is nothing "merely symbolic" about this choice of words. What clinches it for option A is the close agreement between option A and the stem wording compared to option B.

Putting it all together: the critical path
Pick the option whose language mirrors the words used to describe the discovery mentioned in the stem: option A.

CHAPTER 2

Question Discussion Using Standard Highlighting (HL) Analysis

Option B is incorrect. Option B is found in paragraph 2 as option A and additionally as "early Hellenistic age", "slighting ... powers," and "merely

symbolic" are found. So, this can be interpreted as a true statement that is possibly correct as well.

Option C is incorrect. Option C is also found in paragraph 2 as "Stoics" and then the statement that follows relates to "Divine Providence", even though this was not underlined. This would support a belief in Divine Providence and not the reverse.

Option D is incorrect. Option D is found in the reference from option A and as "slighting references to the Olympian powers". This fact logically does not eliminate other "slighting references" which could still be numerous.

Option A is correct. The reference is found in paragraph 2 as "Stoics", "reinterpreted", "many individual deities", "allegorical ... natural". This shows the interpretation of a god as related to the natural phenomena of thunder, which is why it is a better choice than option B.

Question Discussion Using Option Elimination Analysis

Q88   Pre-Study Suggestions

Review the following if needed:
1) Dichotomy of Options **SB A.2.3**
2) Guess Question **SB A.2.4**

Solution Discussion
Please review the AAMC solution for this problem.

Test Taking Skills Comment
This is a Dichotomy of Options **(SB A.2.3)** question with 'support' and 'weaken'. With a dichotomy, you must use Basic Knowledge

(study, passage, general knowledge) **(SB A.2.2)** to select between the two sets. There is no quick or easy way to do this, so it is not wise to try to use this dichotomy. Also, this is a Guess Question **(SB A.2.4)**. This is based on the length of its Stem **(SB A.1)** and Options **(SB A.1.2)** more than its difficulty. You have to determine which of the claims in the options is correct and then determine how the new information in the stem affects it.

QUESTION 3R.VR.VII.89

Question Discussion Using Holistic Approach

This is a direct passage reference question. The stem refers to the concluding line of the passage, which follows a description of the cult of divine saviors. So, it is logical to pick option B. What makes this choice a no brainer is the ease with which it can be shown that the remaining options contradict the stem.

For options A and C, St. Paul saw pagan Hellenism as a world "without God," and the writings referred to in option C agree that the gods are "indifferent." As for option D, the idea that Olympian gods were once human kings was used to justify atheism.

Putting it all together: the critical path

This is a simple question. *See* explanation given earlier.

Question Discussion Using Standard Highlighting (HL) Analysis

Option A is incorrect. Option A is found in the last sentence of paragraph 3, but this statement does not identify "religion as one of the most vital elements."

Option C is incorrect. Option C is found in paragraph 3 as "Menander ... Epicurus", "traditional ... daily", "Hellenistic life". By reading in this area, it is evident that they did not believe the gods were of any significance as in the non HL associated sentences "gods ... Hellenistic life." This does not suggest that religion was vital.

Option B is correct. Option B is found in paragraph 4, as sentence 4, "distinct ... gifts", "conferment ... holiness", "gift ... death", "religion ... moribund", "vital ... Hellenistic". Reading in this section, you see the "vital elements" which are found in the stem. So, this is a true statement and appears to be correct **(SB A.1.2)**.

So, the Best Option **(SB A.1.2)** is option B which has the specific reference of "vital elements". Notice, as is the general pattern, that each option has a specific reference to a location in the passage. The faster you identify and locate the reference, the faster you can assess its veracity i.e. True or False **(SB A.1.2)**, and can then determine if it is Correct or Incorrect **(SB A.1.2)**.

Option D is incorrect. Option D is found in paragraph 3 as "Euhemerus ... equals". But, as you read in this section, it is not discussing the importance of religion in Greek life.

Question Discussion Using Option Elimination Analysis

Q89   Pre-Study Suggestions

Review the following if needed:
None.

Solution Discussion
Please review the AAMC solution for this problem.

Test Taking Skills Comment
No specific techniques for this question.

QUESTION 3R.VR.VII.90

Question Discussion Using Holistic Approach

This is a direct passage reference question. A reference to the Iliad and the Homeric Hymns is found in the second line of the passage in connection with an attitude to the gods that is described as "familiar flippancy." This attitude matches the irreverence mentioned in option C perfectly; there is no need to look further.

Putting it all together: the critical path
This is a simple question. See explanations given earlier.

Question Discussion Using Standard Highlighting (HL) Analysis

Option A is incorrect. Option A is found in paragraph 1 as "rationalistic movements", "fifth century", "divine ... battering". So, this is a True **(SB A.1.2)** option, but it has nothing to with the "Iliad and the Homeric Hymns".

Option B is incorrect. Option B is found in paragraph 2 as "Callimachus and Theocritus", "old gods were no longer a matter of belief". Reading in this section, you see "the poets Callimachus and Theocritus". This is a true statement but has nothing to do with "Iliad and the Homeric Hymns". Notice that the exact phrasing is not used when comparing the option and the passage, but "matter of serious concern" is equivalent to "no longer a matter of belief."

Option D is incorrect. Option D is found in paragraph 3 as "gods of the city ... indifferent". But, this phrase has nothing to do with "Iliad and the Homeric Hymns".

Option C is correct. Option C appears to be the correct **(SB A.1.2)** option consistent with the previous excerpt as "gods ... flippancy" and

"Iliad and the Homeric Hymns" in paragraph 1. The phrase "familiar flippancy" is equivalent to "irreverently" in the option.

Notice that the HL was valuable in finding the location of the reference in the option. Also, notice that each option has a specific reference. If you could not find them rapidly, you could be easily misled by your attempt to remember the statement and the connection. E.g. you could remember you "read" something about "rationalistic movements" or about "indifferent" gods. And if you could not find the locations rapidly, because you think they are true, and they are, you might think that one of them is the correct option.

Question Discussion Using Option Elimination Analysis

Q90 — Pre-Study Suggestions

Review the following if needed:
None.

Solution Discussion
Please review the AAMC solution for this problem.

Test Taking Skills Comment
No specific techniques for this question.

QUESTION 3R.VR.VII.91

Question Discussion Using Holistic Approach

This is a direct passage reference/inference question. If you locate the named poets in the passage, you will see the wording "much less idealized form than their predecessors." The clear inference is that the predecessors of the named poets depicted the gods in idealized fashion. Option D is correct. We hope you smiled at the absurdity of option A!

Putting it all together: the critical path
This is a simple question. *See* explanation given earlier.

Question Discussion Using Standard Highlighting (HL) Analysis

The reference is found in paragraph 2 as "Callimachus and Theocritus", "old gods were no longer a matter of belief".

The key is the part of the passage which precedes these statements:

• "early Hellenistic age",

• "slighting references … powers",
• "merely symbolic",
• "Stoics",
• "reinterpreted",
• "many individual deities",
• "allegorical explanations of natural",
• "Hellenistic sculptors",
• "much less idealistic forms".

Reading carefully, you find that Callimachus and Theocritus were like the Greek Sculptors who represented in "much less idealistic forms". This means the ones before them had used idealistic forms.

> **Options A, B and C are incorrect.** See previous discussion.

> **Option D is correct.** Again, the HL directs you to the location where the answer is found.

Question Discussion Using Option Elimination Analysis

Q91 — Pre-Study Suggestions

Review the following if needed:
1) Three Out of Four Options **SB A.2.8**

Solution Discussion
Please review the AAMC solution for this problem.

Test Taking Skills Comment
Options B, C and D are similar in being a characteristic/adjective and not a noun/object. They are the three of the Three Out of Four Options **(SB A.2.8)**. Option A is the outlier being an object/thing. Outliers tend to be incorrect.

QUESTION 3R.VR.VII.92

Question Discussion Using Holistic Approach

This is an inference question. Cues in the passage such as "merely symbolic," "merely allegorical," "indifferent," "endure our present life," etc., convey the idea that the Olympian gods no longer met the psychic needs of the people. Frankly, this is rather hard to see and is not the easiest path to the correct option. The effortless route to the correct option is to recognize that the statement for option B is a self evident truth, a generality that is universally applicable (almost like $E = mc^2$). One should not, in general, rely on outside knowledge to determine the correct option, but this question is a clear exception to the rule.

Another approach is to eliminate unsuitable options. Option A can be discarded because the successful cult of divine saviors is based on "miraculous gifts" and the elitist statement in option D can also be discarded. That leaves options B and C.

Option C appears to be a strong candidate because it is a reasonable thesis that the old Olympian religion weakened due to the rationalist challenge. However, the flourishing cults of the divine saviors did not meet the rationalist challenge, leaving option B as the correct option.

Putting it all together: the critical path
The stem statement is general and is a positive statement about religion ("vitality"), so pick the most general option that also reflects favorably on religion: option B.

Question Discussion Using Standard Highlighting (HL) Analysis

Option A is incorrect. Option A is found in paragraph 4 as "no longer … Saviors", "distinct miraculous gifts", "conferment … holiness", "gift … death". This HL suggests "miraculous gifts" were desirable, so abandonment was not the key.

Option C is incorrect. Option C is found in paragraph 1 as "rationalistic movements", "fifth century", "divine ... battering". They were demeaning religion, not making it more "vital".

HL phrase). This is not concerned with "vitality".

Option D is incorrect. Option D is found in paragraph 2 as "Callimachus and Theocritus", "old gods ... belief". This is the only reference to "poets" (*see* the sentences just before the

Option B is correct. Option B is found in the same reference as for option D. Also, in reading in this area, you find "of which ... proportions". And "vital" is found in these phrases which relates to "vitality" in the Stem **(SB A.1)**. So, this option is True **(SB A.1.2)** and is the Correct **(SB A.1.2)** option.

Question Discussion Using Option Elimination Analysis

Q92   Pre-Study Suggestions

Review the following if needed:
1) Three Out of Four Options **SB A.2.8**

Solution Discussion

Please review the AAMC solution for this problem.

Test Taking Skills Comment

This is a Three Out of Four Options **(SB A.2.8)** question with options A, B and C all being an action/activity. Option D is a characteristic and is an outlier. There is a second three out of four with options B, C and D being related to people of some type. Option A is the outlier to this group being related to a thing/object ('gift'). Outliers tend to be incorrect. As is the case when there are two Three Out of Four Options **(SB A.2.8)** sets present, there are two guess options. For this question, you would guess from options B or C.

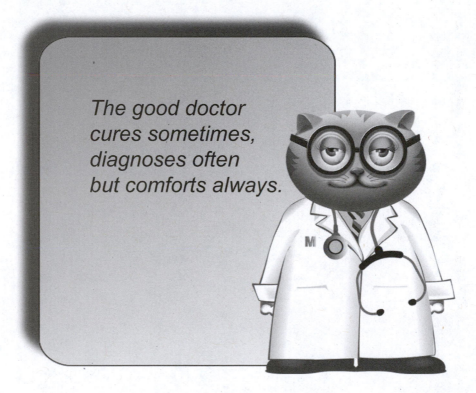

The good doctor cures sometimes, diagnoses often but comforts always.

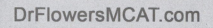

Chapter 3
BIOLOGICAL SCIENCES

AAMC MCAT PRACTICE TEST 3

Chapter 3

AAMC MCAT PRACTICE TEST 3

Explanations and Analysis for
Biological Sciences

Q95 Pre-Study Suggestions

Review the following if needed:
1) Three or More Steps Question **SB A.2.8**
2) Guess Question **SB A.2.4**
3) What are the key pieces of information from the passage?
4) Solve the problem.

Solution Discussion

No prior specific knowledge is needed to solve this problem.

The key information, found in the second paragraph, regarding the Mosaic Hypothesis is:

"killing one cell of each embryo … were independent"

"the fate of the developing … in the embryo."

Option A is incorrect. This is against the Mosaic Hypothesis. The cells, for twins or triplets, divide and each cell results in a complete

identical organism. The Mosaic Hypothesis would predict that only part of the organism should result from the initial divisions. This supports the Regulative Hypothesis.

Option B is incorrect. Again, you need to have some idea that there are divisions of the fertilized egg causing a differential distribution of the determinants among the cells resulting from the division or cleavage for the Mosaic Hypothesis. The Mosaic Hypothesis would only expect one head to be developed. The development of two normal heads suggests some equivalent distribution of determinants in different cells which is against the Mosaic Hypothesis.

Option D is incorrect. This would refute the Mosaic Hypothesis. The genes would certainly be some of the determinants which should be unequally distributed in the divided cells. If all the cells have the same set of genes, but then still develop along different lines, this refutes one possible basis of the theory. The mosaic theory would suggest each of the cells with the same genes, same determinants, should develop the same.

Option C is correct. After any division, the cells are thought to have different sets of determinants and would be expected to develop differently. Note that this does not prove the Mosaic Hypothesis; it is just consistent with it. To obtain more support for the hypothesis, the cells would have to develop the same in a variety of different environmental conditions, in a variety of different relative positions in the developing embryo and the differential distribution of determinants would have to be demonstrated.

Test Taking Skills Comment

This is a reading passage type of question. All the information needed is in the passage. It is up to you to find the key parts of the passage, interpret it and apply it to the question at hand. It is vague as to what determinants mean in this passage. They could have meant 'genes' as we know now. It could mean cytoplasmic components. Because of this we cannot automatically assume it means anything equivalent to our current understandings.

This is a Guess Question **(SB A.2.4)**. This question can fall into this category because it requires a lot of passage reading and interpretation for a science question. The options all involve two lines. If you look at most of the options on the test, they are usually one line only. Two lines mean you have to read and absorb two lines instead of one. If nothing else, this involves more time. Remember time is important on this test. Guess questions should generally be passed over and returned to at the end of the test. This whole passage is more difficult than usual because of the amount of reading and interpretation involved.

This is also a Three or More Step Analysis **(SB A.2.8)** which also makes it difficult. For each option, you have to:

1) determine exactly what the option means;
2) determine how it relates to the Mosaic Hypothesis;
3) determine whether it is true or false; and finally,
4) determine if it is the correct or incorrect answer.

Q96 — Pre-Study Suggestions

Review the following if needed:
1) Embryologic Differentiation **BIO 14.5.1**
2) Dichotomy of Options **SB A.2.3**
3) Internal Inconsistency of Options **SB A.2.5**
4) Complex Sounding Options **SB A.2.2**
5) Three or More Step Analysis **SB A.2.8**
6) What are the key piece(s) of information from the passage?
7) Solve the problem.

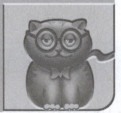

Solution Discussion

The key information from the passage from Biologist 1 is:

"the fate of the developing cells is determined ... in the embryo."

The key information from the passage from Biologist 2 is:

"each cell contained a complete set of determinants," and

"the fate of developing cells depends mainly ... their position in the embryo."

Option A is incorrect. There is no data in the passage or in the question to suggest any environmental factor is responsible for the observation. The radiation was used to kill the nucleus of the frog egg and not activate it - this is Internally Inconsistent **(SB A.2.5)**. The nucleus from the gut was not even exposed to the radiation. If this would have stated the environment of the original frog egg cell (its cytoplasm) was the environment, then this option would have had some plausibility. It does state the

frog egg was activated after the gut nucleus was placed, but it does not state how this was done. Also, the frog egg with the gut nucleus was never 'fertilized' by a sperm.

Option C is incorrect. The question does not suggest the Mosaic Hypothesis at all. In the Mosaic Hypothesis, a gut nucleus should only be able to develop into a gut nucleus because of the distribution of determinants which it should have. Neither the nucleus nor the cytoplasm should have the determinants to develop into any other type of cell. You must also assume the radiation was complete in its job of destroying all the genes in the original frog egg. There is nothing which would suggest anything else. Theoretically, anything can go wrong in any experiment and often does, but in the MCAT, you are not asked to consider a myriad of possibilities unless you are given data or reason to do so. To question whether or not the radiation was complete is to go way beyond the reasonableness and availability of the data. You are told the nucleus of the egg was destroyed and should leave it at that. This option is both internally inconsistent and a Complex Sounding Option **(SB A.2.2)**. It is a complex sounding option because it is not part of your Basic Knowledge (study, passage, general knowledge) **(SB A.2.2)**.

Option D is incorrect. *See* the discussion of option C. This is also Internally Inconsistent **(SB A.2.5)** and a Complex Sounding Option as is option C. Nowhere in the question does it state the frog egg could or could not develop into an adult frog. Since the frog nucleus was destroyed by radiation, the question of the development of the original frog egg is moot. The option is beyond your Basic Knowledge (study, passage, general knowledge) **(SB A.2.2)**.

Bases in DNA

"**A**ll **T**igers and **C**ats **G**rowl"

Adenine bonds to **T**hymine; **C**ytosine bonds to **G**uanine.

BIO 1.2.2

Option B is correct. This option deals with information which is available, your Passage Knowledge **(SB A.2.2)** - the frog egg with the gut nucleus did develop into an adult with the proper activation. This is entirely consistent with the Regulative Hypothesis. What the activation is specifically is irrelevant. The Regulative Hypothesis only requires 'environmental factors and their position in the embryo' for development to occur because 'each cell contained a complete set of determinants'. If the nucleus did not have the complete set of determinants, it could not have developed into an adult as would have been predicted by the Mosaic Hypothesis.

Test Taking Skills Comment

This is a very important question for your test taking wisdom. First of all, you should have eliminated options C and D after carefully reading the passage. If the Mosaic Hypothesis is correct, there is no way for the egg with a gut nucleus to reasonably develop into an adult frog. The Mosaic Hypothesis (MH) clearly states each differentiated cell only has a portion of the total determinants. And that portion of the total determinants determines its characteristics. Since the gut cell could only have a portion of the determinants, there is no reasonable way for it to explain the observation of a differentiated cell nucleus, the gut cell's, giving rise to an adult. Additionally, you must make your choices within the data provided in the passage combined with your prior knowledge.

Option A is tricky but out of bounds. From the passage you read that environmental factors are part of the Regulative Hypothesis (RH), then the option notes the radiation, which is discussed in the question, is the environmental activator. This all sounds superficially plausible. But, in the passage the radiation occurred before the gut nucleus was placed in the frog egg, so how could it be the activator? Secondly, if the radiation destroyed the frog egg nucleus, shouldn't it destroy the gut nucleus as well? You are given no data to suggest that the cytoplasm is somehow activated by the radiation and this is what causes the gut nucleus to develop. This may be possible, but where is the data in the passage. If it is not in the passage, i.e. Passage Knowledge **(SB A.2.2)**, or derivable from information in the passage, then how would you know this? You wouldn't. This is not the kind of information you are expected to know from your study i.e. your Study Knowledge **(SB A.2.2)**.

Option C also gives you some possible reason, 'some genes were retained in the nucleus of the frog egg'. How would you know that or determine that? There is no way from the data given to you. If you cannot reasonably determine this from the passage data (passage knowledge), you are not expected to know it (study knowledge) and the option cannot be correct. As noted above, you have to take at face value that the radiation completely destroys the frog nucleus. This makes this possibility improvable based on the information you have and it must be an incorrect option. Option D is an exercise in logic and reading. There is nothing in the passage which demonstrates there was any attempt to allow the radiated frog egg to develop into an adult before the nucleus was destroyed. So, how can this even be determined based on the data you have? In fact the experimental design would not allow that particular frog egg to even attempt to grow into an adult. Again, watch out for statements or reasons which sound plausible or scientific but go beyond the data you have and are not reasonably known from your basic studies.

This question demonstrates well the concepts of Internal Inconsistency of Options (A and D) **(SB A.2.5)** and Complex Sounding Options (C and D) **(SB A.2.2)**. See the previous discussions in options C and D and in the last paragraph.

Finally, this is a Dichotomy of Options **(SB A.2.3)**. Options A and B is one dichotomy dealing with the Regulative Hypothesis and options C and D is the other dichotomy dealing with the Mosaic Hypothesis. In a dichotomy, you must use some information or fact from Study Knowledge **(SB A.2.2)** or Passage Knowledge **(SB A.2.2)** (occasionally General Knowledge **(SB**

A.2.2) to determine which half of the dichotomy is correct. The passage clearly states the Regulative Hypothesis believes a certain cell has all determinants and therefore the potential to develop into a complete organism. This fact suggests A and B are correct and C and D are not. Then you only have to decide between A and B.

This is also a Three or More Step type question. This makes it more difficult and possibly a Guess Question **(SB A.2.4)**. The steps are:

1) to read the passage and know what the Regulative or Mosaic hypotheses mean;
2) to read the option, the second half, and determine that it applies to the Regulative or Mosaic;
3) to determine if the second half, as it relates to the hypothesis is true or false;
4) to determine if the option is correct or incorrect.

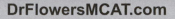

Q97 — Pre-Study Suggestions

Review the following if needed:
1) Embryology **BIO 14.5**
2) What are the key piece(s) of information from the passage?
3) Solve the problem.

Solution Discussion

The key information from the passage from Biologist 1 (MH) is:

"the fate of the developing cells is determined ... of a cell in the embryo."

The key information from the passage from Biologist 2 (RH) is:

"each cell contained a complete set of determinants," and

"the fate of developing cells depends ... their position in the embryo.

Option A is incorrect. The Mosaic Hypothesis (MH) would be consistent with this option.

The Regulative Hypothesis (RH) suggests that complete embryos could develop from separated cells with the proper activation or the proper positioning in the embryo.

Option B is incorrect. This is also most consistent with the MH. That hypothesis states it is the determinants, which differ from cell to cell, which are within the cell which determines cell fate and not the external factors of environment and positioning. The RH notes the cell has the same set of determinants and this alone could not determine cell fate.

Option C is correct. This is one the critical factors of the RH and is almost verbatim from the passage as in the previous quote.

Option D is incorrect. This again is consistent with the MH and inconsistent with the RH as discussed in option B.

Test Taking Skills Comment

Each of these options is a nearly direct statement or a simple modification of the premises of the two hypotheses. The only one consistent with the RH is the option C. This is a reading type question.

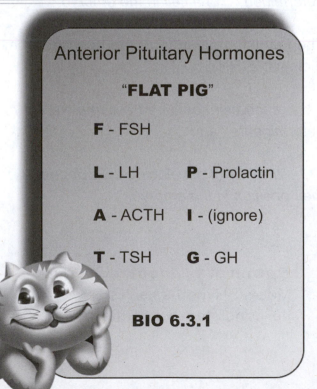

Anterior Pituitary Hormones

"FLAT PIG"

F - FSH

L - LH   **P** - Prolactin

A - ACTH   **I** - (ignore)

T - TSH   **G** - GH

BIO 6.3.1

Q98 — Pre-Study Suggestions

Review the following if needed:
1) Embryonic Differentiation **BIO 14.5.1**
2) Embryonic Determination **BIO 14.5.1**
3) Meiosis **BIO 14.2**
4) Dichotomy of Options **SB A.2.3**
5) Three or More Steps Question
6) What are the key piece(s) of information from the passage?
7) Solve the problem.

Solution Discussion

The key information from the passage from Biologist 1 (MH) is:

"the fate of the developing cells is determined ... of a cell in the embryo."

The key information from the passage from Biologist 2 (RH) is:

"each cell contained a complete set of determinants," and

"the fate of developing cells depends ... position in the embryo."

Option A is incorrect. The Mosaic Hypothesis (MH) and the Regulatory Hypothesis (RH) both involve the development from the fertilized egg. Germ cells do not lose any information during meiosis **(BIO 14.2)**. The purpose of meiosis is to develop gametes **(BIO 14.2)** with one half of the genetic **(BIO 15)** information. Then when Fertilization **(BIO 14.5)** occurs, the genetic material is not duplicated over and over.

The loss of genetic material or determinants as in the MH is not the same as the process of meiosis.

Option C is incorrect. Both the modern theory of embryologic differentiation and embryologic determination and the RH recognize the importance of position in differentiation.

Option B is incorrect. The MH doesn't deal with activation of genes, it states the determinants are either present or absent. It is possible the meaning could be construed to mean activated genes to replace the 'determinants' but this is not clearly stated in the passage.

Option D is correct. This is correct as previous noted and the Regulative Hypothesis is consistent with the modern theory of differentiation/ determination.

Test Taking Skills Comment

This does require you to know the modern idea of differentiation/determination which is quite similar to the Regulative Hypothesis (RH). If you know the current concepts of differentiation/determination, options A and B should be immediately eliminated leaving the choice of C and D as discussed - this is a Dichotomy of Options **(SB A.2.3)**. Then option D is the correct choice by simply reading the passage and knowing the current theory of determination/differentiation.

This is also a Three or More Steps Question which would usually make this a difficult question, but it was not, as 80% or more of the students got it correct. The steps would be:

1) to know the tenets of the Regulative and Mosaic theories;

2) to determine if the 'because' phrase was true or false as relates to the current theories and to the Regulative or Mosaic (actually two steps);

3) to determine if the option was then true or false;

4) to determine if the option was correct.

Q99 — Pre-Study Suggestions

Review the following if needed:
1) Homologous Chromosomes **BIO 15.1**
2) Gametogenesis **BIO 14.2**
3) Mitosis **BIO 1.3**
4) Meiosis **BIO 14.2**
5) Camouflage and Distraction **SB A.1.3**
6) Similar Pair Options **SB A.2.7**
7) Three Out of Four Options **SB A.2.8**
8) Internally Inconsistent **SB A.2.5**
9) What are the key piece(s) of information from the passage?
10) Solve the problem.

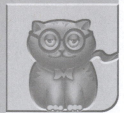

Solution Discussion

There is no information from the passage needed to answer this question. The diagram shows a two cell stage which represents the fertilized egg **(BIO 14.5)** meaning the cell is diploid **(BIO 14.2)**. There are three pairs of homologous chromosomes with one chromosome **(BIO 1.2.2, 14.2)** from the mother and the other from the father. This means the cells are somatic cells and not gametes **(BIO 14.2)**. At each subsequent

Biological Sciences PASSAGE 3.BS.I

division by mitosis **(BIO 1.3)**, each daughter cell will have the same genetic make-up of the parent cells. Only in the germ tissues **(BIO 14.2)** where gametes are formed by meiosis **(BIO 14.2)**, will the number of chromosomes be changed to ½ of each parental cell.

Notice how the "O" in hyp-O-tonic looks like a swollen cell. The O is also a circle which makes you think of the word "around." So IF the environment is hypOtonic AROUND the cell, then fluid rushes in and the cell swells like the letter O.

BIO 1.1.1

Option A is incorrect. This would be a gamete **(BIO 14.2)** of the organism because one half of the chromosomes are present. *See* option B for the other gamete formed.

Option C is incorrect. This cell is 4N, tetraploidy **(BIO 14.2)**, and would result if mitosis occurred but there was no cytokinesis **(BIO 1.3)**.

Option B is incorrect. This could also be a gamete. Notice that there are other possible gametes – *see* option A for another gamete. Can you draw others?

The ***correct option is D*** because the genetic content of all cells, except the gametes, is always the same.

Test Taking Skills Comment

Notice this requires no information from the passage. This is a Camouflage/Distraction question **(SB A.1.3)** because the passage has dealt with embryonic issues and the question is presented as an embryonic question. It is really a question dealing with mitosis and the cell division in somatic cells. If the question was rephrased to ask 'how does the chromosome content change due to mitosis **(BIO 1.3)**, there would be no problem because nearly everyone will know that mitosis does not change the genetic/chromosomal content.

This could be viewed as a Similar Pair Option **(SB A.2.7)** as A and B are similar. It could also be viewed as Three Out of Four **(SB A.2.8)** as options A, B and C all represent a change and option D does not and is the outlier. Generally, the outlier will be incorrect and the no change or zero option will be wrong. In this question, neither skill will help you but overall, if you truly had to guess, you would still be better off taking the guess.

The best knowledge based assessment is that options A and B are Internally Inconsistent **(SB A.2.5)** because they are haploid **(BIO 14.2)** and the 64 cell stage will need to be diploid **(BIO 14.2)**. This would eliminate A and B. Remember knowledge/good logic always takes precedence over guessing (like the similar pair above).

Q100   Pre-Study Suggestions

Review the following if needed:
1) What are the key piece(s) of information from the passage?
2) Solve the problem.

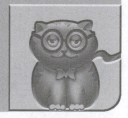

Solution Discussion

The key information from the passage from Biologist 1 (MH) is:

"the fate of the developing cells is determined ... of a cell in the embryo."

cellular determinants are important. Nothing external to the cell matters in its development. This would be evidence against MH.

Option A is incorrect. This is in direct opposition to the Mosaic Hypothesis (MH). This would mean any cell could develop into any other cell given the right conditions. The MH argues that once a cell has taken a certain path of differentiation, it can never go back.

Option C is incorrect. Same as option B. Notice that A, B and C would describe the Regulative Hypothesis.

Option D is correct. Once the cell has its particular set of determinants, it can only become one type of cell regardless of external circumstances - this is what the MH states.

Option B is incorrect. This is counter to the MH. Only the

Test Taking Skills Comment

This is really a reading question based on the passage.

Q101
Pre-Study Suggestions

Review the following if needed:
1) Steroid Hormones **BIO 6.3**
2) Steroid Biochemistry **ORG 12.4.1**
3) Proteins **BIO 3, ORG 12.2.2**
4) What are the key pieces of information from the passage?
5) Solve the problem.

Solution Discussion

There is no specific information required from the passage.

Cholesterol is the precursor of all of the steroid hormones including estrogen and testosterone. The steroid hormones are found in the testis, the ovary and the adrenal cortex. *Option D is correct.*

Option A is incorrect. Insulin is a protein made in the pancreas **(BIO 9.4.2)**.

Option B is incorrect. Gastrin **(BIO 9.3)** is a protein found in the stomach **(BIO 9.3)**.

Option C is incorrect. Thyroxin **(BIO 6.3.3)** is a modified amino acid **(ORG 12.1)** found in the thyroid gland **(BIO 6.3.3)**.

CHAPTER 3

Biological Sciences PASSAGE 3.BS.II

Test Taking Skills Comment

This is simply Study Knowledge **(SB A.2.2)**. There are no skills which will help get this problem right. This is the type of question you want to 'bank' some time on and get through it very quickly.

Q102 — Pre-Study Suggestions

Review the following if needed:
1) Proteins **BIO 3**
2) DNA **BIO 1.2.2**
3) Genes **BIO 15**
4) Genetics **BIO 15**
5) Dichotomy of Options **SB A.2.3**
6) Three or more step Options **SB A.1.4**
7) Complex Sounding Options **SB A.2.2**
8) Internally Inconsistent **SB A.2.5**
9) What are the key pieces of information from the passage?
10) Solve the problem.

Solution Discussion

The key pieces of information from the passage:

Third paragraph:

"HC is relatively common in some families and absent from others."

"no significant difference … in affected and unaffected families."

Fourth paragraph:

"individuals with HC lack … cholesterol containing particle (LDL)."

Although it is not one of the true options, the key to determining that this is a genetic linked condition (BIO 15) is the fact in the fourth paragraph that a protein (BIO 3) defect is tied to the condition. Proteins are made from DNA (BIO 1.2.2, 15) which makes up the genes (BIO 15).

Option B is incorrect. This is suggestive of a genetic basis. This is a Complex Sounding Option (SB A.2.2). There is no passage information, Passage Knowledge (SB A.2.2), that supports this statement. You are told the condition is independent of diet, you are not told that the condition is 'common' in families with a low cholesterol diet. You are told the disease occurs in 1/500 which is hardly 'common'. Since this is not Study Knowledge (SB A.2.2), there is no way for you to know if this is true or not.

Option C is incorrect. If this statement was correct, then this would decrease the likelihood of the disease being genetic. Again, the HC should be relatively

independent of environmental factors to have a significant genetic component. This statement also contradicts the information in the passage as stated above. This is an Internal Inconsistency of Options (SB A.2.5) as the passage states there is no relation to diet.

Option D is incorrect. For a disease to be genetic, at some point, it must be traced back to changes in DNA (BIO 1.2.2). If there are no changes in DNA, then it cannot be genetic (BIO 15). Since DNA determines proteins (BIO 3), if a disease is traceable to a protein, this becomes strong evidence for a genetic basis. This option is Internally Inconsistent (SB A.2.5) because a defective protein would suggest a problem with DNA.

CHAPTER 3

Option A is correct. Since the HC is independent of diet, and since it is more common in certain families than others, this is suggestive of a genetic condition. The strongest evidence would be if an option had related it to a defective protein or the membrane protein or to DNA.

Test Taking Skills Comment

Options B and D are Internally Inconsistent **(SB A.2.5)** as discussed. Option C is a Complex Sounding Option **(SB A.2.2)** as discussed.

This is a Dichotomy of Options question **(SB A.2.3)** with A and B, as yes and C and D as no. For dichotomies you use Basic Knowledge **(SB A.2.2)** to determine which set is correct. As discussed above, there is information which is consistent with this being a genetic condition from the Passage Knowledge **(SB A.2.2)** primarily. So, you can confidently select A and B and then just decide between them. This is very important in this question because the options are two or more lines each.

This is also a Three or More Step Analysis **(SB A.2.8)** question which makes it more difficult. The steps are:

1) to determine if the phrase after the yes or no is valid;
2) to determine if the phrase is consistent with the yes or no;
3) to determine if the option is true or false; and,
4) to determine if the option is correct **(SB A.1.2)**.

This question was very easy, 90% of students got it correct, which is unusual for questions with this structure.

Q103 — Pre-Study Suggestions

Review the following if needed:

1) Digestion of Lipids, Carbohydrates, Proteins **BIO 4, 9.3-9.5**
2) Membranes **BIO 1, 1.2.1**
3) Similar Pair Options **SB A.2.7**
4) What are the key pieces of information from the passage?
5) Solve the problem.

Solution Discussion

The key piece of information is from paragraph 4:

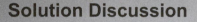

"HC is caused by a malfunction … cholesterol-containing particle (LDL)."

Option A is in incorrect. The hypothesis of the mechanism of the disease has nothing to do with the small intestinal absorption of lipids **(ORG 12.4)**. And, it is stated that diet, which would require absorption, has nothing to do with the disease.

Option C is in incorrect. The hypothesis has nothing to do with bile **(BIO 9.4.1)** directly. But, since bile is important for the absorption of lipids, which cholesterol is, there could be a connection. As for option A, diet has nothing to do with the condition.

Option D is in incorrect. This would result in death. Receptors are specific molecules for specific functions - only that receptor needs

CHAPTER 3

to be affected for a certain effect to be observed.

Option B is correct. The defect is hypothesized to be the absence of the LDL receptor on the plasma membrane. If a drug blocks that receptor, that is equivalent to removing that receptor from the membrane. The binding of the drug to the plasma membrane proteins would prevent the binding of the LDL. This would mimic the condition in HC.

Test Taking Skills Comment

The reasoning needed is discussed previously. You will not be tricked by the test. Since option A and C were not discussed, it is unlikely they will relate to the question unless you make a Study Knowledge **(SB A.2.2)** connection as was discussed. You are given information about membranes and must trust that the question will center around them. This is a Similar Pair Options **(SB A.2.7)** as options B and D both deal with membranes. This is a reasonable similar pair option.

Q104 — Pre-Study Suggestions

Review the following if needed:
1) Dominance and Recessive Relationships **BIO 15.1**
2) Alleles **BIO 15.1**
3) Pedigrees **BIO 15**
4) Camouflage and Distractions **SB A.1.3**
5) Dichotomy of Options **SB A.2.3**
6) Similar Pair Options **SB A.2.7**
6) What are the key pieces of information from the passage?
7) Solve the problem.

Solution Discussion

The key information from the passage:

From paragraph 1:

"The typical blood cholesterol level of healthy humans is about 1.8 mg/mL."

From paragraph 2:

"The cholesterol level of moderately … cholesterol levels around 7.0 mg/mL."

Option A is incorrect. A recessive gene would only be expressed if it was homozygous **(BIO 15.1, 15.3)**. There is some expression of the condition in the parents as their cholesterol level is between the normal and the severely affected child. The child must be homozygous for the condition. For the child to be homozygous and to have parents which are not equally affected, the parents must be heterozygous **(BIO 15.1, 15.3)** for the condition. Since they have some expression of the condition and are heterozygous, the gene cannot be recessive.

Option C is incorrect. In a completely dominant **(BIO 15.1, 15.3)** gene, only one of the chromosomes, only one of the two allelic positions, has to have the dominant gene. In this case, the gene will be expressed to the fullest and should reflect the most severe form of the condition. Since each parent has a higher than normal cholesterol, each has a form of the disease. With a dominant gene, this should be the maximal form of the disease, which it is not because the son has a more severe form. So, the gene cannot be completely dominant as discussed in option A as the parents have to be heterozygous and they are not severely affected. Remember a completely dominant gene will show the full phenotype **(BIO 15)** whether it is heterozygous or homozygous.

Option D is incorrect. If the gene was completely dominant, each parent would express the condition fully as does the child. *See* discussion in options A, C and B. Both parents do carry the allele and are heterozygous.

Option B is correct. The gene is co-dominant **(BIO 15.1)** or incompletely dominant **(BIO 15.1)**. This is also consistent with the information from the passage. A co-dominant gene means both alleles will be expressed. The best example of a co-dominant gene is the ABO blood group **(BIO 15.2)**. So, in this question, this would mean the defective allele would result in a severe level, but the normal allele would result in normal levels and these could average out to the 3.0 mg/dL noted for the parents.

In incompletely dominant genes, shown best by a white allele and a red allele for flower color, the presence of both alleles (the heterozygous state) results in a pink genotype and not red or white. If the red and white alleles were co-dominant, there would be patches of red and white but no pink. So, this question could be either co-dominant or incompletely dominant. If the alleles were co-dominant, there would be normal cells which could take up some of the cholesterol but there would be abnormal cells that could not and the net cholesterol could be somewhere in between.

The same would be true if they were incompletely dominant. This is the case here with the normal cholesterol being 1.8 mg/mL and the mild form being 3.0 mg/mL, in the parents, and the severe form being 7.0 mg/mL, in the child. This means the parents are each heterozygous in the gene, with only one copy, and the child is homozygous, with two copies of the gene. What is the risk of the parents having another child with the severe form? (Answer: 25%). Can these parents have a normal child? (Answer: yes, a 25% chance).

Test Taking Skills Comment

Sometimes you and I are tempted to think that since there are Similar Pair Options **(SB A.2.7)**, such as C and D, that one of them must be correct. This may be true in some situations, but as is the case here, it is not always so. Remember similar pair options have less reliability when there is more than one similar pair present or when there are other test skills present as in this question; this is especially true for dichotomies.

This question is also a Dichotomy of Options **(SB A.2.3)**. You use your Basic Knowledge (study, passage, general knowledge) **(SB A.2.2)** to determine which half of the dichotomy is correct. Your study knowledge should tell you that for a dominant relationship, the phenotype should be all or none and not half-way or blending. The fact that you have three states (normal, severe and intermediate) precludes purely dominant

relationships of the alleles. When an allele is dominant, the genotype **(BIO 15)** does not matter as long as one dominant allele is present you get the full phenotype **(BIO 15)**. So, heterozygous and homozygous **(BIO 15.1, 15.3)** completely dominant **(BIO 15.1)** give the same phenotype. This means you should eliminate options C and D.

The question has a mild Camouflage and Distractions **(SB A.1.3)** with the different levels of cholesterol for the different conditions. You just have to refocus the question to your understanding of dominance-recessive relationships.

Q105 Pre-Study Suggestions

Review the following if needed:
1) Digestion of Lipids, Carbohydrates, Proteins **BIO 4, 9.3-9.5**
2) Dichotomy of Options **SB A.2.3**
3) Best Option **SB A.1.2**
4) What are the key pieces of information from the passage?
5) Solve the problem.

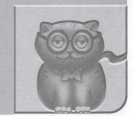

Solution Discussion

There is no information from the passage needed to solve this problem. In fact, there is no answer given for this problem.

Option B is incorrect. These capillaries **(BIO 7.5.2)** would only affect the smooth muscle and peristalsis **(BIO 9.2)** and does not directly affect absorption.

Option D is incorrect. Same as for the other incorrect options.

Option C is incorrect. Again vessels in this area have nothing directly to do with absorption of fats.

Option A is correct. By elimination, this option is correct but it is really not correct either. This question has no correct answer. *See* the following discussion.

Test Taking Skills Comment

This is a rare mistake by AAMC. This will or has been corrected I'm sure. Capillaries **(BIO 7.5.2)** do not constrict. It is the pre-capillary arterioles which constrict and control blood flow to a capillary bed. Lymphatic vessels **(BIO 7.6)** do not constrict either and lacteals are part of the capillary system. Neither capillaries nor lymph vessels contain smooth muscle which is necessary for them to contract. The only way to get the answer they want you to get is to realize that the absorption of nutrients takes place in the intestinal villi **(BIO 9.5)** and this is the only option with this possibility. It is in the lacteals where the fats do go when they enter the body across the intestinal wall. So, it may have been possible to use a Dichotomy **(SB A.2.3)** choice with A or C, the lacteals. Although options C and D would be a Similar Pair **(SB A.2.7)**, remember it is best not use this when there are more than one similar pair or other test skills available.

This is definitely a situation where you have to choose the Best Option **(SB A.1.2)** even when there are no truly correct options available.

Q106 — Pre-Study Suggestions

Review the following if needed:
1) Genetics **BIO 15**
2) Membranes **BIO 1, 1.2.1**
3) Best Option **SB A.1.2**
4) What are the key pieces of information from the passage?
5) Solve the problem.

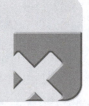

Solution Discussion

The key piece of information from the passage:

"no significant difference between the dietary habits of individuals in affected and unaffected families."

Option A is incorrect. This may be suggestive of a genetic disorder but is not adequate. There are a lot of environmental differences between families which could account for the difference.

Option C is incorrect. This is also not specific enough. It is again suggestive. If a specific protein could be identified, then this would be strong evidence because proteins are indirectly from DNA.

But membranes also contain lipids and this could be the problem. Or an external inhibitor could be affecting the membrane.

Option D is incorrect. This is the same as option C.

Option B is correct. Of the options given, this would still present the strongest case for a genetic basis because one would expect the diet to make a difference in cholesterol levels. Since it has no effect on the disease, this is suggestive

CHAPTER 3

of genetic influences.

Test Taking Skills Comment

The fact that the membrane protein is missing is not stated as one of the options even though the passage mentioned it. An abnormal or a missing protein is much stronger evidence for a genetic basis than the circumstantial evidence of diet. I'm not sure

I wouldn't select option D based on the passage - I do feel a little confused because the endocytotic vessel statement was so closely tied to the membrane protein statement in the passage. This is determination of the Best Option **(SB A.1.2)**

Q107 — Pre-Study Suggestions

Review the following if needed:
1) Genetics **BIO 15**
2) Monohybrid Crosses **BIO 15.3**
3) Dominance and Recessive Relationships **BIO 15.1**
4) Three Out of Four **SB A.2.8**
5) Solve the problem.

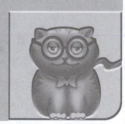

Solution Discussion

This is a monohybrid cross **(BIO 15.3)** (one trait with two alleles **(BIO 15)** in dominant-recessive **(BIO 15.1, 15.3)** relationship. This is equivalent to the second cross (F2) which is of the offspring from a first cross (F1) of pure dominants and pure recessives. The offspring of the second cross, which will be F3 will always be in the ratio of 3:1

phenotypes **(BIO 15)** of dominant:recessive. The genotypes **(BIO 15)** will be 1:2:1 and are DD, Dd, dd with D=dominant, d=recessive. The monohybrid cross and the dihybrid cross **(BIO 15.3)** are specifically required which started with the 2003 revisions of the MCAT. This means option B is correct which is approximately 1/3 of the 787.

Test Taking Skills Comment

This is a Three Out of Four **(SB A.2.8)** question with options B, C and D being the three and option A being the outlier which has a value of zero. Generally, the outlier will be incorrect and zero or no-change options will generally be incorrect.

Q108 Pre-Study Suggestions

Review the following if needed:
1) Aerobic Respiration **BIO 4.5**
2) Anaerobic Respiration **BIO 4.5**
2) Glycolysis **BIO 4.5, 4.6**
3) Krebs Cycle **BIO 4.7**
4) Electron Transport Chain **BIO 4.9**
5) Oxidative Phosphorylation **BIO 4.8**
6) Fermentation **BIO 2.2, 4.5**
7) Cell Organelles **BIO 1.1, 1.2.1**
8) Camouflage and Distractions **SB A.1.3**
9) Three Out of Four Options **SB A.2.8**
10) Solve the problem.

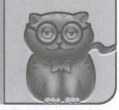

Solution Discussion

The glucose is metabolized as discussed in the energy metabolism. This means the molecules of glucose start in glycolysis, go through the Krebs cycle and then down the electron transport chain. The atoms of glucose may also end up in some of the fermentation reactions. Glycolysis takes place in the cytoplasm **(BIO 1.2)** as does fermentation. The Krebs cycle, electron transport and oxidative phosphorylation are all mitochondria **(BIO 1.2.1)** associated. The C14 label will be detected anywhere glucose is, or where any of the breakdown products of glucose may be found. The cell nucleus **(BIO 1.2)** is the site of DNA transcription to RNA **(BIO 1.2.2, 3)** and DNA duplication **(BIO 1.2.2)**. The ribosomes **(BIO 1.2.1)** are the site of protein biosynthesis **(BIO 3)**.

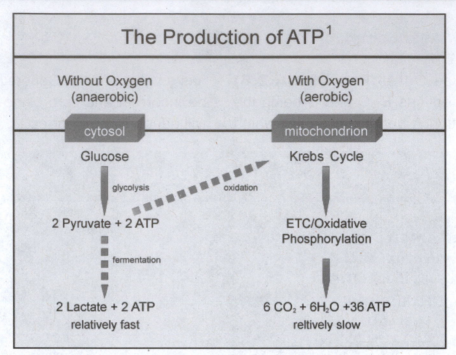

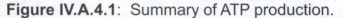

Figure IV.A.4.1: Summary of ATP production.

Option A is incorrect. The glucose is broken down in the cytoplasm before its breakdown product (pyruvate) goes to the mitochondrion.

Option C is incorrect. The glucose has no metabolism associated with the ribosomes.

Option B is incorrect. The glucose may go into the nucleus, but this is not part of the metabolic process. At any rate, it would still pass through the cytoplasm first before it would appear in the mitochondrion.

Option D is correct. This is as previously described.

Test Taking Skills Comment

There are many ways of asking or determining your understanding of a concept without directly asking it. In this case, all the question is really testing is your knowledge of the metabolic breakdown of glucose and the main cycles/processes of this in the cell. If you can restate a question, including its Camouflage and Distractions **(SB A.1.3)**, into another simple, more obvious or more familiar one, the answer may become easier.

In this case, an alternative question is where is glucose metabolized in the cell? The answer is via glycolysis and the Krebs cycle. The answer should be more obvious. This is a Three Out of Four **(SB A.2.8)** question. Options B, C and D all have two locations. Option A is the outlier with only one location. In general, outliers will be incorrect and may be ignored.

Q109 — Pre-Study Suggestions

Review the following if needed:
1) Carbohydrates, Lipids and Proteins Metabolism **BIO 4, 9.3-9.5**
2) Kidney's handling of Carbohydrates, Fats and Proteins and General Kidney Function **BIO 10**
3) Complex Sounding Options **SB A.2.2**
4) Camouflage/Distractions **SB A.1.3**
5) Solve the problem.

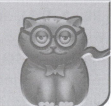

Solution Discussion

Option A is incorrect. Glycogen is a carbohydrate. Its final metabolic products will be carbon dioxide and water. It cannot account for the nitrogen in urine.

Option C is incorrect. The fats will be metabolized mainly to carbon dioxide and water. Ketone bodies may appear in the blood or urine, but no nitrogen is found in the typical fats.

CHAPTER 3

Option D is incorrect. The kidney always excretes some nitrogenous wastes; it does not reabsorb large amounts of nitrogenous wastes. An increase of nitrogen in the urine means that more protein (amino acids) is being metabolized. In kidney failure, nitrogen is retained in the body and is a key clinical indicator of kidney failure.

Option B is correct. During prolonged starvation, the body's proteins are broken down and the nitrogen, as urea, would be excreted in the urine.

Test Taking Skills Comment

This is a Camouflage/Distractions question **(SB A.1.3)**, and it can be rephrased to ask what are the breakdown products of the key nutrients **(BIO 3, ORG 12.2-12.4)** in the body. The primary major nutrients that have nitrogen are the proteins.

Option D is also a Complex Sounding Option **(SB A.2.2)**. You cannot assess this option based on your Basic Knowledge (study, passage, general knowledge) **(SB A.2.2)**. Your study did not require you to understand kidney failure and its effect on reabsorption of substances. The question (passage) did not describe any effect or even the presence of kidney failure. So, there is no way you can assess this option.

Addition of an Amine to a Carbonyl Group

"**SE PI**" (or "**SE**a **PI**e")

- **S**econdary amine produces an **E**namine

- **P**rimary amine produces an **I**mine

Note: tertiary and quaternary amines do not react with the C=O group **(ORG 7.2.3)**.

Q110   Pre-Study Suggestions

Review the following if needed:
1) Intermolecular Forces **CHM 4.2**
2) Boiling Points, General **CHM 5.1.2**
3) Boiling Points in Organic Molecules **ORG 3.1.1, 6.1, 8.1, 9.2, 10.1, 11.1.2**
4) Distillation **ORG 13.3**
5) Dichotomy of Options **SB A.2.3**
6) Three or More Step Analysis **SB A.2.8**
7) Internal Inconsistency of Options **SB A.2.5**
8) What piece(s) of information are important from the passage?
9) Solve the problem.

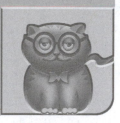

Solution Discussion

The information needed from the passage is the following (from the second paragraph) and the two structures as shown in the passage:

"A chemist attempted ... entirely of (+)-carvone and limonene".

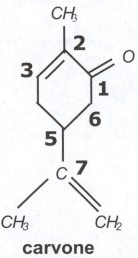

carvone

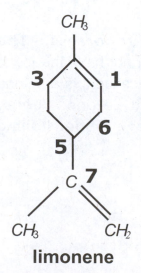

limonene

CHAPTER 3

Boiling points depend on the intermolecular forces **(CHM 4.2)** in molecules. Polar molecules **(CHM 3.3)**, e.g. those with a carbonyl group **(ORG 7.1)**, will have stronger intermolecular forces than those with only carbon and hydrogen. This means their boiling points will be higher. In distillation **(ORG 13.3)**, the compound with the lowest boiling point will distill off first.

points than corresponding alkenes **(ORG 4)**, which limonene is. If the carbon chain is very long, of course, this effect and difference becomes minimal.

Option B is incorrect. The higher boiling point substance will not distill off first. The lowest boiling point substance will always distill off first. This option is an excellent example of Internal Inconsistency of Options **(SB A.2.5)** because of the facts discussed previously.

Option D is incorrect. This is for the same reason as B and is an example of Internal Inconsistency of Options **(SB A.2.5)**.

Option A is correct. Limonene will have the lower boiling point of the two because it is a hydrocarbon which is also an alkene. The lower boiling point substance will distill off first. *See* option C.

Option C is incorrect. The (+)-carvone will not have the lower boiling point because it is a ketone **(ORG 7)** and ketones, being carbonyls, have higher boiling

Test Taking Skills Comment

First, you should realize that this is really a question about your knowledge of boiling points of organic molecules - every option contains a reference to boiling point. You should also, immediately, eliminate options B and D because they are Internal Inconsistency of Options **(SB A.2.5)** with the fact that lower boiling point substances will distill off first. It is always the lowest boiling point substance which will distill off first. The remainder of the analysis is as above. Generally, for organic comparisons look for the functional group differences and apply what you know about them to the problem at hand.

This is also a Dichotomy of Options **(SB A.2.3)** times two. The first dichotomy is carvone or limonene. Remember you must use Basic Knowledge (study, passage, general knowledge) **(SB A.2.2)** to select the correct half of the dichotomy. The study knowledge is that oxygen is polar and its compounds will have a higher boiling point than non-polar compounds. This means you will select the lower boiling point compound which is limonene and options A and B. This is because the study knowledge regarding distillation is that the lower boiling point substance will always come out first. This means for the second dichotomy of lower (options A and C) or higher (options B and D) boiling points, you would select options A and C. Also, in a double dichotomy, if you select both correctly you are left with the answer. This means only option A is left from your choices.

Finally, this is a Three or More Step Analysis **(SB A.2.8)** and these are usually, but not always, more difficult. The steps are:

1) to determine if the phrase after the compound applies to the compound;
2) to determine if the option is true or false as relates to the question;
3) to determine if the option is correct or incorrect.

Q111 — Pre-Study Suggestions

Review the following if needed:
1) Distillation **ORG 13.3**
2) What piece(s) of information are important from the passage?
3) Do you know what an ebulliator does? Does it matter?
4) Solve the problem.

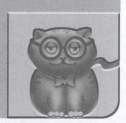

Solution Discussion

The pieces of information from the passage which are helpful are:

"An ebulliator was lowered ... small bubbles into the system."

"The contents of the distillation flask were heated"

"and the apparatus was connected to a vacuum source."

Option A is incorrect. The ebulliator is placed into the distillation flask. Only bubbles are coming from the ebulliator. How can this keep the condensing flask cool? It cannot. Remember a condensed vapor is a liquid anyway. This is what you want in the receiving flask of a distillation.

Option B is incorrect. The vacuum is established by the vacuum source attached to tubing near the receiving flask. Since bubbles, which are gas, are being introduced into the solution via the ebulliator, how can added gas decrease a pressure to reach a vacuum? It cannot.

Option D is incorrect. Since the system is operating under a vacuum pump, any loss of pressure will be through the vacuum source operation. Since the ebulliator is introducing bubbles, this means the tip is under the liquid. How can the gas pressure, which is what is being discussed, be decreased by an object introducing bubbles under the surface of the liquid? It cannot.

Option C is correct. An ebulliator is a device for introducing small bubbles into the liquid. By doing this, large bubbles and pockets of superheated fluid do not build up and result in bumping or explosion of the liquid. This keeps the liquid heating uniformly and smoothly. Other ways of introducing small bubbles and preventing superheating and bumping are porous stones or wood chips.

Regular stones only work for a non-vacuum situation. Also, the distilling flask can have a stirrer to get the liquid moving and preventing excessive local heating/ superheating.

Test Taking Skills Comment

To solve this problem, you did not need to know what an ebulliator actually does. Given the information in the passage, it is possible to eliminate all the other options. This type of knowledge is of the general type you should have gained from your general lab work in organic chemistry. It should not be necessary to specifically study what an ebulliator is to deduct what it does. You should remember the importance of introducing small bubbles into your solutions which were being heated. Ebullient is defined as to bubble or boil, boiling or agitated.

Q112 — Pre-Study Suggestions

Review the following if needed:
1) Distillation **ORG 13.3**
2) Boiling Points, General **CHM 5.1.2**
3) Boiling Points of Organic Molecules **ORG 3.1.1, 6.1, 8.1, 9.2, 10.1, 11.1.2**
4) What are the key pieces of information from the passage?
5) Solve the problem.

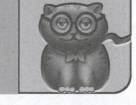

Solution Discussion

There is no information from the passage necessary to solve the problem.

Option B is incorrect. A lower pressure would only decrease the boiling points of each of the components. This would be a proportionate decrease, so no increased separation would be expected.

Option C is incorrect. The condenser is an after-the-fact effect on the separation of the liquids. The separation occurs in the fractionating column, not in the condenser. Whatever vapors are present in the condenser will condense; decreasing the temperature, by using ice, will not affect the composition of the vapor which presents to it.

Option D is incorrect. This would certainly make the separation less efficient. There are different levels of temperature at different levels of the fractionating column. The temperature will decrease progressively as the vapor rises in the column. If the column is short, there may not be adequate temperature steps or gradations to allow the separation of liquids with close boiling points.

Option A is correct. Rapid heating can result in liquids with close boiling points to boil at the same time. This would decrease the efficiency of the separation. By increasing the temperature in the distilling flask very slowly, this will allow each component to boil at a distinct temperature. This will increase the efficiency of the separation.

Test Taking Skills Comment

There is nothing from the passage to help with this problem. Some thought and especially experience in the lab are best to answer this problem. Options C and D should be able to be eliminated with your knowledge of distillation. Also, an understanding that vacuum is used to allow the distillation to occur at lower temperatures and not specifically for the efficiency of the separation could help eliminate option B.

Q113 — Pre-Study Suggestions

Review the following if needed:

1) Optical Isomerism **ORG 2.3.2**
2) Hybrid Orbitals (sp-2: linear; sp^2-3:planar; sp^3-4:tetrahedral; sp^{3}d-5:triangular bipyramidal; sp^{3}d^2-6:octahedral or square bipyramidal) **ORG 1.2, CHM 3.5**
3) Camouflage and Distractions **SB A.1.3**
4) Three Out of Four type question **SB A.2.8**
5) Internal Inconsistency of Options **SB A.2.5**
6) What information is needed from the passage?
7) Solve the problem.

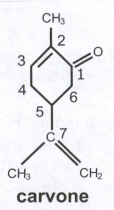

Solution Discussion

The only information needed from the passage is the structure of the compound, (+ or -)-carvone which is given:

The critical feature of an optical isomer is that it has an asymmetric carbon. The asymmetric (chiral) carbon must:

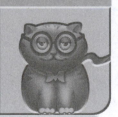

carvone

Biological Sciences PASSAGE 3.BS.VI

- be sp^3 hybridized (tetrahedral, 4 orbitals, 109.5 degrees) **(ORG 1.2)**
- have four different substituents attached.

This is the Basic Knowledge (study, passage, general knowledge) **(SB A.2.2)** you have to know.

Option A is incorrect. Carbon #2 is sp^2 hybridized (planar, 3 orbitals, 120 degrees) **(ORG 1.2)**.

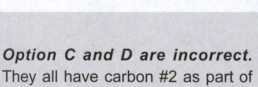

Option C and D are incorrect. They all have carbon #2 as part of the answer which is known to be incorrect. Also, carbon #7 is sp^2 hybridized.

Option B is correct. Carbon #5 is sp^3 hybridized **(ORG 1.2)** and it has four substituents attached. Also, all four substituents are different:

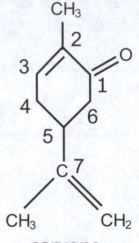

carvone

- three of the substituents of carbon 5 are shown and labeled 1, 2 and 3 (1 and 2 could be changed);
- the fourth substituent is hydrogen;
- all four of the substituents are different.

Test Taking Skills Comment

There is nothing from the passage required to solve this problem except the structure which is data. This is actually a straight forward application of Basic Knowledge (study, passage, general knowledge) **(SB A.2.2)**, yet, only half of the students got it correct. You are not usually given the basic knowledge you are required to apply. In this question, you are not asked to identify the asymmetric carbon. You are told that the plus and negative compounds differ in the orientation about some atom.

Yet, all that is being asked is to identify the asymmetric carbon atom. This is a Camouflage and Distractions **(SB A.1.3)** in which you have to rephrase the question to make more obvious or simpler. The steps you must make are to look for the following features:

- the carvone compounds are optical isomers,
- optical isomers differ in orientation about certain atoms only,
- the atoms which distinguish optical isomers are called asymmetric carbons and have the following features (see previous information).

You are given a clue in the "differ in orientations of the substituents". This is an elimination question. Since you should be able to identify carbon 2 as sp^2 hybridized and know

this carbon cannot be asymmetric. Then all options with carbon 2 cannot be correct. Carbon #2 is a type of Internal Inconsistency of Options **(SB A.2.5)** as it is known that a multiply bonded carbon cannot be asymmetric.

This could also be a Three Out of Four **(SB A.2.8)** type question as options A, C and D all have #2 and options B, C and D have #5. Usually, when there are two Three Out of Four's **(SB A.2.8)**, you can guess from the common options which would be C and D - most of the time your answer will be from these common options.

But, no test skill is 100% as demonstrated in this example. Using your Basic Knowledge (study, passage, general knowledge) **(SB A.2.2)** should always take precedence. The basic knowledge here is knowing that optical isomers are distinguished at the asymmetric carbons and knowing that a double/triple bonded **(ORG 1.3.1)** carbon cannot be asymmetric.

CHAPTER 3

Biological Sciences PASSAGE 3.BS.VI

Q114 — Pre-Study Suggestions

Review the following if needed:

1) Boiling Points in Organic Compounds **ORG 3.1.1, 6.1, 8.1, 9.2, 10.1, 11.1.2**
2) Effects of Pressure and Vapor Pressure on the Boiling Point **CHM 5.1.1, 5.1.2**
3) Phase Diagrams **CHM 4.3.3**
4) Three Out of Four type question **SB A.2.8**
5) Camouflage and Distractions **SB A.1.3**
6) Similar Pair Options **SB A.2.7**
7) What information is needed from the passage?
8) Solve the problem.

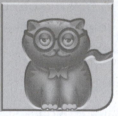

Solution Discussion

There is no critical information from the passage other than the vacuum present in the system.

Options B, C and D are incorrect. The boiling points always decrease as pressure is decreased, as in a vacuum.

Option A is correct. The pressure will increase if there is a leak in the apparatus. Increasing external pressure means the boiling points will both increase. Review boiling points and phase diagrams to understand this very important point.

Test Taking Skills Comment

There is nothing from the passage required to solve this problem. This is actually a straight forward application of Basic Knowledge (study, passage, general knowledge) **(SB A.2.2)**, yet, only half of the students got it correct. The concepts are as discussed previously - remember to know the basic concepts very well and how to apply them.

This is a Camouflage and Distractions **(SB A.1.3)** as you could have rephrased the question to ask what the effect of pressure on boiling point is which is the real question. The vacuum and set-up are distractions and camouflage.

This is also a Three Out of Four **(SB A.2.8)** type question that may not be very obvious. Options A, B and D are similar in that all are a change of some type. Option C is the outlier which has no change: outliers and no change/zero options tend to be incorrect. A reasonable guess would have been from options A, B or D.

This is also a Similar Pair Options **(SB A.2.7)** with options A/B being similar as they result in a specific change. They are also the mirror image/opposite type of similar pair that seems to carry more weight.

Q115 — Pre-Study Suggestions

Review the following if needed:
1) X-linked traits **BIO 15.3**
2) Dominance-Recessive Relationships **BIO 15.1**
3) Three Out of Four type question **SB A.2.8**
4) Dichotomy of Options **SB A.2.3**
5) Similar Pair Options **SB A.2.7**
6) Negative Question **SB A.1.2**
7) What piece(s) of information are important from the passage?
8) Solve the problem.

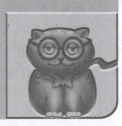

CHAPTER 3

Solution Discussion

The key piece of information from the passage is from paragraph 1:

"families in which many males ... ability to respond to Hormone X."

This piece of information means the trait is an X-linked recessive trait **(BIO 15.3)**. If it was autosomal recessive **(BIO 15.1, 15.3)**, females would have been affected equal to males. If it was dominant **(BIO 15.1, 15.3)** and on the X chromosome, females would have been affected equal to males. Since an affected male has the trait on his X chromosome, this can only be passed to his daughter and not to any male offspring. A daughter will only have the disease if the mother is also a carrier (a 50% chance of being affected) or affected (a 100% chance of being affected).

Option A is incorrect. A father cannot pass an X-linked recessive allele **(BIO 15.3)** or a dominant allele to the son, because the son gets the father's Y chromosome and not the X chromosome (that comes from the mother). A daughter will be a carrier but will *not show the disease unless she also received the allele from her mother.*

Option B is incorrect. Same as for option A. Half of the females will be expected to be affected only if the mother is a carrier (heterozygous **(BIO 15.1, 15.3)**) for the trait.

Option C is incorrect. Same as for option B. The 'none of the males' is correct. You do not have enough information to evaluate the outcome for the daughters. But, just based on the information you do have, no daughter will have the disease just based on the father. The mother would have to be a carrier or have the disease for the daughter to get it.

Option D is correct. Based on the information given, no data on the mother, this is the best answer.

Test Taking Skills Comment

This is a difficult question. Yet, it only requires the application of very basic information as presented in the problem. It is very important that you understand genetics **(BIO 15)** very well. The discussion on genetics is exceedingly complete and we suggest that you study it very carefully and with maximal understanding.

This is a good Dichotomy of Options **(SB A.2.3)** problem. Based on your knowledge of sex-linked genes, you should immediately eliminate any options that have the males affected. This eliminated the dichotomy of options A and B that have the males affected. This makes your work much easier as you only have to consider C and D. If you guess from C or D, you will have done better than the rest of the students as only 40% of them got the correct answer.

This could also be a Similar Pair Options **(SB A.2.7)** as options C and D both have none for the males, but options B and C have half of the females. When there is more than one similar pair, or when there are other test skills present, the similar pairs approach should take the back seat.

This could also be a Three Out of Four **(SB A.2.8)** type question as options A, B and C all have someone being affected and option D, the outlier, has none being affected. Usually the outlier or negative or no-change or zero option will be incorrect. But, this is a negative type question and in negative type questions, the outlier may be correct and you have to be more careful. This is not the typical negative question (with 'except' or 'not'), but the 'unable' is a qualifier that makes it a negative question.

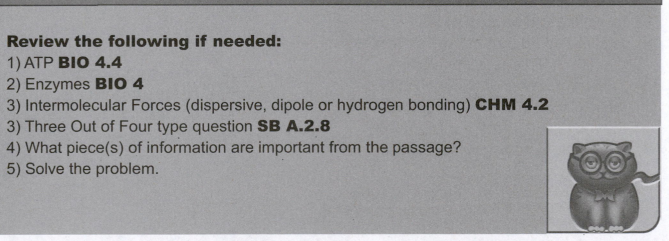

Q116 — Pre-Study Suggestions

Review the following if needed:
1) ATP **BIO 4.4**
2) Enzymes **BIO 4**
3) Intermolecular Forces (dispersive, dipole or hydrogen bonding) **CHM 4.2**
3) Three Out of Four type question **SB A.2.8**
4) What piece(s) of information are important from the passage?
5) Solve the problem.

Solution Discussion

The key piece of information found in the passage is from second paragraph, item 4:

"Protein R phosphorylated Protein P."

When an enzyme phosphorylates another molecule, the phosphate cannot come from the enzyme. Why? Because an enzyme is a catalyst **(CHM 9.7)** and a catalyst is unchanged in the reaction. Enzymes use cofactors or coenzymes which may be changed in a reaction, but you are not given any information in this regard. In this case, the phosphate comes from the ATP which is hydrolyzed and will end up as ADP or AMP depending on the exact mechanism of the enzyme.

Option A is incorrect. Hormone X is stated to only bind to protein R. Nothing else is stated about its mechanism of action. There is no requirement of ATP for one molecule to bind to another molecule. This is a spontaneous process determined by noncovalent interactions **(CHM 4.2)** between the molecules involved. The major noncovalent forces are the van der Waals, the dipole and hydrogen bonding. The van der Waals forces may be considered the hydrophobic forces. All of these are electrostatic **(CHM 4.2)** in nature and require no input of energy from ATP.

Option C is incorrect. Phosphorylated protein P is required to cause the calcium influx. There is no clue as to how this occurs. It may or may not require any additional energy - if it does, you have no way of determining this. You don't know if the phosphorylated protein P is high or low energy in terms of the phosphate group. You don't know if the phosphorylation resulted in a conformational change or opened or closed some ion channel or not. Although, these may be possible, you are not given the information to decide.

Option D is incorrect. Since A and C are incorrect, option D must be incorrect.

Option B is correct. The passage states protein R phosphorylates protein P. To do this, ATP is a reasonable co-reactant.

Test Taking Skills Comment

This question is testing basic understanding of cell metabolism and protein, enzyme function. ATP should be well known to all. It only does limited functions within the cell and is only generated by a limited number of mechanisms. Knowing this and the clue from the passage gives the answer. It should have been possible to eliminate hormone X because only binding is required. This would have left a 50% guess of option B or C.

This is a Three Out of Four **(SB A.2.8)** type question as options A, B and C only contain one possibility. Option D contains two possibilities and is the outlier; outliers are usually incorrect and can be eliminated.

CHAPTER 3

Q117   Pre-Study Suggestions

Review the following if needed:
1) Membranes **BIO 1**
2) Complex Sounding Option(s) **SB A.2.2**
3) What piece(s) of information are important from the passage?
4) Solve the problem.

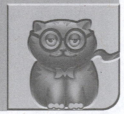

Solution Discussion

The key piece of information is found in paragraph 2, item 6:

> *"Phosphorylated Protein P was necessary … the rate of Ca^{2+} entry."*

Option A is incorrect. Na^+/K^+ pump is used to pump sodium and potassium from one side of a membrane to another. There is no mention of sodium or potassium transport in this problem.

Option B is incorrect. A phosphatase is an enzyme which removes phosphate. You should at least think phosphate is involved in some way. There is no indication that phosphorylated protein P does anything at all to phosphate. The passage only states it allows the influx of calcium ion.

Option D is incorrect. There is nothing in the passage which states that phosphorylated protein P binds to anything whether a hormone or not. It is clear that protein R is a hormone receptor and an enzyme (*see* items 2 and 4 of paragraph 2).

Option C is correct. The statement above states this molecule causes the influx of calcium into the cell. One way for this to occur is for the molecule to result in an ion, membrane channel for the calcium. So, this is possible, but not proven, in the passage, to be the action of phosphorylated protein P.

Test Taking Skills Comment

Your general feeling and understanding of biology is tested in this question. It is difficult to state exactly what you should have studied to be able to solve this problem other than understanding membrane function. Its solution comes about as result of your general study and carefully reading the passage. Note the limitations of the information - don't reach beyond what you are presented without very good and clear

Sounding Option(s) **(SB A.2.2)** which are options A, B and D. You are given no Basic Knowledge (study, passage, general knowledge) **(SB A.2.2)** to determine if A, B or D may be correct. You are told in the passage that phosphorylated protein P allows the entry of calcium ion. Based on your general knowledge of membranes and molecular membrane transport, this is a reasonable option.

Q118 — Pre-Study Suggestions

Review the following if needed:
1) Membrane Transport **BIO 1.1.1, 1.1.2, 1.1.3**
2) Best Option **SB A.1.2**
3) Dichotomy of Options **SB A.2.3**
4) Complex Sounding Option(s) **SB A.2.2**
5) What piece(s) of information are important from the passage?
6) Solve the problem.

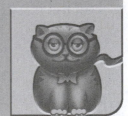

Solution Discussion

The key pieces of information are found in the second paragraph in items 1 through 6 and will not be repeated.

CHAPTER 3

Option A is incorrect. This option is a true statement but is not correct. The binding of hormone X to protein R is the beginning of the cascade. Certainly if there is no bound X to R, the influx of calcium will eventually cease but not immediately. If the only step in the cascade was the binding of the X to R, then the unbinding would result in immediate cessation of the influx. For example, in the situation of a neurotransmitter (could be X) binding to the post-synaptic membrane (could be R), this binding itself can open an ion channel and efflux/influx of ions may result. Then its immediate unbinding would cause cessation of the influx/efflux.

However, in the passage, there are key steps subsequent to the binding of X and R which finally cause the influx of calcium. R must phosphorylate P, and it is only the phosphorylated P which causes the influx of calcium. So, even if the X is removed from the R, there may still be some phosphorylated P allowing the influx of calcium. Eventually, with no X bound to R, the R will stop phosphorylating P and the phosphorylated P will

decrease and return to baseline and this will stop the influx. While this is a true option, it is not the correct option because it is not the Best Option **(SB A.1.2)**.

Option B is incorrect. Where in the passage is it stated or can be deducted that endocytosis occurs? There isn't any. There is no requirement for a molecule which binds to a membrane receptor to undergo endocytosis. You must be given this information in some manner. This is an example of a Complex Sounding Option(s) **(SB A.2.2)**. Remember, for the option to be correct, you must be able to assess its correctness from your Basic Knowledge (study, passage, general knowledge) **(SB A.2.2)**. If you cannot determine the correctness from your study knowledge, passage knowledge or general knowledge, then the option cannot be correct. There is no way for you to determine if endocytosis occurs, so there is no way this option can be seriously considered.

Option C is incorrect. The termination of the synthesis of P would eventually cause the influx to stop. But, there still may be phosphorylated P causing influx. Until the phosphorylated P is removed or blocked, influx may still continue. Also, you are given no means of knowing how protein P is synthesized or not, based on the passage - a Complex Sounding Option(s) **(SB A.2.2)** as in option B. But, even if you assume this happens, you are still left with the protein P that is already phosphorylated as the key qualifier in the stem is 'immediately'. So,

even if it was true, it would still not be the Best Option **(SB A.1.2)** as in option A.

Option D is correct. See the previous discussions of A, B and C. The final step is the phosphorylated P resulting in the influx. If the P was dephosphorylated, the influx would stop immediately. This 'immediate' effect is what makes this the Best Option **(SB A.1.2)**.

CHAPTER 3

Test Taking Skills Comment

Options A and C are not the Best Option **(SB A.1.2)** because they do not address the key word 'immediately' as well as option D does. Options B and C are also Complex Sounding Option(s) **(SB A.2.2)** as discussed previously.

This is also a Dichotomy of Options **(SB A.2.3)** as options A and B deal with hormone X and protein R and options C and D deal with protein P. With a Dichotomy of Options **(SB A.2.3)**, you must use

your Basic Knowledge (study, passage, general knowledge) **(SB A.2.2)** to determine which half of the dichotomy is correct. In this question, the passage provides the information. Since protein P is involved in the final step, it would make most logic that if it was altered in some way, that this would be most 'immediate' reason why calcium transport would stop.

Q119 — Pre-Study Suggestions

Review the following if needed:
1) Mutations **BIO 16.3**
2) Dichotomy of Options **SB A.2.3**
3) What piece(s) of information are important from the passage?
4) Solve the problem.

Solution Discussion

The key pieces of information are found in paragraph 2:

Item 3:

"Protein R was smaller than … normal in all other cells examined."

Item 5:

"When activated Protein R was … Family 1, but not Family 2."

Option A is incorrect. Item 5 suggests that the defect in Family 2 is in protein P and not protein R. Item 3 shows that R from Family 2 is normal in size but does not state it is abnormal. If the defect was, in fact, due to R, a single amino acid could have caused it (the mutation; **BIO 16.3**). A single amino acid replacement can result in a normal size protein, but a malfunctioning protein.

Option C is incorrect. See the previous discussion. If there was a premature stop codon **(BIO 3)**, the protein produced would be smaller than expected. This is typically non-functional. So, the protein would be smaller than expected and non-functional. This fits the description of the mutation possible for Family 1 which has an abnormal protein R.

Option D is incorrect. There is no evidence presented that hormone X is the problem in Family 2. If there was a premature stop codon, hormone X would be expected to be shorter than normal and dysfunctional. Also, hormone X, Item 2, is noted to bind to all protein R's.

Option B is correct. The data supports the proposition that the abnormal molecule in Family 2 is protein P - look at the previous items 3 and 5. Protein P is dysfunctional in Family 2 and one way the mutation could occur is by changing one of the amino acids.

Test Taking Skills Comment

Option D should be eliminated because there is not data to suggest there was any problem with hormone X (it bound to all R's). The correct answer is obtained by correctly assessing that the problem in Family 2 is not with the R but with the P as discussed above. Options C and D, as a Dichotomy of Options **(SB A.2.3)**, should be eliminated because a premature stop codon would result in shorter than expected protein - the protein in

family two is of normal size (for the R except for Family 1). You are not given information on the size of protein P in Family 2. This is why there is only one option for protein P. So, although, there is a dichotomy, it is not as helpful as usual. The key to this problem is to identify that the affected molecule in Family 2 is the protein P. Since there is only one option with protein P, that must be your answer.

CHAPTER 3

Q120 — Pre-Study Suggestions

Review the following if needed:

1) Blood Vessels **BIO 7.3**
2) Capillary Function **BIO 7.5.2**
3) Blood **BIO 7**
4) Camouflage and Distractions **SB A.1.3**
5) Three Out of Four type question **SB A.2.8**
6) Similar Pair Options **SB A.2.7**
7) Solve the problem.

Solution Discussion

Option A is incorrect. The immune response does not increase when a known protein or antigen is added/injected. Albumin **(BIO 7.5)** is a known antigen (actually known molecule) and would not elicit an immune response. If the protein was in anyway foreign and antigenic, then an immune response would be initiated.

Option B is incorrect. There may be a very small leakage of albumin into the tissues. Remember proteins do not normally cross the endothelium **(BIO 7.4)** of the capillaries. The albumin would be carried back to the veins and circulation via the lymphatic system **(BIO 7.6)**.

Option C is incorrect. This would not occur. The effect of added albumin, or any osmoregulatory protein (a protein which increases the oncotic pressure **(BIO 7.5.2)** of the circulation), is to increase the oncotic pressure inside the capillary and draw fluid back into the capillary.

to increase the oncotic pressure within the circulatory system. This shifts the balance in the capillary **(BIO 7.5.2)** such that the oncotic pressure will have a greater effect than the hydrostatic pressure and pull more fluid back into the capillary. The effect of more albumin is to move the balance point between HP and OP to left and result in an earlier influx of fluid into the capillary.

Option D is correct. The effect of added albumin which stays within the circulatory system is

Test Taking Skills Comment

You can only answer this question if you know the previous information. You should be able to eliminate option A. This is a mildly Camouflage and Distractions **(SB A.1.3)** question because the question is about the capillary dynamics **(BIO 7.5.2)** discussed in the link. You are supposed to know that proteins, especially albumin, result in the oncotic pressure which pulls fluid into the capillary.

This is also a Three Out of Four **(SB A.2.8)** type question as options B, C and D all deal with tissue effects. Option A is an outlier and outliers are usually incorrect. Options C and D are a reasonable Similar Pair Options **(SB A.2.7)** as they are part of the Three Out of Four **(SB A.2.8)** and are also a mirror image/similar pair.

CHAPTER 3

Q121   Pre-Study Suggestions

Review the following if needed:
1) Taxonomy **BIO 16.5**
2) Solve the problem.

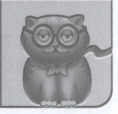

Solution Discussion

An understanding of the general concepts of taxonomy is needed to solve this problem.

Options A, C and D are incorrect. A class is a higher level in the sequence and can have a larger number of differing organisms. The higher the classification, i.e. toward the kingdom end, the less related any two organisms may be. The lower on the list, i.e. toward the genus, means the organisms must be more closely related and contains fewer.

Option B is correct. A genus would contain organisms which are very similar because it is lower in the list as discussed above. Learn the mnemonic in the link given for taxonomy **(BIO 16.5)**.

Test Taking Skills Comment

You can only answer this question if you know the previous information - this is why Study Knowledge **(SB A.2.2)** is still very important.

Q122 — Pre-Study Suggestions

Review the following if needed:
1) Imprinting **BIO 16**
2) Habituation **BIO 16**
3) Conditioning (learning) **BIO 16**
4) Discrimination (learning) **BIO 16**
5) Learning/Behavior **BIO 16**
6) Solve the problem.

Solution Discussion

Option B is incorrect. Habituation means the ducklings would be less likely to follow the large moving object if re-exposed to it repeatedly over time.

Option C is incorrect. Conditioning requires the pairing of some behavior or stimulus with some expected outcome. There is no pairing in this case.

Option D is incorrect. Discrimination is not a type of learning. The word has a number of different meanings. Probably in this case, it refers to the ability to distinguish between stimuli or options.

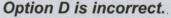

Option A is correct. Imprinting is a set behavior which begins during a critical period of time.

CHAPTER 3

Test Taking Skills Comment

You can only answer this question if you know the previous information - your Study Knowledge **(SB A.2.2)**.

Cyclohexane ring: when you have low energy, you sit down in a **"CHAIR"** to rest (stable). **"BOATS"** can be tippy, so they are less stable. **ORG 3.3**

Q123 — Pre-Study Suggestions

Review the following if needed:

1) Ring Strain **ORG 3.3**
2) Heat of Combustion (ΔH_c) **CHM 8.2, ORG 3.2.1**
3) Enthalpy (ΔH) **CHM 8.4**
4) Combustion Reactions **CHM 8.2, ORG 3.2.1**
5) Camouflage and Distractions **SB A.1.3**
6) Solve the problem.

Solution Discussion

Options A, B and D are incorrect. Each of these rings **(ORG 3.3)** has more strain than the cyclohexane and will have higher heats of combustion.

Option C is correct. The cyclohexane has the lowest heat of combustion because it has the lowest ring strain.

Test Taking Skills Comment

You can only answer this question if you know the previous information. This is a Camouflage and Distractions (**SB A.1.3**)

and you can rephrase the question. What is being asked is which ring has the lowest ring strain.

Q124 — Pre-Study Suggestions

Review the following if needed:
1) Nucleophiles **ORG 1.6, 4.2.1, 5.2, 6.2.3**
2) Lewis Bases **CHM 3.4**
3) Aromatic Compounds **ORG 5** (N.B. previous knowledge of Aromatics is no longer required for the new MCAT CBT)
4) Resonance in Organic Chemistry **ORG 1.4**
5) Inductive Effects **ORG 9.6**
6) Steric Effects in Nucleophilic Reactions **ORG 6.2.3**
7) Dichotomy of Options **SB A.2.3**
8) Best Option **SB A.1.2**
9) Solve the problem.

Solution Discussion

You are told this question is about nucleophiles (**ORG 1.6, 6.2.3**). So, you have to recall your Study Knowledge (**SB A.2.2**) of nucleophiles. The key to a nucleophile is the presence of a free pair of electrons. This means a nucleophile must be a Lewis base (**CHM 3.4**). The more available and polarizable (less held by the atom) the electrons, the better is the The

nucleophile. steric effects are more important for the target of the nucleophile as in nucleophilic substitution reactions (**ORG 6.2.3**). So, molecules with a free pair of electrons on a larger molecule and without strong inductive or resonance effects (**ORG 9.6, 1.4**) decreasing the availability of the electron pair will be stronger nucleophiles.

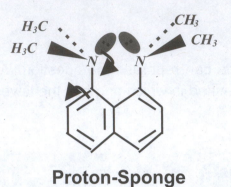

Proton-Sponge

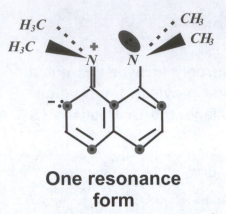

**One resonance
form**

There are certainly steric effects in this molecule but primary, secondary and tertiary **(ORG 3.1)** amines **(ORG 11)** are still good nucleophiles. The key to the strength of the nucleophile is the availability of the electron pair. Aromatic rings **(ORG 5)** do have an inductive effect **(ORG 9.6)** and will withdraw electron density away from the nitrogen electron pair through the sigma bonds **(ORG 1.3)**. This will make the electrons less available and will decrease the nucleophilic

strength of the nitrogens. But, the main effect by the aromatic rings is the resonance effect **(SB ORG 1.4)**, through the pi bonds **(ORG 1.3)**, on the free pair of electrons as shown above. Only one resonance form is drawn, but the negative charge of the pair of electrons will be delocalized to each of the carbons with the blue dot on the second structure. This is a significant removal of electron density and availability of electrons to act as a Lewis base or as a nucleophile.

Option A is incorrect. The molecule shown is not a strong base **(CHM 6.1-6.6)**. amines **(ORG 11)** are the bases of organic chemistry, but they are weak bases **(CHM 6.1-6.6)**. The presence of the electron withdrawal by induction and resonance as discussed above means the compound is an even weaker base than usual.

Option B is incorrect. The electrons on the nitrogen have a significantly decreased electron density as discussed above.

Option D is incorrect. This may have some effect. But major steric effects on nucleophilic attack is the steric effects of the substrate **(ORG 6.2.3)**, the target of the nucleophile. This is a possible option but not the Best Option **(SB A.1.2)**.

Option C is correct. This is the Best Option **(SB A.1.2)** of the ones given as discussed above.

Test Taking Skills Comment

When two or more option(s) are correct, you have to determine which is the Best Option **(SB A.1.2)**. This means you have to look at the question carefully and determine which factor is the most important. For this problem, it is the availability of the electron pair which is the most important determinant of nucleophilic strength. This is why option C is better than option D.

This is also a Dichotomy of Options **(SB A.2.3)**. The dichotomy is either 'yes' or 'no' for the compound being a good electrophile. Besides the analysis given above for each option, if you knew that the possible steric effect and especially the electronic effect would make the compound a poorer nucleophile than the parent amine, you would select the 'no' half and pick your answer from options C or D.

CHAPTER 3

Q125 — Pre-Study Suggestions

Review the following if needed:
1) Excretory System **BIO 10**
2) Dimensional Analysis **SB A.2.5**
3) Dichotomy of Options **SB A.2.3**
4) Complex Sounding Option(s) **SB A.2.2**
5) What piece(s) of information is important from the passage?
6) Solve the problem.

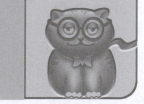

Solution Discussion

The key pieces of information are found in paragraph 2:

"tubular transport maximum (T_m)"

"The T_m is the maximum rate … can be reabsorbed by the kidney."

Option A is incorrect. The passage does not directly talk about the 'rate of concentration'. This term would have to take the form of (mass/volume)/time. The Tm is mass/time; these are two different units. This is inconsistency of dimensions **(SB A.2.5)**. The passage talks about filtration rate but this term is also not directly defined. The Figure 1 only shows the concentration of the plasma and of the urine of substances but no rate is shown. This option is a Complex Sounding Option(s) **(SB A.2.2)**, because the option(s) is not determinable from your Basic Knowledge (study, passage, general knowledge) **(SB A.2.2)**.

Option B is incorrect. See the discussion of option A.

Option D is incorrect. You should know that the bladder **(BIO 10)** has nothing to do with the filtration, secretion and reabsorption processes by the kidney **(BIO 10)**. It is simply a storage tank until emptying to the outside occurs. There is no further processing of the urine in the bladder.

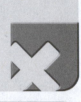

Option C is correct. The T_m is noted to be the tubular transport maximum, so you should expect the tubules to be involved in the process. Then the definition is the maximal rate of reabsorption by the tubules which would be the kidney's capacity.

Test Taking Skills Comment

This question is a matter of interpreting the information provided which is straightforward from the passage. This is as much a simple reading passage as a science passage. You should eliminate options A and B because of unit differences which make them incongruous with T_m. Option D makes no anatomic or physiologic sense.

There is an inconsistency of dimensions **(SB A.2.5)** as discussed for options A and B.

This is Complex Sounding Option(s) **(SB A.2.2)** for options A and B as discussed above.

This is a Dichotomy of Options **(SB A.2.3)** with one set being A and B, for rate of concentration, and the other being C and D, for capacity. This could be tricky to pick because the T_m is defined as a 'maximum rate of transport (mg/min)'. If you are not careful, you may select A or B because of the 'rate of concentration' noted. But as discussed above, a rate of concentration would have to have concentration/time which is not the same as mg/min, which is a mass/time. If you are not certain about which half of the dichotomy to pick based on your Basic Knowledge (study, passage, general knowledge) **(SB A.2.2)**, then you should not use the Dichotomy of Options **(SB A.2.3)** skill.

Q126   Pre-Study Suggestions

Review the following if needed:
1) Excretory System **BIO 10**
2) Three Out of Four type question **SB A.2.8**
3) What piece(s) of information is (are) important from the passage?
4) Solve the problem.

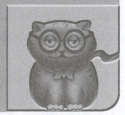

Solution Discussion

No prior information is needed to solve this problem.

The key pieces of information are found in paragraph 2:

"tubular transport maximum (T_m)"

"The T_m is the maximum rate … can be reabsorbed by the kidney."

"The T_m for glucose averages 320 mg/min in an adult human."

Options B, C and D are incorrect. The T_m means the maximal load presented to the tubules which will be completely reabsorbed by the

tubules. If the T_m is 320mg/min, this means that all loads of glucose filtered up to 320 mg/min will be completely reabsorbed by the tubules. For glucose to appear in the urine, the amount presented to the kidneys must exceed 320 mg/min.

Option A is correct. Since the load presented to the tubules is less than the T_m, no glucose will appear in the urine.

Test Taking Skills Comment

This question is a matter of interpreting the information provided which is straightforward from the passage. This is as much a simple reading passage as a science passage.

This is a Three Out of Four **(SB A.2.8)** type question with options B, C and D being similar. In this case, the outlier, option A, is the correct one. Generally, the outlier and options that are no change or zero are incorrect; in the rare occasions they are correct, you just want to be sure they are.

Q127

Pre-Study Suggestions

Review the following if needed:
1) Kidney **BIO 6.3, 10**
2) Blood Pressure on the Kidney Function **BIO 10.3**
3) Role of ADH in Kidney and Fluid Function **BIO 10**
4) Dichotomy of Options **SB A.2.3**
5) Similar Pair Options **SB A.2.7**
6) Internal Inconsistency of Options **SB A.2.5**
7) What piece(s) of information are important from the passage?
8) Solve the problem.

Solution Discussion

The key pieces of information are:

From paragraph one:

  "Plasma clearance refers to ... a substance from the plasma."

From paragraph two:

  "Plasma clearance is affected ... will begin to appear in the urine."

The blood pressure and blood volume help to determine the filtration rate of the kidney **(BIO 10.3)**. The higher either one is, the greater the amount of filtered blood at the glomerulus. This means as blood pressure or blood volume increases, a greater filtered load is presented to the tubules of the kidney. The reverse occurs for a low blood pressure or low blood volume. So, when the blood pressure is low, the mass of substance presented to the tubules will decrease (decreased mg/min). This means it is more likely for the tubules to clear the urine of the substance and more is reabsorbed back into the plasma and there is less plasma clearance of the substance.

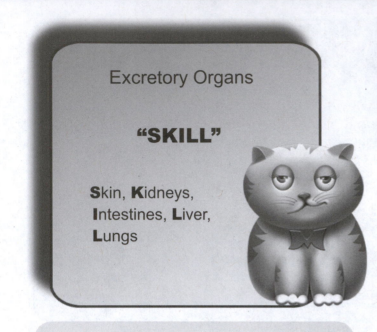

Excretory Organs

"SKILL"

Skin, **K**idneys,
Intestines, **L**iver,
Lungs

is lower. This is an Internal Inconsistency of Options **(SB A.2.5)**.

Option D is incorrect. The ADH will be high, but this by itself does not best explain the reason for the decrease. In fact, as ADH increases, the blood volume will increase. As blood volume increases, the filtered load will increase delivering more of the substance to the kidney and this might cause an increased plasma clearance and not a decreased.

Option A is incorrect. This statement is a True Statement **(SB A.2.2)**, in and of itself, because an increased concentration in the urine would be consistent with a greater plasma clearance as one of the possibilities. But, it is not Correct **(SB A.2.2)**, because a lowered blood pressure would not result in a greater filtered load to be excreted.

Option C is correct. The effect of a lowered BP results in a lowered filtered load. If the load is lower, there can be more complete reabsorption of the filtered load. This would result in less of the substance being cleared from the plasma and means there would be less in the urine as well.

Option B is incorrect. The ADH levels will tend to be higher and not lower when the blood pressure

Test Taking Skills Comment

This is a difficult question which requires a sophisticated understanding of renal physiology as discussed. With some basics, option B should be eliminated as noted. The others are difficult to sort out unless the physiology is understood as discussed. I would consider this a Guess Question **(SB A.2.4)**.

This is an Internal Inconsistency of Options **(SB A.2.5)** for option B and also for D as discussed previously.

This is also a Dichotomy of Options **(SB A.2.3)** with A and B being an increase and options C and D being a decrease. Since a dichotomy requires the use of Basic Knowledge (study, passage, general knowledge) **(SB A.2.2)** to determine which half of the dichotomy is correct, this may be very difficult to do in this question. When is not obvious based on your basic knowledge which half of the dichotomy is correct, it is best not to use this skill. If you did remember from your study knowledge that decreased blood pressure would decrease the filtered load, then you could select C or D for your guess.

You could also evaluate this as a Similar Pair Options **(SB A.2.7)** with options B and D both having ADH. But, remember to be very careful when more than one similar pair is present, which is always the case in dichotomy questions, and when other skills are also evident.

Q128   Pre-Study Suggestions

Review the following if needed:
1) Graphs and Charts **GS A.3**
2) Dichotomy of Options **SB A.2.3**
3) Internal Inconsistency of Options **SB A.2.5**
4) Mutually Excluding Options **SB A.2.6**
5) What piece(s) of information are important from the passage?
6) Solve the problem.

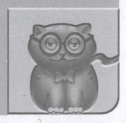

CHAPTER 3

Biological Sciences PASSAGE 3.BS.V

Solution Discussion

The key pieces of information from the passage are:

"tubular transport maximum (T_m)"

"The T_m is the maximum rate … can be reabsorbed by the kidney."

And the Figure 1:

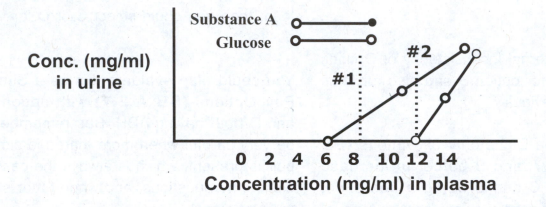

Option A is incorrect. The slope **(GS A.3)** of the line for glucose is greater than the slope for substance A. This is an Internal Inconsistency of Options **(SB A.2.5)**. If this is not clear, review the information on graphs. Also, the slope does not give a rate of clearance value. The slope is the change in the vertical axis divided by the change in the horizontal axis. This gives the concentration in urine over the concentration in plasma which would be a unitless quantity. A rate would have to have a time factor in the denominator. This is also an Inconsistency of Dimensions **(SB A.2.5)**. *See* option D for further discussion.

Option C is incorrect. This is precisely the reason the glucose will be cleared at a slower rate. The T_m of Substance A is reached first and it will be removed from the plasma and appear in the urine first. This is an Internal Inconsistency of Options **(SB A.2.5)** which is determined by understanding the definition of T_m and the Graph **(GS A.3)** in Figure 1.

Option D is incorrect. *See* the discussion in option A. Option A stated the slope of Substance A is higher than glucose. This option states the slope of glucose is lower than that of substance A. These

are identical statements. They are Mutually Excluding Options **(SB A.2.6)**. These types of options are not common, but when you can recognize them, you eliminate two options immediately.

Option B is correct. Since the T_m of the substance A is lower than that of glucose, Substance A will appear in the urine first. At line #1, the concentrations given in the problem, it is clear that only Substance A is appearing in the urine. No glucose is being removed from the plasma. Glucose would not begin to appear in the urine until line #2 plasma concentration is reached.

Test Taking Skills Comment

The reasoning is as discussed previously.

See the previous discussions in options A, C and D for Internal Inconsistency of Options **(SB A.2.5)** and Mutually Excluding Options **(SB A.2.6)**.

This is also a Dichotomy of Options **(SB A.2.3)** as options A and B have Substance A and options C and D have glucose. In a dichotomy, you must use Basic Knowledge (study, passage, general knowledge) **(SB A.2.2)** to select the correct half. Passage

CHAPTER 3

knowledge here tells you that a substance will not be cleared from the plasma until its filtration rate exceeds its T_m. Since this is only possible for Substance A, your answer must come from A or B.

Q129 — Pre-Study Suggestions

Review the following if needed:

1) Excretory System **BIO 10**
2) Graphs and Charts **GS A.3**
3) Three Out of Four Type question **SB A.2.8**
4) What piece(s) of information are important from the passage?
5) Solve the problem.

Solution Discussion

The key pieces of information from the passage are:

"tubular transport maximum (T_m)"

"The T_m is the maximum rate ... reabsorbed by the kidney."

And the Figure 1:

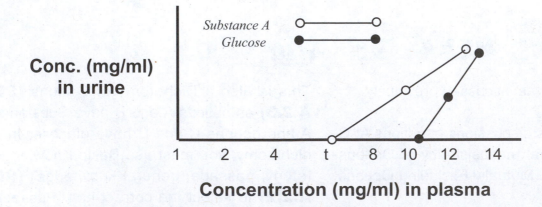

Options A, C and D are incorrect. The T_m will correspond to the plasma concentration at which the substance first appears in the urine. For the glucose, none of these are correct. For A, the glucose has not even appeared in the urine. For C and D, the glucose has already appeared in the urine.

reabsorption of the substance from the urine. When this maximum is exceeded, the substance appears in the urine. So, the value of T_m would correspond to the plasma concentration at which the substance first appeared in the urine. From Figure 1 for glucose, this is 10 mg/mL. For the substance A, the T_m would correspond to the value of 6 - 7 mg/mL.

Option B is correct. The T_m represents the maximal rate of

Test Taking Skills Comment

The reasoning is as discussed previously. This could be a Three Out of Four (**SB A.2.8**) type question, although a weak one.

Options B, C and D are all greater than 10. Option A is less than 10 and is the outlier. Outliers are usually incorrect.

Q130 Pre-Study Suggestions

Review the following if needed:
1) Kidney Function **BIO 6.3, 10**
2) Hormonal Effects on Fluids/Kidney **BIO 10**
3) Effect of Blood Pressure on Kidney Function **BIO 10.3**
4) What piece(s) of information are important from the passage?
5) Solve the problem.

Solution Discussion

The description of Experiment 2 is found in the passage, but this is not even required to solve the problem. There is enough information in the question itself to solve it.

Option B is incorrect. The T_m is a relatively fixed characteristic of the substance and the tubules are not directly affected by blood pressure. Certainly the T_m is affected by hormones and other substances like aldosterone and ADH, e.g. you are not given any data to evaluate this.

Option C is incorrect. Water reabsorption is increased by ADH, but this effect is in the collecting ducts **(BIO 10)**. Most of the reabsorption of other substances occurs before the collecting ducts and are not directly affected by ADH.

Option D is incorrect. The purpose of the Loop of Henle (LOH) **(BIO 10)** is to help maintain the osmolar gradient of the medulla to regulate the reabsorption of water and it is not directly concerned with absorption of other substances other than NaCl. ADH does not directly affect the LOH ion transport.

Option A is correct. The elevated blood pressure increases the glomerular filtration rate which increases the filtered load of substance A. This means more will be available for filtering and the T_m may be exceeded and the remainder will appear in the urine.

Test Taking Skills Comment

This question does require a good understanding of the workings of the renal system and hormones and blood pressure as discussed. It is clear this is a very difficult question, as the number of students who got it correct was barely above the guess rate.

Q131 — Pre-Study Suggestions

Review the following if needed:
1) Complex Sounding Option(s) **SB A.2.2**
2) Similar Pair Options **SB A.2.7**
3) What piece(s) of information are important from the passage?
4) Solve the problem.

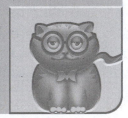

Solution Discussion

No prior knowledge is required to answer this question.

No specific information is found in the passage.

Option B is incorrect. Males and females contain the same number and types of bones. This should be something you know from your General Knowledge **(SB A.2.2)**.

Option C is incorrect. This cannot be determined from the passage. You can either recall this information or determine, since it was not discussed in the passage, it is not something you are expected to know either way. Both of these are weak arguments. It would have been best to know the basics of calcium metabolism and that for absorption, there are not major differences between males and females. This is a Complex

Sounding Option(s) **(SB A.2.2)**, because the question cannot be answered with Basic Knowledge (study, passage, general knowledge) **(SB A.2.2)**.

production which are apparently equal. This is also a Complex Sounding Option(s) **(SB A.2.2)** as in option C.

Option D is incorrect. This is found in the passage as noted above. The passage does not note any difference between the sexes. It notes that both sexes have age related declines in vitamin D

Option A is correct. It is General Knowledge **(SB A.2.2)** that women have less dense bones than men. Since the bones are thinner, they have less reserve to protect them when bone loss begins.

Test Taking Skills Comment

There will be questions which rely upon your General Knowledge **(SB A.2.2)**. Fortunately these are rare as most questions will either require prior specific knowledge or have adequate information in the passage to solve the problem. This is really an in between problem. Also, this is one of those questions which will test your ability to determine the limits of what you should know from your studies. For options C and D, you would have to know some fairly specific details about calcium and vitamin D metabolism and physiology. The AAMC MCAT manual does not require this. If you are not required to bring these details to the test, then the only way you can know them

is to have the details given in the passage. These are Complex Sounding Option(s) **(SB A.2.2)**. Your ability to distinguish between required science and extreme science will help you eliminate options such as C and D above. To do this, you must have prepared well and be confident in your preparation.

Similar Pair Options **(SB A.2.7)** are present as options C and D. If you did not have a clue, it would be reasonable to guess C or D. Remember that these test skills are not 100%, but on the average you will come out better than the 25% baseline guess. But, this is weak because it is based on 'less efficient' which is soft and is a pure guess. Your

Complex Sounding Option(s) **(SB A.2.2)** are based on logic and knowledge and should take precedence. So you would eliminate options C and D.

Q132 — Pre-Study Suggestions

Review the following if needed:
1) Effects of Estrogen in Women **BIO 6.3, 14.1**
2) Female Anatomy **BIO 14.1**
3) Menstrual Cycle **BIO 14.3**
4) What piece(s) of information are important from the passage?
5) Solve the problem.

Solution Discussion

There is nothing from the passage which will help solve the problem.

Option A is incorrect. Breast development is one of the effects of estrogen. By replacing estrogen, the breasts should be maintained and not atrophy.

Option B is incorrect. Estrogen is needed for vaginal wall integrity and secretions. In menopause, one of the problems is a fragile vaginal wall and dryness. Estrogens are added to increase integrity of the wall and lubrication.

Option D is incorrect. Estrogens do not cause the milk production. They allow breast growth and development. It is prolactin, from the anterior pituitary, which results in milk production. Oxytocin, from the posterior pituitary, allows 'milk letdown'.

Option C is correct. Post-menopausal women often hesitate in taking estrogen/progesterone combinations because of the return of menstrual periods.

CHAPTER 3

Biological Sciences   PASSAGE 3.BS.VI

Test Taking Skills Comment

There is nothing from the passage to solve this problem. If you do not know the functions of estrogens in females, you will not get this problem correct except by guessing.

Q133 Pre-Study Suggestions

Review the following if needed:
1) Calcium Metabolism **BIO 7.5**
2) Growth Hormone **BIO 6.3.1**
3) Thyroid Hormone **BIO 6.3.3**
4) What piece(s) of information are important from the passage?
5) Solve the problem.

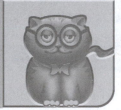

Solution Discussion

Option A is incorrect. Although GH may affect bones, its levels are not directly affected by calcium.

Option B is incorrect. Calcitonin is stimulated by high calcium levels.

Option C is incorrect. Thyroid hormone is not regulated by calcium levels. It is noteworthy, beyond the scope of the MCAT, that hyperthyroidism is associated with osteoporosis.

Option D is correct. PTH is inhibited by high serum calcium and stimulated by low serum calcium.

Test Taking Skills Comment

There are no tricks. You either have the knowledge or you guess. There is nothing in the passage which will help you:

Q134 — Pre-Study Suggestions

Review the following if needed:
1) Similar Pair Options **SB A.2.7**
2) What piece(s) of information are important from the passage?
3) Solve the problem.

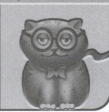

Solution Discussion

The pieces of information from the passage are found in paragraph 2:

"Aging-related abnormalities in parathyroid ... to estrogen deficiency"

And in paragraph 3:

"Currently, hormone replacement ... estrogen therapy."

Options A, B and D are incorrect.
In men the only factors identified are the PTH, calcitonin and vitamin D. Estrogens are not identified as a key player in the decline in bone mass in men. The paragraph only identifies estrogen as being important in women. The individual

is receiving estrogen therapy and would be expected to have an increased level of bone at any rate - this means option A would be definitely eliminated. It is possible, based on the information, to consider option B seriously because estrogen replacement decreases the risk in women, but estrogen is not identified as a critical factor in males. Option D would be less likely because of the protective effect of estrogen supported by the passage and again that estrogen is not identified

as a factor in males. Generally, longer more complicated appearing options/explanations will be incorrect.

Option C is correct. Since estrogen is not identified as a key factor of bone loss in men, its decline or increase should not affect what happens in men.

Test Taking Skills Comment

This is a very difficult question. You have to rely on the fact that you have done a good preparation and do recall what you are supposed to know regarding the pertinent endocrinology. This means you do not have to know all the intricacies of estrogen effects in males. Therefore, you must base your answer on the information in the passage and do not have to recall some minutia of information from your study. Then using the information in the passage, you can reach the best answer. Option A can be eliminated as discussed previously. Option D should be eliminated for the same reason, all you know is that estrogen replacement can

decrease the risk of osteoporosis in women, so the disease should appear at a later age, because he is receiving estrogen, rather than earlier age. This leaves options B and C. You have no information that males have any effect either way from the female hormone, estrogen. This is a guess question.

This could also be a Similar Pair Options **(SB A.2.7)** as options C and D both have 'approximately the same'. If you guessed from these two, your guess percentage would be better than the percentage of all students on the question as only 35% of all students got it correct.

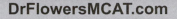

Q135   Pre-Study Suggestions

Review the following if needed:
1) Bone **BIO 11.3**
2) Dichotomy of Options **SB A.2.3**
3) Internal Inconsistency of Options **SB A.2.5**
4) What piece(s) of information are important from the passage?
5) Solve the problem.

Solution Discussion

The key piece of information is from the first sentence in the first paragraph:

"*Osteoporosis is a pathological … person's bone mass*".

Option A is incorrect. Increased osteoblast would increase bone mass, and decreased osteoclast would increase bone mass which would result in more bone. This option is Internal Inconsistency of Options **(SB A.2.5)** with the information given in the stem.

Option B is incorrect. Increased osteoblast would increase bone

mass, and increased osteoclast would decrease bone mass, which would result in an indeterminate state. This is an Internal Inconsistency of Options **(SB A.2.5)**.

Option C is incorrect. Decreased osteoblast would decrease bone mass, and decreased osteoclast would increase bone mass which would result in an indeterminate state of bone change. This is an Internal Inconsistency of Options **(SB A.2.5)**.

CHAPTER 3

Option D is correct. Decreased osteoblast would decrease bone mass, and increased osteoclast would decrease bone mass which would result in less bone as found in osteoporosis.

Test Taking Skills Comment

This is totally from the passage and is analyzed as previously shown. Most students got it correct. As noted previously, this question is another example of Internal Inconsistency of Options **(SB A.2.5)**.

It is also a Dichotomy of Options **(SB A.2.3)** type question. The correct answer must contain decreased osteoblast and/or increased osteoclast activity to decrease bone mass. The correct dichotomies to pick are decreased osteoblast, which are options C and D, and increased osteoclast activity which are options B and D. Since this is double dichotomy, by picking the common option of the dichotomy, which is D, you should have your answer. But, the Internally Inconsistent **(SB A.2.5)** as discussed above are knowledge based and should take precedence, but both lead to only one option as possible because they use similar logic/knowledge. This reinforces your choice.

Q136   Pre-Study Suggestions

Review the following if needed:
1) Carbonyl Group **ORG 7.1**
2) Aldol Condensation **ORG 7.2.4**
3) What is the structure and molecular weight of acetone?
4) What piece(s) of information is important from the passage?
5) Solve the problem.

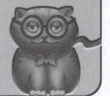

Solution Discussion

The structure of acetone is (information in paragraph 1 from passage):

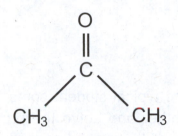

Its molecular weight is 58 g/mole

= 3x12 + 1x16 + 6x1

= 36 + 16 + 6

= 58.

Other important information from the passage is from the structure isolated and paragraph 1 (*see* previous structure):

"*NaOH in the solvent acetone [(CH3)2CO]*"

"*a small amount of Product A (shown below).*"

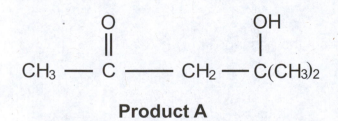

Product A

"*The chemist determined that Product A ... self-condensation of acetone.*"

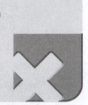

Options A, C and D are incorrect. See the following.

Option B is correct. This could be determined by using the passage only or by understanding the aldol condensation **(ORG 7.2.4)**. From the previous discussion and studying the reactions shown, it should be evident that in the formation of the beta-hydroxy intermediate, that no atoms are lost in the reaction step. This means the beta-hydroxy alcohol contains twice the number of atoms of the original compound and its molecular mass will be twice that of the original compound. If the beta-hydroxy intermediate has a molecular weight of 144, then the original molecule must have been 1/2 of that or 72. Based on the paragraph above, you should be able to determine that the Product A is exactly twice the molecular mass of the acetone as shown previously. Then you should assess that

CHAPTER 3

the same holds for the molecule discussed in this question.

Test Taking Skills Comment

This is totally from the passage and is analyzed as previously shown. But by knowing the aldol condensation, the solution should be even more evident and easier. This is a situation in which the test makers will argue that the answer can be derived from the passage without any prior knowledge, which is correct. But the missing point is that it will take the typical student some 'time' to put this together and solve the problem in the absence of that prior knowledge. With a decent understanding of the knowledge behind the problem, an understanding of the aldol condensation, the process is much quicker and less stressful. Adverse stress and time constraints will lower test scores.

Q137 — Pre-Study Suggestions

Review the following if needed:
1) Aldol Condensation **ORG 7.2.4**
2) Le Chatelier Principle **CHM 9.9**
3) Similar Pair Options **SB A.2.7**
4) Camouflage and Distractions **SB A.1.3**
5) Internally Inconsistent **SB A.2.5**
6) What piece(s) of information are important from the passage?
7) Solve the problem.

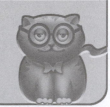

Solution Discussion

The full equation is:

$$2\ acetone \underset{\longleftarrow}{\overset{NaOH}{\longrightarrow}} Product\ A$$

No other information is given to you nor derivable by you.

Option A is incorrect. Catalysis has no effect on equilibrium. Catalysts determine the rate of the reaction. This is Internally Inconsistent **(SB A.2.5)** and should be eliminated.

Option B is incorrect. Same as option A.

Option D is incorrect. You are given no information to assess the effect of temperature. If you were given the energy of the reaction, you could answer this question as true or false. As it stands you cannot even address it. If acetone was boiling away, it could not react and would pull the reaction to the left.

Option C is correct. If Product A is removed, this is the same as decreasing it. The equilibrium is shifted to the side of the decrease and more Product A will be formed.

Test Taking Skills Comment

See the previous analysis. Remember, whenever you have an equilibrium condition and are asked to determine shifts or the effects of perturbations to it, use the Le Chatelier Principle **(CHM 9.9)** as a first attempt to solve it. Also, very importantly, Le Chatelier is classified as a Physical Sciences concept, yet it is very appropriate for use here. This is why links to all other subjects are provided in this review.

This is a Camouflage and Distractions type

question **(SB A.1.3)** because you were not told to use Le Chatelier but you were given the conditions which should alert you to use the Le Chatelier Principle.

This is a Similar Pair Options **(SB A.2.7)** if you truly have to guess. Options A and B are similar enough to choose one of them without any other information. As you can see, if you don't have adequate knowledge, which would eliminate options A and B as a similar pair, guessing is still guessing. Overall, the use of the test skill of similar pair will give you a better guess rate than 25%. Always go with knowledge, when available, over a true guess skill. *See* the previous Internally Inconsistent **(SB A.2.5)** discussion.

Q138   Pre-Study Suggestions

Review the following if needed:
1) Stoichiometry **CHM 1.5**
2) Chemical Formulas/Structures **CHM 1.5**
3) Internal Inconsistency of Options **SB A.2.5**
4) Three Out of Four type question **SB A.2.8**
5) What piece(s) of information are important from the passage?
6) Solve the problem.

Solution Discussion

The key pieces of information are observations 1 and 2:

"consisted only of carbon, hydrogen and oxygen."

"Molecular weight of 116 g/mole."

Since option A does not contain O, it is eliminated. Since the other 3 options all contain C, H and O, then the issue is the molecular mass of 116. Whichever has this mass is the potential product. The masses of options B, C and D are:

option B: $= 2 \times 16 + 7 \times 12 + 14 \times 1$
$= 32 + 84 + 14$
$= 32 + 98$
$= 130.$

option C: = 1x16 + 6x12 + 12x1
                 = 16 + 72 + 12
                 = 16 + 84
                 = 100.

option D: = 2x16 + 6x12 + 12x1
                 = 32 + 72 + 12
                 = 32 + 84
                 = 116.

Options B and C are incorrect. Each has the wrong molecular mass.

Option D is correct. Has the correct molecular mass and contains C, O and H.

Option A is incorrect. Does not contain oxygen and is an Internal Inconsistency of Options **(SB A.2.5)** type question and does not have the right molecular mass.

Cis/trans (Geometric) Isomers
"**Z**: **Z**ame **Z**ide,
E: **E**pposite"
Z for same side and **E** for opposite sides **ORG 2.3.4**

Test Taking Skills Comment

Notice, you could have also solved this by comparing the atoms in Product A with each of the options. Since the only option with 6 carbons, 2 oxygens and 2 H's lost to saturation **(ORG 12.4)** (a double bond or ring), as in Product A, you would select option D.

This is a Three Out of Four **(SB A.2.8)** type question. Options B, C and D are similar in having oxygen in them. Option A is an outlier with no oxygen. Outliers tend to be incorrect and can be ignored. Similar Pair Options **(SB A.2.7)** should not be used because there is more than one similar pair (options B and C with a straight chain and oxygen, and options B and D with two oxygens).

Q139   Pre-Study Suggestions

Review the following if needed:
1) Aldol Condensation **ORG 7.2.4**
2) Reactions of Double Bonds **ORG 4**
3) Dichotomy of Options **SB A.2.3**
4) Internal Inconsistency of Options **SB A.2.5**
5) What piece(s) of information are important from the passage?
6) What is the structure of Product B?
7) Solve the problem.

Solution Discussion

The key piece of information is from the last paragraph:

    "structure of Product A was ... dehydration product, Product B."

The structure of product B would be:

$$CH_3 - \overset{\overset{\displaystyle O}{\|}}{C} - CH_2 = C(CH_3)_2$$

Your basic study of carbonyls and aldol condensation **(ORG 7.2.4)** informs you that the preferred product in the aldol condensation is the conjugated **(ORG 1.3.1)** dehydration product. This means a double bond **(ORG 1.3.1)** is formed as shown. The bromine adds to the double bond and is decolorized from red to colorless in the dark.

Option A is incorrect. Product B does contain a double bond. This is Internal Inconsistency of Options **(SB A.2.5)**. Decolorization occurs if a double bond (aliphatic not aromatic) is present when bromine is added.

Option C is incorrect. Product B does contain a double bond.

Option D is incorrect. The solution will turn colorless as the bromine is added to the double bond. A situation in which a molecule will have a double bond but will not decolorize bromine is when the double bond(s) is aromatic **(ORG 5)**. This is Internal Inconsistency of Options **(SB A.2.5)**.

Option B is correct. When the aldol hydroxy ketone is dehydrated, the carbon containing the OH group forms a double bond with the adjacent carbon, therefore the molecule can undergo the addition of bromine.

Test Taking Skills Comment

This is a more difficult problem which requires you to combine several components of organic chemistry as discussed. This is really a Knowledge and Application **(SB A.2.2)** question and not a passage reading question. You should eliminate options A and D because they are Internal Inconsistency of Options **(SB A.2.5)** - one of the dichotomies you can use.

This is a Dichotomy of Options **(SB A.2.3)**. There is a double dichotomy present. If you know the compound B has a double bond and you would know this if you studied the aldol condensation reaction, then you would know options A and C are incorrect as one of the dichotomies (and either B or D is correct). And, since you know that bromine reacts with double bonds to go from red to colorless, you know options C and D are incorrect (and either A or B is correct). In a double dichotomy, if you know both dichotomies, the option common to both is the correct option which is option B.

Q140 — Pre-Study Suggestions

Review the following if needed:

1) NMR **ORG 14.2**
2) What piece(s) of information are important from the passage?
3) Solve the problem.

Solution Discussion

The key information from the passage is the formula and structure of acetone:

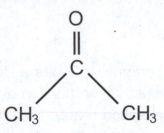

Option A is correct. The only issues are the peaks generated from acetone. Since all six hydrogens are equivalent, only one peak will be generated. This peak will not be split because there are no neighboring hydrogens to the methyl groups.

Options B, C and D are incorrect. All six of the hydrogens on the acetone are equivalent. Only one NMR peak will result (not counting splitting, which should not occur in this structure!).

Test Taking Skills Comment

This is a knowledge question about NMR. Notice that as usual, you are not asked to interpret an NMR spectrum. What you are quired to know are the basic principles and how they are applied to a given structure.

Q141 — Pre-Study Suggestions

Review the following if needed:
1) Carbonyl **ORG 7.1**
2) Three Out of Four type question **SB A.2.8**
3) What piece(s) of information are important from the passage?
4) What are the structures of acetone, Product A and Product B?
5) Solve the problem.

Solution Discussion

The key piece of information from the passage is from observation 4:

"Product A was a methyl ketone because it gave a positive iodoform test."

The structure of product A is in the passage. The other structures were discussed in previous questions and are as follows:

Options A, B and C are incorrect.
See the following.

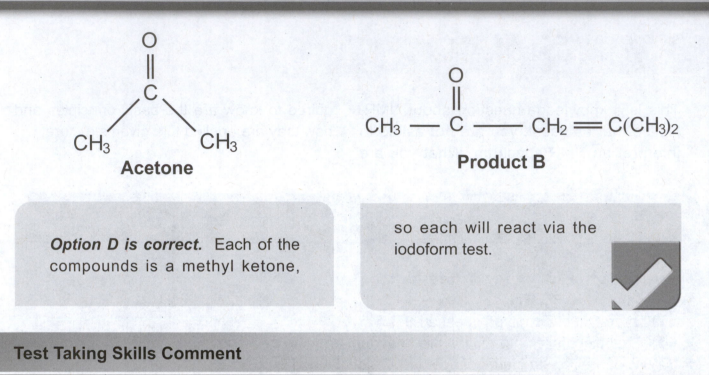

Acetone

Product B

Option D is correct. Each of the compounds is a methyl ketone,

so each will react via the iodoform test.

Test Taking Skills Comment

This is purely a passage question. It apparently was very difficult because only 40% of students got it correct. The iodoform reaction is given in the passage, so there is no reason not to know that. A possible problem could have been knowing what a methyl ketone was. If this is the case, you should review the structures and functional groups of organic molecules and familiarize yourself with them. Since the formula of acetone was given, one would be expected to be able to draw the structure from it and realize it is also a methyl ketone and would react. If you missed this, again, you need to restudy functional groups and structures and get more familiar with them. It would seem these two choices would be 'obvious' but they were not. If they were, even guessing between C and D, because A and B options would be eli-

minated would give 50% of students getting the answer correct.

The structure of Product B would be more difficult, but has been discussed in other questions. In general, spend time just familiarizing yourself with organic structures and terminology as this seems to be a general deficit. This could be viewed as a Three Out of Four **(SB A.2.8)** type question; options B, C and D all have multiple choices and option A is an outlier with only one choice. Generally, the outlier will be **incorrect**. This could also be a Similar Pair Options **(SB A.2.7)** with B and C as a similar pair, C and D as a similar pair, and B and D as a similar pair. Remember when you can identify more than one legitimate similar pair, it is best not to use the skill.

Q142 — Pre-Study Suggestions

Review the following if needed:
1) Cell Structure and Function **BIO 1**
2) Bacteria Structure **BIO 2.2**
3) Energy Metabolism **BIO 4.4-4.10**
4) Three Out of Four type question **SB A.2.8**
5) Camouflage and Distractions **SB A.1.3**
6) Similar Pair Options **SB A.2.7**
7) Internally Inconsistent **SB A.2.5**
8) Best Option **SB A.1.2**
9) Solve the problem.

Solution Discussion

Option A is incorrect. The cell wall **(BIO 2.2)** plays no role in metabolism, it is outside of the bacterial cell (that portion within the plasma membrane) itself.

Option B is incorrect. The ribosome **(BIO 1.2.1)** is the site of protein synthesis **(BIO 3)** using mRNA **(BIO 3)** as a template. Even though the ribosomes are different in prokaryotes and eukaryotes, the functions are still the same. This is Internally Inconsistent **(SB A.2.5)** based on your Study Knowledge **(SB A.2.2)**.

Option C is incorrect. A bacterium **(BIO 2.2)** does not have a nuclear membrane **(BIO 1.1)**. This is Internally Inconsistent **(SB A.2.5)**.

CHAPTER 3

Option D is correct. Even though this is not explicitly stated, by elimination this is the Best Option **(SB A.1.2)**.

Test Taking Skills Comment

The test is not trying to fool you or penalize you for your Basic Knowledge (study, passage, general knowledge) **(SB A.2.2)**. You are required to know that knowledge and not be afraid to apply it and go beyond it if asked and if logical. Your basic knowledge should eliminate options B and C as previously noted . Additionally, you should know the cell wall is an 'external appendage' of the bacterium and its purpose is for structure and osmotic protection and not metabolism. Even if you did not know the cell membrane was the site, it remained the Best Option **(SB A.1.2)** as the others were eliminated. Also, you know that oxidative phosphorylation in eukaryotes occurs in the mitochondrion **(BIO 1.2.1)** on its inner membrane, and the mitochondrion has some homology or is an 'ingested' bacterium.

This is also a Three Out of Four **(SB A.2.8)** type question as options A, C and D all deal with membrane like structures. Option B is an outlier, and outliers can usually be eliminated. Also, this is a legitimate Similar Pair Options **(SB A.2.7)** as options C and D are similar, since both refer to membrane and there are no other obvious similar pairs in the options.

Q143 — Pre-Study Suggestions

Review the following if needed:
1) Cell Organelles **BIO 1.2.1**
2) DNA **BIO 1.2.2, 15**
3) RNA **BIO 3**
4) Camouflage and Distractions **SB A.1.3**
5) Solve the problem.

Solution Discussion

Option B is incorrect. The Golgi **(BIO 1.2.1)** is involved with the processing of proteins and not RNA.

Option D is incorrect. The endoplasmic reticulum **(BIO 1.2.1)** is the site of synthesis of proteins, steroids and performs other functions, but RNA is not made there.

Option C is incorrect. The ribosomes **(BIO 1.2.1)** use mRNA and tRNA and rRNA **(BIO 3)** but do not incorporate UTP into any RNA. They are the site of protein synthesis **(BIO 3)**.

Option A is correct. All the nucleic acids **(BIO 1.2.2)**, in eukaryotes, are made in the nucleus **(BIO 1.2)** (neglecting the small amount made in mitochondria). The UTP is used by the nucleolus to make the RNA's.

CHAPTER 3

Test Taking Skills Comment

The knowledge and reasoning is as discussed previously.

This is a mildly Camouflage and Distractions **(SB A.1.3)** question typical of these types of questions. The real question being asked, that you rephrase the question to, is: what is the role of UTP and what contains it? The answer to this is RNA. Then you know that RNA is made from DNA in the nucleus by transcription **(BIO 3)**.

Q144 — Pre-Study Suggestions

Review the following if needed:
1) Protein Structure and Function **BIO 3, ORG 12.2**
2) Enzyme Function **BIO 4.1-4.3**
3) Complex Sounding Option(s) **SB A.2.2**
4) Camouflage and Distractions **SB A.1.3**
5) Solve the problem.

Solution Discussion

Option A is incorrect. Pepsin may be feedback inhibited. However, there is nothing provided in the passage to suggest that the substance causing this feedback inhibition will increase its presence or inhibition due to a drop in pH, which is the variable changing. Feedback inhibition means the product of the enzyme feeds back and stops the action of the enzyme. An external factor such as pH would just be an enzyme inhibition of some type.

Option B is incorrect. There is nothing presented to suggest that the lowering of pH decreases the synthesis of pepsin. This may or not occur; there is just no evidence to support it. This is a Complex Sounding Option(s) **(SB A.2.2)** because you have no Basic Knowledge (study, passage, general knowledge) **(SB A.2.2)** to determine if it is True or False **(SB A.1.2)**. Notice this is different than option A because you are supposed to have the study knowledge of what feedback inhibition is and what inhibitors of proteins are.

Option C is incorrect. The stability of the peptide (amide) bonds per se does not directly affect the catalysis. The catalysis is due to the catalytic site. The bonding here does not directly involve the peptide bonds which are the bonds between amino acids **(ORG 12.1)**. At any rate, how would pH make the peptide bond more stable? What evidence or knowledge do you have to support or refute this? There is no Basic Knowledge (study, passage, general knowledge) **(SB A.2.2)** for this so this is a Complex Sounding Option(s) **(A.2.2)** that you cannot assess either way. Therefore, it is incorrect. You should be aware of the amide bond **(ORG 14.1)** which includes the peptide bond.

Option D is correct. What you are expected to know is that each protein has an optimal range of function and one of the factors affecting this is the pH. Since the pH optimum is 1.5, any deviation up or down will decrease the activity and function of the protein. Proteins depend upon their protein structure (tertiary and quaternary) for function. Changes in variables like the temperature and pH can affect the tertiary/quaternary structures and function.

Test Taking Skills Comment

The MCAT does not require you to have advanced knowledge in a subject unless it is presented in passage or question. Knowing if options B or C are correct in relation to a pH change would be considered advanced knowledge and this is why these are Complex Sounding Option(s) **(SB A.2.2)**. Since no data is presented in the passage/ question to assess it, they cannot be correct options. Option D, on the other hand, takes basic knowledge about the structure of proteins and their functions, gives you some conditions and asks you to make the connection or inference. Option A is also within your basic knowledge as you are supposed to know what feedback inhibition means. This is well within the scope of your knowledge and is what the MCAT expects you to do.

This is also a Camouflage and Distractions

(**SB A.1.3**) question as you should rephrase it to get to the real question, which is knowing what affects the protein/enzyme and what the functions depend upon - i.e. tertiary and quaternary structures.

Q145 Pre-Study Suggestions

Review the following if needed:
1) Arrangement of Objects **GS A.1.4, SB A.2.9**
2) Camouflage and Distractions **SB A.1.3**
3) Solve the problem.

Solution Discussion

In this problem, you are given three amino acids which must be combined in a linear sequence and each may be used only one time. This is calculated as follows:

X = 3 and each is not reused and order is important. The number of ways these may be sequenced = 3 x 2 x 1 = 6.

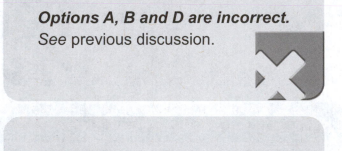

Options A, B and D are incorrect. *See* previous discussion.

Option C is correct. *See* previous discussion.

Test Taking Skills Comment

This problem has nothing of essence to do with the amino acids; they are mere x's and y's. The problem is testing your basic understanding of probability and combinations/permutations. This is why this is a Camouflage and Distractions **(SB A.1.3)** and you must rephrase or simplify it to basic probability problem as discussed.

Q146   Pre-Study Suggestions

Review the following if needed:
1) Meiosis **BIO 14.2**
2) Mitosis **BIO 1.3**
2) Camouflage and Distractions **SB A.1.3**
3) Complex Sounding Option(s) **SB A.2.2**
4) Internal Inconsistency of Options **SB A.2.5**
5) Solve the problem.

Solution Discussion

Option A is incorrect. The offspring could have 4n, 8n, etc. because of the lack of migration of chromosomes due to no spindles **(BIO 1.3)**. This could result in greater genetic variability **(BIO 15.5)** only because there are more copies of the same chromosomes.

This could depend on your interpretation of genetic variability. Review the link to clarify what genetic variability is.

Option C is incorrect. Cell walls are made from different proteins than tubulin. The spindle does not refer to the cell wall. Also, if the drug blocks the assembling of spindle microtubules, what is the effect on other microtubule assembling? You don't know. And, if there is excess tubulin, how do you know it would be used, if it was to be used, for this purpose? This option has problems with being Internally Inconsistent **(SB A.2.5)** and a Complex Sounding Option(s) **(SB A.2.2)** type question and should therefore be eliminated.

aspect of the cell. And how do you know the excess tubulin will be used for this purpose? You don't. This option is also a Complex Sounding Option(s) **(SB A.2.2)** and should be eliminated. It is potentially Internal Inconsistency of Options **(SB A.2.5)** because a drug that blocks tubulin assembly may not be selective enough not to block cilia/flagella assembly - you just don't have enough information to determine this.

Option D is incorrect. Movement may be related to tubulin like proteins as in cilia **(BIO 1.2)** and flagella **(BIO 1.2)**. This would result in poorer movement if these were not made but could result in more movement if they were. But again, spindles do not refer to this

Option B is correct. Spindle relates to the processes of cell division and mitosis and/or meiosis **(BIO 14.2)**. In either one, there will be a lack of movement of the chromosomes at anaphase. This will result in some cells with duplicate chromosomes or more.

Test Taking Skills Comment

In this problem, you must stick to the issue presented which is spindle microtubules. This should make you think of issues dealing with mitosis or meiosis.

This is a potential Similar Pair Options (**SB A.2.7**), but there are more than one similar pair present: options A and B are a similar pair as both relate to genetics/chromosomes, and options C and D are similar as both relate to excess tubulin. When more than one similar pair is identified, it is best not to use the skill.

There is also Internal Inconsistency of Options (**SB A.2.5**) and Complex Sounding Option(s) (**SB A.2.2**) as discussed previously.

MCAT biology often involves experiments so it's important to be able to identify the main components. For example, to determine the effect of a barking dog on the heart rate of cats, one group of cats would be exposed to that loud pest (experimental group)!

The researcher will then compare the average cat heart rate in the experimental group against another group of cats exposed to non-barking dogs (the control group).

All other variables, such as pet size and fleas, will remain the same for each group. So, generally, "treatment" is given to the experimental group but not to the control group.

GS C.1, C.2

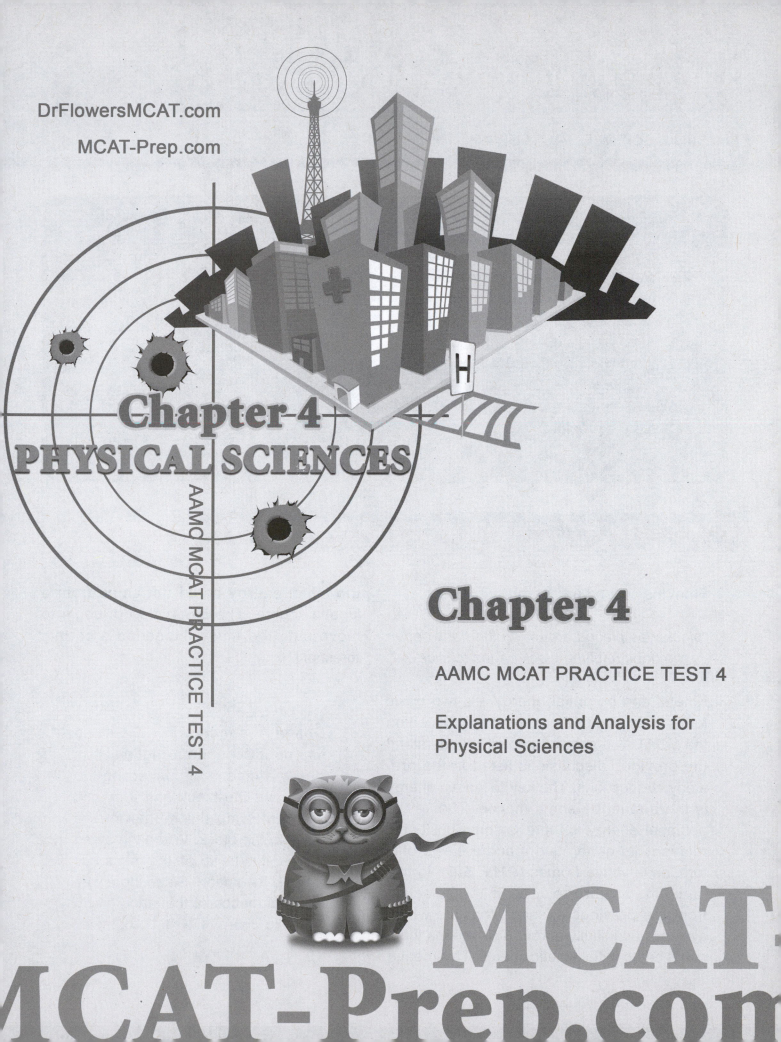

Chapter 4
PHYSICAL SCIENCES

AAMC MCAT PRACTICE TEST 4

Chapter 4

AAMC MCAT PRACTICE TEST 4

Explanations and Analysis for
Physical Sciences

MCAT-Prep.com

Q01 — Pre-Study Suggestions

Review the following if needed:

1) Kinetic Energy **PHY 5.3**
2) Potential Energy **PHY 5.4**
3) Conservation of Energy **PHY 5.5**
4) Dichotomy of Options **SB A.2.3**
5) Camouflage and Distractions **SB A.1.3**
6) What information is needed from the passage?
7) Solve the problem.

Solution Discussion

From the second paragraph:

"block was placed at rest on the flat wooden … the hook until the block began to slide …"

Kinetic and potential energy are two basic forms of energy that are commonly tested on the MCAT. You should thoroughly understand the previous discussions listed in the pre-study suggestions. The key to kinetic energy is there must be some motion. The key to potential energy is there is some positional relationship generating it and it exists only for Conservative Forces (**PHY 5.6**). In this problem, you are told, as in the selection from the previous passage that the whole system was initially at rest. This means there could be no initial kinetic energy. This means

the initial energy could not come from a kinetic source. The block did not begin to move until the mass exceeded a certain threshold.

Option A is incorrect. The string has no independent motion. It is simply a means of connecting the mass and the block and a means of transferring the motion of the mass to the block. When the string moves, it is because the mass has initiated its motion. Since there was no initial motion of the string giving it Kinetic Energy (**PHY 5.3**), there can be no transfer of its kinetic energy to the block.

Did you hear about the industrialist who had a huge chloroform spill at his factory?

His business went insolvent.

Option B is incorrect. The board does not move so it cannot have any kinetic energy at any time.

Option D is correct. The mass has a certain gravitational potential energy (U_B) at rest given by $m_M gh_{Mo}$, where m_M = mass of the mass, h_{Mo} = original height of the mass above the reference. As the m_M exceeds the forces holding the block in place it will begin to move downward and its height will now become equal to h_{M1}. Since h_{Mo} > h_{M1}, there is a change in potential energy of the mass (ΔU_M) of $m_M g(h_{Mo} - h_{M1})$. This loss of potential energy is converted to kinetic energy of the mass. The loss of potential energy of the mass is also the reason that the forces on the block are overcome and the block begins to move giving it kinetic energy. The moving mass has to overcome the Frictional Forces (**PHY 3.2**) on the block.

Option C is incorrect. The block does have gravitational Potential Energy (**PHY 5.4**) and this could be converted to kinetic energy. Gravitational potential energy (U) takes the form of $U_B = m_B gh$, where m_B = mass of the block, g = gravity acceleration and h_B = height of block above a reference. To change the U_B, one of the factors must change. As long as the block is on the board, the m_B and the h_B do not change. Since the g is a constant, there is no way for the U_B to change and be converted to kinetic energy.

CHAPTER 4

Test Taking Skills Comment

This could be viewed as a Conservation of Mechanical Energy (**PHY 5.5**) problem and, as such, is a Camouflage and Distractions (**SB A.1.3**) question. The kinetic energy of the block has to come from some other form of energy. That other form of energy then must lose energy to the block. Notice that the total energy lost to the block from the mass, would include heat, sound, then the kinetic energy of the block combined with the work will overcome the force of friction.

This is also a Dichotomy of Options (**SB A.2.3**). Since there was no initial motion of any of the components, there could be no initial kinetic energy. There was initial potential energy of the mass as discussed previously. This means you could have eliminated options A and B.

Q02 · Pre-Study Suggestions

Review the following if needed:
1) Friction **PHY 3.2**
2) Graphs and Charts **GS A.3**
3) Three Out of Four Options **SB A.2.8**
4) Similar Pair Options **SB A.2.7**
5) Complex Sounding Option(s) **SB A.2.2**
6) What information is needed from the passage?
7) Solve the problem.

Solution Discussion

The following information is needed:

    The data in Table 1:

    "Table 1 shows the threshold mass, M_T, necessary to initiate sliding of each block."

You have to assess that the threshold mass, M_T, is the measure of the static friction. The greater the threshold mass, M_T, the greater the static friction and vice-versa. This means you can substitute the M_T for static friction.

Option C is incorrect. The reasoning is presented in option B. This option would require M_T to increase as the square of the base area. So, for wood, if the base area doubled going from Set 1 to Set 2 (2x), then M_T should have increased four times (2^2 = 4x). This did not occur.

Option B is incorrect. If static friction is directly proportional to the base area, the M_T that initiates movement of the block should increase as the surface area increases. Looking at the wood blocks, it is evident that as the surface area increased, second column, the M_T, fourth column, did not change. This option would require the M_T to increase as the base area did - this did not happen.

Option D is incorrect. The reasoning is presented in option B. This option would require M_T to vary inversely as the base area changes. For wood, if the base area doubled going from Set 1 to Set 2 (2x), the change in M_T should be the reciprocal or 1/2 of its initial value. But, this did not occur.

CHAPTER 4

Option A is correct. Table 1 shows, as explained in option B that for wood, as the surface area increased from Set 1 to Set 3, the M_T did not change in value. This means the M_T, which is the stand-in for static friction, is independent of the surface area.

Test Taking Skills Comment

This can be solved using the passage as described.

Also this can be viewed as a Three Out of Four Type Question **(SB A.2.8)** with two different sets of three out of four. The primary three out of four is for options A, B and D all with base area as opposed to option C which has square of base area. This is the better of the two three out of fours. Guessing from A, B or D would give you a chance for the correct option. The other three out of four is options B, C and D which are change options versus option A which is a no change option.

In general, no change or zero options will be incorrect and should usually be ignored. In any of these test taking skills techniques, there are no absolutes. When you have two of them present you should either choose not to apply them or apply a consistent rule to use them. For this type of three out of four, the more specific 'base area' options are better than the no-change options. So, I would suggest you pick your guess from the A, B or D group rather than from the B, C or D group related to no-change.

This is also a Similar Pair Options (**SB A.2.7**) as options B and C both use directly proportional and a guess from these two would not be unreasonable - but would be wrong. They also conflict with the three out of four; this is another reason to ignore a similar pair.

Finally, this question illustrates extremely well the concept of Basic Knowledge (study, passage, general) (**SB A.2.2**). In the discussion on Friction (**PHY 3.2**), you are told that friction is independent of the area of base contact. This is then basic knowledge. Many test preparers will tell you that this question is a passage related question and can be solved only with information from the passage which is correct as explained previously. We want you to have this very basic knowledge to make questions like this simpler.

By knowing the basic knowledge of friction, you would know that friction is independent of the area of contact. This will help you decrease the amount of time to solve this problem by recognizing that option A is probably correct. Then if you wanted to be more certain, you could quickly go over the chart to verify your conclusion. This will save you a lot of time. If you do not have this basic knowledge, then you must go through a more time consuming analysis as presented previously. Remember if you cannot determine the answer from basic knowledge, then the option is wrong and is a Complex Sounding Option(s) (**SB A.2.2**).

Q03   Pre-Study Suggestions

Review the following if needed:
1) Friction **PHY 3.2**
2) Three Out of Four type question **SB A.2.8**
3) Similar Pair Options **SB A.2.7**
4) Camouflage and Distractions **SB A.1.3**
5) What information is needed from the passage?
6) Solve the problem.

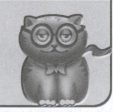

Solution Discussion

Information from the passage:

Table 1 shows the M_T, threshold mass, needed to begin motion for each block interacting with the wood board (see paragraph two). The greater the M_T, the greater the friction between the block and the wood board. Note the board is always wood and does not change. So, the lowest friction and the weakest forces would be for the lowest value of M_T. The key to solving this question is making the connection between the M_T, Threshold Mass, and the value of the static friction. Then you should use your Basic Knowledge (study, passage, general) (**SB A.2.2**) about Friction (**PHY 3.2**).

Option A is incorrect. There is no experiment that measures the motion of metal against metal.

Option D is incorrect. The M_T's between the wood and steel are intermediate between the stone and wood blocks. This means the steel on wood are of intermediate strength.

Option C is incorrect. The M_T's for the stone block are the greatest of all. This means the strongest forces are between the wood and the stone.

Option B is correct. The M_T's for the wood on wood are the lowest of all the experiments. This means the weakest forces are between the wood and wood.

Test Taking Skills Comment

You have to recognize the concept being tested, so this is a Camouflage and Distractions (**SB A.1.3**) type question. In this case, the concept is Friction (**PHY 3.2**). The MCAT does not always declare what is being tested. When it doesn't, you have to use the clues to determine what the concept is. In this passage, you are told that friction is important. In this question, though, you are asked about attractive molecular forces between surfaces. By knowing your Basic Knowledge (study, passage, general) (**SB A.2.2**) about friction, you should connect that friction involves attractive molecular forces, so this question is actually about friction.

Basic knowledge means that you must use information from your basic study, as discussed in the reference - either study knowledge or passage knowledge. A combination of both should lead you to understand that the M_T is a proxy, i.e., a stand in, for static friction. So, your study knowledge should tell you that increasing static friction means increasing attractive molecular forces between the surfaces. Your passage knowledge tells you that increasing M_T means increasing static friction. So, looking at the Table, you are able to determine which surface will have the lowest static friction, i.e., the lowest M_T, and the weakest intermolecular forces.

This is also a Three Out of Four Type Question (**SB A.2.8**). Options B, C and D all have wood as one of the options. Option A is an outlier without wood. Outliers are usually incorrect and can be ignored.

This is also a Similar Pair Options (**SB A.2.7**) with two sets of similar pairs. Options A and B are similar being between one type of surfaces and options C and D are similar in being between two types of surfaces. Remember, when there is more than one similar pair present, it is best not use this technique.

Q04 — Pre-Study Suggestions

Review the following if needed:
1) Friction **PHY 3.2**
2) Newton's Laws (First, Second, Third) **PHY 2.2, 2.3, 4.2**
3) Uniformly Accelerated Motion **PHY 1.5**
4) Graphs and Charts **GS A.3**
5) Relationships of Variables
6) Complex Sounding Option(s) **SB A.2.2**
7) Three Out of Four type question **SB A.2.8**
8) Camouflage and Distractions **SB A.1.3**
9) What information is needed from the passage?
10) Solve the problem.

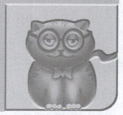

Solution Discussion

The information needed from the passage is the description of the experiment found in paragraph two - refer to that if needed.

The Forces Acting On the Block (**PHY 3.2, 3.2.1**) are:

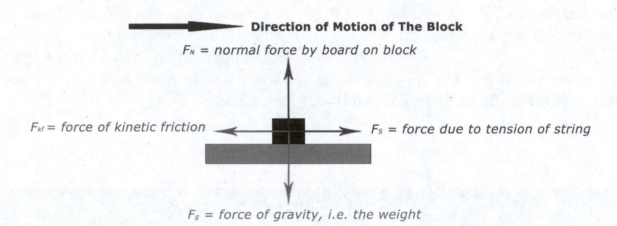

Direction of Motion of The Block

F_N = normal force by board on block

F_{kf} = force of kinetic friction

F_s = force due to tension of string

F_g = force of gravity, i.e. the weight

Since the object is in motion along the board, the following is true from Newton's Laws (First, Second) (**PHY 2.2, 2.3, 4.2**):

$$F_{net} = F_S - F_{kf} = m_b a_b$$

F_{net} = net force acting on the block

m_b = mass of the block

a_b = acceleration of the block.

If there is a net force that is constant, and the motion is in a straight line, then the equations of Uniformly Accelerated Motion (**PHY 1.5**) are valid, and the equation of importance, since Speed (**PHY 1.3**) is at issue, is:

$$v_b = v_{ob} + a_b t = a_b t$$

v_b = the speed of the block at any given time = t

v_{ob} = the original speed of the block = 0.

Since a_b is a constant, the following relationship holds between v_b and t:

$$v_b \; \alpha \; t.$$

This means they are Linearly Related (**GS A.3.1**) - the speed will increase linearly with time. In a plot of v (y-axis) versus t (x-axis), the **a** (acceleration) is the slope and is positive. This means they are Linearly Related (**GS A.3.1**) - the speed will increase linearly with time. In a plot of v (y-axis) versus t (x-axis), the a (acceleration) is the slope and is positive.

Option A is incorrect. As shown previously, the speed will increase with time. Just because the forces were constant doesn't mean the speed or velocity would be constant. Remember any constant force has a constant acceleration (**PHY 1.3**). Any acceleration means the velocity (or speed if linear path) is also changing due to the acceleration.

Option B is incorrect. The speed is proportional to the first power of t (time). If it was proportional to time raised to a power, then the relationship would be exponential (**GS A.4**). For example, if the question had asked about distance or displacement, the following equation would have been used:

$$d = d_0 + v_0 t + at^2/2$$

since, $d_0 = 0$ and $v_0 = 0$

$$d = at^2/2$$

this means,

$$d \propto t^2.$$

This would be an exponential relationship; in this case a Direct Square Relationship (**GS A.3.1**).

Option C is incorrect. Since there is a net force acting, the acceleration is acting and will cause the speed to increase immediately at a constant rate.

Option D is correct. As shown previously, the speed is proportional to the first power of the time. This makes it a linear relationship.

CHAPTER 4

Test Taking Skills Comment

This was a more difficult problem. It is possible the statement that the forces were constant served as a distraction and set the thought constant in the mind. The problem is solved by drawing it out and analyzing the forces as shown. The rest is the application of basic information.

This is a Camouflage and Distraction (**SB A.1.3**) type question. This is an application of the concepts of Uniformly Accelerated Motion (**PHY 1.5**) and the understanding of Forces (**PHY 5.6**) acting on objects. These are explained previously.

This is a multiple Three Out of Four (**SB A.2.8**) question. The first set are Options A, B and D are straight forward effects. Option

C is more complicated and is the outlier. Outliers tend to be incorrect. The second three out of four options are B, C and D which all have 'increasing' in them and option A is the outlier being 'constant'. Outliers tend to be incorrect. By applying both of these, you could eliminate options A and C by purely guessing.

This is also a Complex Sounding Option (**SB A.2.2**) question. Option C is a complex sounding option compared to the others. When options appear more complex than others, they will usually be incorrect. This is slightly different than the usual complex sounding option which depends on your Basic Knowledge (study, passage, general) (**SB A.2.2**).

Q05 — Pre-Study Suggestions

Review the following if needed:
1) Friction **PHY 3.2**
2) What information is needed from the passage?
3) Solve the problem.

Solution Discussion

The situation described in the question is as follows:

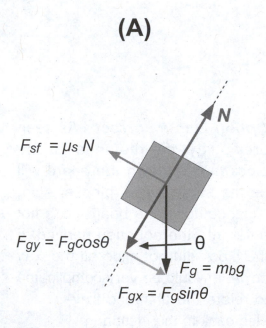

(A)

(B)

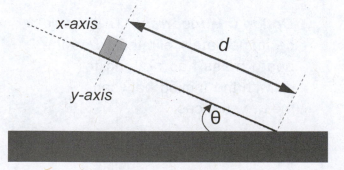

F_{sf} = force of static friction

μ_s = coefficient of static friction

N = normal force of board on the block

F_g = weight of the block

F_{gx} = component of weight along the x-axis (or along the board)

F_{gy} = component of weight along the y-axis (or perpendicular to the board)

m_b = mass of the block

g = gravitational acceleration

d = distance the object slides down the board

t = time moving down the board

θ= the angle at which the block begins motion down the board

The block will begin to slide when the force down the ramp (F_{gx}) becomes greater than the force of Coefficient of Static Friction (F_{sf}) **(PHY 3.2)** holding the block in place. So, the static friction at the onset of motion is found as follows:

$$F_{sf} = F_{gx}$$

$$\mu_s N = F_g \sin\theta$$
$$= m_b g \sin$$

$$\mu_s = m_b g \sin\theta / N.$$

The only factor that changes here is the angle of the board with the horizontal.

If the block did not slide down the whole board length, the calculation calculation would be more difficult and certainly beyond anything required by the MCAT.

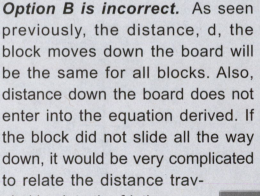

Option A is incorrect. The time it takes the block to slide down the board is not a factor in the equation derived and would not affect the coefficient of static friction. The time may be found as follows using Uniformly Accelerated Motion (**PHY 1.5**):

F_{net} = net force acting down the board on the block
$$= F_{gx} - F_{sf} = m_b a_b$$

a_b = acceleration of block down the board
$$= (F_{gx} - F_{sf})/m_b$$

$$d = a_b t^2 / 2$$

$$t^2 = 2d/a_b.$$

Option B is incorrect. As seen previously, the distance, d, the block moves down the board will be the same for all blocks. Also, distance down the board does not enter into the equation derived. If the block did not slide all the way down, it would be very complicated to relate the distance traveled back to the friction.

Option C is incorrect. This should be immediately eliminated as the board mass has nothing to do with the friction between the two surfaces.

Option D is correct. Based on simple physics principles as shown previously, you can relate the angle of the board directly to the friction.

Q: Why are chemists great for solving problems?

A: They have all the solutions.

Test Taking Skills Comment

This was a simple problem as more that 90% got it correct. I doubt the reasoning as shown previously was used in getting this question correct - you wouldn't have time to do it as it is shown previously. Probably many students remembered this from their basic physics as this technique is mentioned in basic texts. The previous analysis is more complete and could be helpful it to review important principles in physics. It may have been sufficient to take the question literally using the phrase 'To determine the static friction force on the block when sliding began' and assess each option on it. Then options A and B would be incorrect because the time and distance down the board would reflect kinetic friction and not static friction. Again the mass of the board would be irrelevant.

Q06 — Pre-Study Suggestions

Review the following if needed:
1) Lewis Acids and Bases **CHM 3.4, 6.1**
2) Intermolecular Forces **CHM 4.2**
3) Acids and Bases **CHM 6.1, 6.2**
4) Oxidation States **CHM 1.6**
5) Covalent Bonds **CHM 3.2**

CHAPTER 4

6) Three or More Step Analysis **SB A.1.4**

7) Camouflage and Distraction **SB A.1.3**

8) What information is needed from the passage?

9) Solve the problem.

Solution Discussion

The information from the passage is found in paragraph #2:

"NH₃ has a tendency to form coordination … NH₃ forms covalent bonds with a transition metal ion."

Option C is incorrect. The ammonia is a weak base in water solution. But it is not its basic strength in water that causes it bind to the transition metal. The reason for the base characteristics is the free pair of electrons on the nitrogen and this is the same reason it bonds to the transition metal.

Option B is incorrect. Nitrogen in ammonia can form hydrogen bonds. But, the statement in the passage is that a covalent bond is formed. Hydrogen bonds are non-covalent bonds.

Option D is incorrect. The N in ammonia is –3:

Oxidation state of ammonia is determined as follows,

$NH_3 : N + 3H = 0$

$N = -3H = -3 (+1) = -3$

Each H is a +1 oxidation state.

It is not the oxidation state of N that is important in the bonding to the transition metal.

Option A is correct. The N forms a coordinate covalent bond with the transition metal's empty orbitals. Both electrons come from the ammonia nitrogen. The ammonia is acting as a Lewis Base (**CHM 3.4, 6.1**) and the transition metal is a Lewis Acid (**CHM 3.4, 6.1**).

Test Taking Skills Comment

Remember that True or False (**SB A.1.2**) answers, as options, may not be the Correct or Incorrect (**SB A.1.2**) answer for the question. In this problem, each of the previous options are true statements. You certainly have to determine if the option is true to even consider it as a possible option. The next step is to determine if the true option answers the question being asked. This is why this is a Three or More Step Analysis (**SB A.1.4**) question; you have to do the following: 1) determine if the statement is true or false as a property of ammonia; 2) determine if the option then answers the question being asked about coordination compounds and ammonia (is it true or false in relation to the question at hand); and, finally, 3) determine if it is the correct answer. This is a mild Camouflage and Distractions (**SB A.1.3**) type question. The 'coordination compound' is not that essential to the concept being tested, the ability of ammonia to act as a Lewis Base (**CHM 3.4, 6.1**), nor is the concept of Lewis Base clearly evident in the Stem (**SB A.1**) of the question. Also, notice how many different concepts may be brought into play in a single question.

Q07 — Pre-Study Suggestions

Review the following if needed:
1) Boiling Points **CHM 5.1.2**
2) Electronegativity **CHM 3.3**
3) Periodic Trends **CHM 3.3**
4) Double and Triple bonds **CHM 3.2, ORG 1.3**
5) Bond Polarity **CHM 3.5, ORG 1.5**
6) Molecular Polarity **CHM 3.5**
7) Three Out of Four Options **SB A.2.8**
8) Internally Inconsistent **SB A.2.5**
9) What information is needed from the passage?
10) Solve the problem.

Solution Discussion

Both N_2 and O_2 are linear molecules. Both N_2 and O_2 are very electronegative (**CHM 3.3**) elements. But, because the molecules are linear and symmetric, the molecules are non-polar (**CHM 3.5, ORG 1.5**):

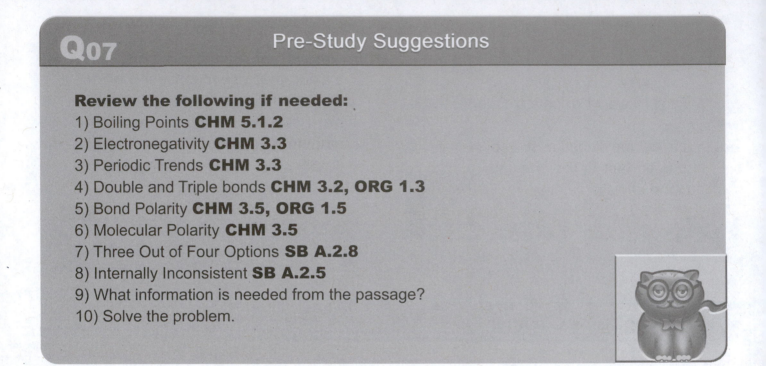

Dipole moment is zero.

The dipoles cancel.

Dipole moment is zero.

The dipoles cancel.

The only contribution to the dipole **(CHM 3.3)** is from the free pairs of electrons. There are no dipole Forces **(CHM 3.3)** between the nitrogens or the oxygens within each molecule because both atoms (in each molecule) have the same electronegativity.

Option A is incorrect. The nitrogen is less reactive than the oxygen. Reactivity can only be compared in the same row or the same column **(CHM 2.3)**. Reactivity will relate to how vigorously an atom will lose or gain electrons (only the Valence Electrons **CHM 3.5**). On the left side of the chart, it is the loss of electrons that determine the reactivity. This is measured by the Ionization Potential (Energy, IP or IE, **PHY 12.5**). On the right side of the chart, it is the gain of electrons and electronegativity that determines reactivity. In the location of N and O, the O will have the greater electronegativity and is expected to be more reactive. But, it is not the chemical reactivity that determines the Boiling Points (BP) **(CHM 5.1.2)** of substances. It is the presence of Intermolecular Forces **(CHM 4.2)**.

Option B is incorrect. This is not a correct way of stating this. Molecules do not have electronegativity, atoms or elements have electronegativity. Essentially, the statement is false - it is Internally Inconsistent (**SB A.2.5**). If it was meant that N is less electronegative than O, then this would be a correct statement. In any row, electronegativity would tend to increase as one goes from left to right. Even if this is true, the electronegativity by itself is not a determining factor in boiling points. It would be the effect of the electronegativity of the individual atoms on the Polarity **(CHM 3.5)** of the molecule that would affect the boiling point. See option A that demonstrates that neither molecule has a net dipole moment - therefore each molecule is non-polar. More polar molecules would have higher BP's.

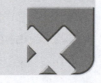

Option D is incorrect. As shown previously, this is a correct statement. But, the presence or absence of a Multiple Bonds (**CHM 3.2**) is not one of the major factors affecting boiling points.

Option C is correct. The Molar (Molecular) Mass (Weight, MM, MW) (**CHM 1.3**) is important because it affects the Dispersive (van der Waals, London) Forces (**CHM 4.2**) between molecules. The major factor affecting boiling points of substances is the Intermolecular Forces (**CHM 4.2**). The stronger the intermolecular forces the higher the boiling point. Intermolecular forces increase from dispersive, to Dipole Moment Forces (**CHM 4.2**) to Hydrogen Bonding (**CHM 4.2**). Since this molecule cannot form hydrogen bonds, and since it is non-polar as described previously, the only important intermolecular force left is the Dispersive (van der Waals, London) Forces (**CHM 4.2**). Van der Waals forces will increase as the polarizability or as the molecular weight of the element or molecules increase. Since oxygen has a greater molecular weight than nitrogen, (*see* the Periodic Chart or Table **CHM 2.3**), then oxygen will have stronger van der Waal forces. Since oxygen has stronger van der Waal forces, it will have a higher boiling point.

Test Taking Skills Comment

This is a problem in recognizing the key concept. This problem is all about understanding that boiling points are determined by intermolecular forces and you need to assess which of the factors listed affect the intermolecular forces. It is not a Camouflage and Distractions (**SB A.1.3**) because you are told the concept is boiling point. Again notice that options are True (**SB A.1.2**), but may not be the Correct (**SB A.1.2**) answer. This is also a mild Three Out of Four Type Question (**SB A.2.8**) if you understand the concept of boiling points. Reactivity, option A, has nothing to do with boiling points leaving B, C and D as the possible options. Also, as discussed in option B, it is Internally Inconsistent (**SB A.2.5**).

Q08 — Pre-Study Suggestions

Review the following if needed:
1) Le Chatelier's Principle **CHM 9.9**
2) Camouflage and Distractions **SB A.1.3**
3) What information is needed from the passage?
4) Solve the problem.

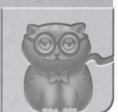

Solution Discussion

This is a Le Chatelier's Principle (**CHM 9.9**) problem and should be recognized as such. The Reaction IV is needed from the passage:

$$N_2(g) + 3H_2(g) \longleftrightarrow 2NH_3(g)$$

$$\Delta H = -92 \text{ kJ/mol.}$$

This should be rewritten as:

$$N_2(g) + 3H_2(g) \longleftrightarrow 2NH_3(g) + volume + energy$$

Volume is on the right side because there are fewer gas molecules on that side.

Energy is on the right because the reaction is Exothermic ($-\Delta H$), Enthalpy (ΔH) is negative (**CHM 7.5, 7.6**).

Option B is incorrect. A decrease in pressure would cause the volume to increase. This would shift the reaction to the left and decrease the amount of NH_3.

Option D is incorrect. A Catalyst (**CHM 9.7**) has no effect on the Equilibrium

Option C is incorrect. If the temperature is increased, the energy would increase and this would shift the equilibrium to the left. This would decrease the amount of NH_3.

Option A is correct. If the H_2 is added, the equilibrium will shift to the right. This will cause an increase in the NH_3.

Test Taking Skills Comment

This was an easy problem because a molecule in the reaction was the correct answer. If the temperature or the pressure were the correct answer, which either could have been, then the problem would have been more difficult. But, if you study and learn the technique discussed, none of the variations will be a problem for you. This is a mild Camouflage and Distractions (**SB A.1.3**) type question because the word Equilibrium (**CHM 9.8**) was mentioned. Any time equilibrium is mentioned and some type of change is occurring, always determine if you need to use Le Chatelier's Principle (**CHM 9.9**); most of the time you will.

Q09 — Pre-Study Suggestions

Review the following if needed:
1) Stoichiometry **CHM 1.5**
2) Limiting Reagents **CHM 1.5**
3) Moles **CHM 1.3**
4) Three Out of Four Options **SB A.2.8**
5) Internally Inconsistent **SB A.2.5**
6) What information is needed from the passage?
7) Solve the problem.

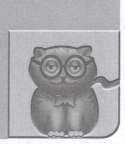

Solution Discussion

The equation for Reaction I is:

$$S(s) + O_2 \rightarrow SO_2(g)$$

$$\Delta H = -296.8 \text{ kJ/mol}$$

Since the equation is balanced, this means it will take one mole of S to react with one mole of O_2 (basic Stoichiometry **CHM 1.5**). The Moles (**CHM 1.3**) of each substance present is:

For S: Molar Mass (Molecular Weight) = 32 (**CHM 1.3**) moles
= grams/molar mass
= 36/32 = 9/8
= 1.125 moles

For O_2: molar mass = 32 moles
= grams/molar mass
= 32/32 = 1 mole.

The substance not in the ratio required in the equation is the limiting reagent. Since there are 1.125 moles of S present, there should be 1.125 moles of O_2 to use up the entire S. So, the O_2 is the Limiting Reagent (**CHM 1.5**).

CHAPTER 4

Option A is incorrect. There is excess sulfur present - *see* previously.

Option C is incorrect. SO_2 is not a reactant, so it cannot be a limiting reagent. This is an Internally Inconsistent (**SB A.2.5**) option and should be eliminated based on the equation previously.

Option D is incorrect. There would not be a limiting reagent if all reactants were in the exact ratios present in the Balanced Equation (**CHM 1.5**). This is not the case in this reaction.

Option B is correct. Oxygen is the limiting reagent, because there are 1.125 moles of S, there should be the same number of moles to have a reaction use up all of the reactants.

First Law of Energy Conservation

Cats know that energy can neither be created nor destroyed and so we will, therefore, use as little energy as possible.

Test Taking Skills Comment

Nothing of substance is needed from the passage other than the equation. This has an Internally Inconsistent (**SB A.2.5**) option as discussed in option C. This is also a Three Out of Four Options (**SB A.2.8**) where options A, B and C all have a specific optionand option D is an outlier having a no change/zero type option. In general, outliers will be Incorrect (**SB A.1.2**) and can be ignored. Also, unless you have a compelling reason and are not guessing, you should not select zero/no change options.

Q10   Pre-Study Suggestions

Review the following if needed:
1) Doppler Effect **PHY 8.5**
2) Vectors **PHY 1.1**
3) Three Out of Four Options **SB A.2.8**
4) Similar Pair Options **SB A.2.7**
5) Solve the problem.

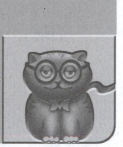

Solution Discussion

Initial Motions: The receiver (R) and the source, the jet, (S) have the following relative speeds:

	R (ground)	S (jet)
	•	•→
Actual Speeds:	0 m/s	+300 m/s
Relative Speeds:	+300 m/s (moving away from each other)	

The actual speed to the right is taken as positive and to the left as negative. Since the Velocities **(PHY 1.3)** are in a straight line, the Speed **(PHY 1.3)** can be used, and added as a Scalar **(PHY 1.1)**, instead of using Vectors **(PHY 1.1)**, but it is still better understood by using vectors. The relative speed will be negative if they are approaching each other, and it will be positive if they are moving away

from each other. The frequency detected by the receiver in this situation, moving away from each other, will be less than that emitted by the source; this frequency change will be negative or decreasing because the R and S are moving apart.

Option A is incorrect. The relative and actual speeds are:

	R (ground)	S (jet)
	←•	•→
Actual Speeds:	-900 m/s	+600 m/s
Relative Speeds:	+1500 m/s (moving away from each other)	

CHAPTER 4

Since the net motion is away from the receiver, the frequency should decrease and will be different than the initial motions discussed; the decrease will be greater in this instance. The frequency change in this situation will be negative and will change much faster than in the initial motion previously.

Option B is incorrect. The relative and actual speeds are:

	R (ground) ←•	S (jet) •→
Actual Speeds:	-300 m/s	+600 m/s
Relative Speeds:	+900 m/s (moving away from each other)	

Since the net motion is away from the receiver, the frequency should decrease and will be different than the initial motions discussed. The frequency change in this situation will be negative and the change will be greater than in the initial motion previously.

Option C is incorrect. The relative and actual speeds are:

	R (ground) •	S (jet) •→
Actual Speeds:	0 m/s	+600 m/s
Relative Speeds:	+600 m/s (moving away from each other)	

The receiver and source are moving apart at a speed greater than in the initial motion. This means the frequency will decrease faster than for the original motion.

Option D is correct. The relative and actual speeds are:

	R (ground) •→	S (jet) •→
Actual Speeds:	+300 m/s	+600 m/s
Relative Speeds:	+300 m/s (moving away from each other)	

The receiver and source are moving apart at a speed equal to the initial motion. This means the frequency will decrease at the same rate as for the initial motion.

Test Taking Skills Comment

This is a straightforward application of the Doppler Effect (**PHY 8.5**). It is also a Three Out of Four Options (**SB A.2.8**) type question that is a zero change type. Options A, B and D are all change options. Option C is the no change and is the outlier. Generally, the outlier will be incorrect with one exception being in change questions like this - you have to be more careful; but you should generally not accept the zero/no change option unless you have compelling reasons – i.e., you are not guessing.

This is also a Similar Pair Options (**SB A.2.7**) type question that would lead you astray - options A and B are both similar in that the receiver is moving opposite to the jet. This is actually a good guess bet for a similar pair type question. But, these are only techniques and are not guarantees! It is always best to know what is going on than to guess - but, when you have to guess, take your best educated shot using these techniques.

Q11 — Pre-Study Suggestions

Review the following if needed:
1) Graphs and Charts **GS A.3**
2) Relationships of Variables **GS A.3.1**
3) Slope **GS A.3**
4) Three Out of Four Options **SB A.2.8**
5) Similar Pair Options **SB A.2.7**
6) Internally Inconsistent **SB A.2.5**
7) What information is needed from the passage?
8) Solve the problem.

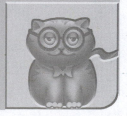

Solution Discussion

The key information is found in Table 2 which shows the movement of the plane away from the source at different speeds along with changes in frequency and wavelength. The critical observation, from Graphs and Charts (**GS A.3**) interpretation, is that as the speed away from the source is increasing, the wavelength change is increasing. This means a plot of the speed vs. change in wavelength, which is found in the options, should have a positive Slope (**GS A.3**). The only graph with a positive slope is option A. This means option A must be correct.

The problem could have been made more difficult by giving other options with positive slopes such as:

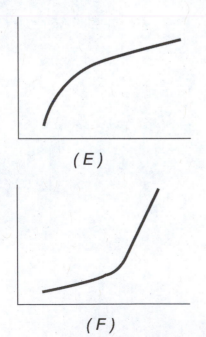

(E)

(F)

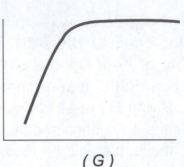

(G)

When this occurs, you will have to get an estimate of the slope to determine if it is constant, meaning the line is straight, or if it is not constant and how it is changing. For the correct option A, the slope would not change between two different sets of points. For letter E above, the slope would be decreasing as goes from left to right. For letter F, the slope will be increasing as goes from left to right. For letter G, the slope is positive and then goes to zero as goes from left to right. You would have to determine the slope at two points, one on the left side and one on the right side of the graph. For this problem, the slopes at two different points are determined as follows:

Using Table 2 data:
$$\text{Slope} = \Delta y/\Delta x$$
$$= \Delta \text{speed}/\Delta \text{wavelength}$$

Point on left side of graph:
$$\text{Slope} = (322-246)/(16-12)$$
$$= 76/4 = + 19$$

Point on right side of graph:
Slope = (671-447)/(34-22)
       = 224/12 = +18.7 ≈ +19

Within the error of measurement, the slope is constant and would be a Straight Line (**GS A.3.1**). Then you could eliminate letter E because the slope would decrease to the right. You would eliminate letter F because the slope should increase to the right. You would eliminate letter G because the slope should be near zero to the right.

Option B is incorrect. This means the slope is zero. The speed should be the same and the wavelength change would be increasing.

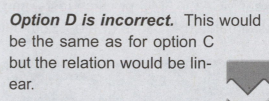

Option C is incorrect. If this graph was true, this would mean the wavelength change should be decreasing as the speed is increasing.

Option D is incorrect. This would be the same as for option C but the relation would be linear.

Option A is correct. See the previous discussion.

Test Taking Skills Comment

This is a Graphs and Charts (**GS A.3**) type problem. You have to interpret the information in the table. This is a Three Out of Four Options (**SB A.2.8**) question. Options A, B and D are all straight lines. Option C is an outlier as it is curvilinear. Generally, outliers will be incorrect and should be ignored when in the guess mode. This is also a Similar Pair Options (**SB A.2.7**) type question. But, the problem is there are two similar pairs present, options A and D are similar and options C and D are similar. When there is more than one similar pair present, you should not use this technique (how can you pick the correct similar pair to guess from! Note: this is not the same as a Dichotomy of Options (**SB A.2.3**).

This is also a soft Internally Inconsistent (**SB A.2.5**) type question because the Table 2 clearly shows the relation of speed and change in wavelength has to be a positive slope - this observation should eliminate options B, C and D immediately as internally inconsistent. *See* previously for how the problem could have been made more interesting and difficult. But, even this is a very important illustrative point as relates to the real MCAT, AAMC practice tests, and the mock/simulated MCAT's of most commercial companies. The real MCAT, AAMC practice tests, has to test out their whole exam. It's not a simple matter of making difficult questions, anyone can do that, it's a matter of making a spectrum of questions consistent with the overall requirements of the real test. But, for now, we can play 'what if' as previously for educational purposes.

Q12 — Pre-Study Suggestions

Review the following if needed:
1) Doppler Effect **PHY 8.5**
2) Wave Characteristics **PHY 7.1**
3) Wavelength **PHY 7.1**
4) Graphs and Charts **GS A.3**
5) Three Out of Four Options **SB A.2.8**
6) Complex Sounding Option(s) **SB A.2.2**
7) What information is needed from the passage?
8) Solve the problem.

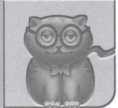

Solution Discussion

The information needed from the passage is found in Table 2. (*See* Graphs and Charts **GS A.3**).

The problem wants to know about the distance between adjacent peaks of the The problem wants to know about the distance between adjacent peaks of the transmitted waves at the receiver. The adjacent peaks are nothing more than the crests of the Waves (**PHY 7.1**). The distance between any two adjacent crests is the Wavelength (**PHY 7.1**) of the wave. So, if the crest separation is increasing, then the wavelength is increasing and vice-versa. Table 2 shows the effect on the wavelength when the jet is flying away from the receiver at different speeds. It shows the wavelength is increasing as the speed is increasing. This means the separation between crests, or peaks, will also be increasing.

Option A is incorrect. The distance between the peaks will increase and not decrease. If the jet was moving toward the receiver then this would happen.

Option B is incorrect. When there is relative motion between the source and the receiver, the Frequency (**PHY 7.1**) and wavelength will be changing.

Option D is incorrect. The changing part is correct. But, the change in peak separation is dependent upon the relative movement of the source and the receiver. If the receiver is stationary, then the speed of the source relative to the receiver becomes critical in the frequencies and wavelengths picked up by the receiver. This option is also a Complex Sounding Option(s) (**SB A.2.2**). This is one of the very important observations for you to make. The other three options, A, B and C, are very simply stated, but option D is much more, relatively, complexly stated. This is one of the aspects of this concept.

Complex sounding options will generally be incorrect - if you are in a guess mode, and even if you are not, you should eliminate them. Remember the key concept here is your Basic Knowledge (study, passage, general) (**SB A.2.2**). How are you going to determine 'it changes, but is not dependent on the speed'? You have to make this determination from your Study Knowledge (**SB A.2.2**) of which there is none for this. If you can-

CHAPTER 4

not determine it from your study knowledge, then you have to get it from your Passage Knowledge (**SB A.2.2**) – there is nothing in the passage which will allow you to assess 'is not dependent on the speed'.

Option C is correct. *See* the previous explanation.

Test Taking Skills Comment

This is another application of the Doppler Effect (**PHY 8.5**) with some basic Wave Characteristics (**PHY 7.1**) knowledge added and with some interpretation from the table in the passage. This is also a Complex Sounding Option(s) (**SB A.2.2**) as discussed in option D. It is also a Three

Out of Four Options (**SB A.2.8**) type question as options A, C and D all involve some type of change whereas option B is no/zero change type option. Remember, unless you have compelling reasons; do not select no/zero change type options. Outliers are usually incorrect.

Q13 — Pre-Study Suggestions

Review the following if needed:
1) Doppler Effect **PHY 8.5**
2) Sound **PHY 8.1**
3) Electromagnetic Waves **PHY 9.2.4**
4) Wavelength **PHY 7.1**
5) Frequency **PHY 7.1**

7) Three Out of Four Options **SB A.2.8**

8) Mutually Excluding Options **SB A.2.6**

9) Complex Sounding Option(s) **SB A.2.2**

10) What information is needed from the passage?

11) Solve the problem.

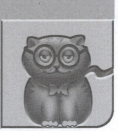

Solution Discussion

No information is needed from the passage. The equations that determine the shift in Frequency (**PHY 7.1**) as relates to Doppler Effect (**PHY 8.5**) are as follows (you are not given this formula in the passage and I doubt you have to know it; you do have it in your review; it is being used here for illustrative purposes):

$$f_o = f_s (1 \pm v_o /v)/(1 \pm v_s /v)$$

f_o = frequency at the observer,

f_s = frequency emitted by the source,

v = the speed of the wave,

v_o = the speed of the observer,

v_s = the speed of the source.

The percentage change in frequency would be as follows:

% change frequency

$= [(f_s - f_o)/f_s] \times 100\%$

$= [(f_s - f_s (1 \pm v_o /v)/(1 \pm v_s /v)]/f_s$

$= 1 - (1 \pm v_o /v)/(1 \pm v_s /v).$

From this equation, it should be clear it is the ratio of v_o/v and the v_s/v that will determine the value of the change in frequency. The impact of the ratio of v_o/v or v_s/v will be the greatest if the value of the v, the speed of the wave, is smaller. As the frequency of the wave increases, the ratio becomes smaller and will have a smaller impact on the frequency change.

Option B is incorrect. The frequency of the wave is not in the equation - it cancels out when percentage is considered. How do you determine the frequency of the sound waves? Do you know that sound waves have a higher frequency than radio waves? What information do you need to determine this? Were you required to memo-

CHAPTER 4

rize that information? The answer is no. Then if not, where would you need to find that information? Answer - in the passage and it is not in the passage. This makes it a Complex Sounding Option(s) (**SB A.2.2**). But there is another problem with this option as discussed in option C. This one type of a complex sounding option - *see* option D discussion for another.

Option C is incorrect. This is the same reasoning as in option B. You should have a test taking skills clue combined with basic knowledge that options B and C cannot be correct. Since the frequency is inversely related to the wavelength, options B and C are essentially equivalent - a high frequency means a shorter wavelength. So, if one is correct, the other is correct. Since there can be only one correct answer, neither can be correct. This is a classic Mutually Excluding Options (**SB A.2.6**) and you should study it carefully. *See* option B.

Option D is incorrect. Although options B and C subtlety presents you with information you do not have, this one is glaring in terms of its scientific sounding without adequate information to support - it is a Complex Sounding Option(s) (**SB A.2.2**). Remember the key to recognizing and eliminating complex sounding options is your appreciation and grasp of Basic Knowledge (study, passage, general) (**SB A.2.2**). Nowhere in your study is it required that you know the relative interference of the atmosphere with sound and radio waves. Even if you did know that, how does that affect the frequency change?

It would be reasonable to assess that radio waves, since they are Electromagnetic Waves (**PHY 9.2.4**), would be less affected than sound, which are mechanical waves, by the atmosphere generally. But, there are magnetic and electric fields and other objects in the atmosphere that also interfere with radio waves as well. So, how are you to distinguish the relative effects? You are not. This is why you cannot reasonably assess this option.

Option A is correct. You should know radio waves are electromagnetic waves and travel at the speed of light. Sound waves are mechanical waves and travel much slower. Then using the previous Doppler relationship, you can determine the importance of the relative speeds. But you should be able to arrive at this option without knowing the previous complicated equation. *See* the following discussions.

Test Taking Skills Comment

This was a difficult question as only 45% got it correct. You can use some test taking skills to eliminate all options except A as discussed previously. This is also a Three Out of Four Options (**SB A.2.8**) question. Options A, B and C are similar in having some characteristic of sound waves in the option. Option D is the outlier with a totally different topic. Outliers tend to be incorrect and can often be ignored. This gets your guess percentage up to 33%.

This is an example of Mutually Excluding Options (**SB A.2.6**). This opportunity does not arise often. There must be parameters involved in different options that are connected to each other in some manner. The test maker will give the same net effect of each parameter but the options will appear different. If you can determine that the effect of the parameter is identical between the options, then those options cannot be correct - they are mutually excluding. This question provides a good example.

You know the wavelength (λ) and frequency (f) are intimately connected by the wave Equation ($v = \lambda f$, **PHY 7.1**). If one increases, the other must decrease. So, if one of the options has higher frequency and another has shorter wavelength as the effect, then neither can be correct because both are

CHAPTER 4

the same effect. This is found in options B and C in this problem. There is also a Complex Sounding Option(s) (**SB A.2.2**) as discussed in option D previously. With the application of these test skills, you eliminate options B, C and D and are left with option A as 100% bet - much better than the 45% average correct.

Q14 — Pre-Study Suggestions

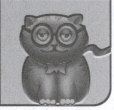

Review the following if needed:
1) Doppler Effect **PHY 8.5**
2) Three Out of Four Options **SB A.2.8**
3) What information is needed from the passage?
4) Solve the problem.

Solution Discussion

No information is needed from the passage.

The equations that determine the shift in frequency are as follows (which again, you probably do not have to know):

$$f_o = f_s (1 \pm v_o /v)/(1 \pm v_s /v)$$

f_o = frequency at the observer,
f_s = frequency emitted by the source,
v = the speed of the wave,
v_o = the speed of the observer,
v_s = the speed of the source.

Since the relative speeds are the same $v_o = 0$ and $v_s = 0$ because they are not moving relative to each other. The equation now becomes:

$$f_o = f_s (1 \pm 0/v) / (1 \pm 0/v)$$
$$= f_s (1 \pm 0)(1 \pm 0)$$
$$= f_s (1)(1) = f_s.$$

This means there is no shift in the frequency. You could have put 268 m/s in for both v_o and v_s and the results would have been the same.

Options B, C and D are incorrect. *See* the previous discussion.

Option A is correct. You could have also reasoned if there is no relative motion, there is no shift in frequency.

Test Taking Skills Comment

This is a straightforward application of the Doppler Effect **(PHY 8.5)**. This is a Three Out of Four Options **(SB A.2.8)** as options B, C and D are all positive options. Option A is a zero/no change option. Remember outliers and no change/zero options are usually incorrect. You should not take this type of option unless you have a compelling reason. In this question, your compelling reason should be the fact that you understand Doppler.

Q15 — Pre-Study Suggestions

Review the following if needed:
1) Doppler Effect **PHY 8.5**
2) Dichotomy of Options **SB A.2.3**
3) Complex Sounding Option(s) **SB A.2.2**
4) Mutually Excluding Options **SB A.2.6**
5) What information is needed from the passage?
6) Solve the problem.

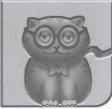

CHAPTER 4

Solution Discussion

Nothing is needed from the passage but you can use the information in Table 3 if needed. There is a decrease in the wavelength at the receiver, which means there was an increase in the Frequency (**PHY 7.1**) consistent with Doppler Effect (**PHY 8.5**). This means the objects are moving closer. In this case, it means the star is moving toward the earth. From Table 3, you see the effect of a source approaching the receiver - there is a decrease in the wavelength. This corresponds to the decrease in wavelength in this problem, so the objects are moving closer together.

a Complex Sounding Option(s) (**SB A.2.2**) and is a Mutually Excluding Options (**SB A.2.6**) along with option C.

Option C is incorrect. How do you know this? Also, this option and option B are essentially the same. This information is beyond your study and the passage. This is a Complex Sounding Option(s) (**SB A.2.2**) and is a Mutually Excluding Options (**SB A.2.6**) along with option B.

Option A is incorrect. If the star was moving away from earth, the wavelength would be increasing. This is also shown in Table 2.

Option B is incorrect. How do you know this? Also, this option and option C are essentially the same. This is information beyond your study and the passage. This is

Option D is correct. This is the most reasonable explanation and it is consistent with your studies of the Doppler Effect (**PHY 8.5**).

Test Taking Skills Comment

This is one of those rare questions where two options are essentially the same - options B and C are Mutually Excluding Options (**SB A.2.6**). This is also a Complex Sounding Option(s) (**SB A.2.2**) question for options B and C. This is also a Dichotomy of Options (**SB A.2.3**) question as options A and D versus B and C is the dichotomy.

Your Basic Knowledge (study, passage, general) (**SB A.2.2**) tells you that the Doppler deals with changes in wavelength and frequency that are opposite and you can use this information to determine if objects are moving closer together or farther apart. So, the most reasonable half of the dichotomy to choose is A or D. Since there is nothing from your study knowledge or from your passage knowledge to allow you to even consider options B or C, these cannot be correct.

Q16 — Pre-Study Suggestions

Review the following if needed:
1) Acids and Bases **CHM 6.1, 6.2**
2) Acid Strength **CHM 6.1-6.6**
3) Base Strength **CHM 6.1-6.6**
4) Salts **CHM 6.7**
5) pH **CHM 6.1, 6.2**
6) Dichotomy of Options **SB A.2.3**
7) Three or More Step Analysis **SB A.1.4**
8) Solve the problem.

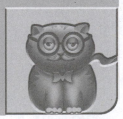

CHAPTER 4

Solution Discussion

Salts (**CHM 6.7**) result from the combination of an Acid and a Base (**CHM 6.1- 6.6**). The salt may then have acid or base properties depending on what is combined-review the section if you are familiar with these possibilities. The lowest pH will result when the acid is the strongest or the base is the weakest. Strong acids or bases have neutral salts and therefore result in a neutral pH. To get an acid as a salt, the base must be a weak base. So, the lowest pH would result when the acid results in a neutral Conjugate Acid (**CHM 6.3**) and the base part results in an acidic, weak, Conjugate Acid (**CHM 6.3**), weak. So, the answer would be option A.

Option C is incorrect. This is the same as B. In addition to more acid than base being added, the pH could also be acidic if the pK_a of the acid is smaller than the pK_b of the base. This would mean that more H^+ is dissociated from the acid than OH^- from the base leaving a net of H^+ in solution lowering the pH. The salt would not be neutral, but you need more information, the pk_a's (**CHM 6.8**) to determine the resultant pH (**CHM 6.1, 6.2**).

Option B is incorrect. A strong acid and a strong base would neutralize each other and should be neutral if began with equal amount of each. The only way this could be correct is if there was more acid than base. But, it is very reasonable to assume that equal amounts of acid and base are being added to form the Salt (**CHM 6.7**) which would be neutral.

Option D is incorrect. This one will definitely be eliminated as the strong base would neutralize all of the H^+ from the acid and the pH would rise and not fall. There would have to be a great excess of the weak acid over the strong base to get a lowering of the pH. Also, the weak acid would result in a salt which is weakly base and this is the main reason the pH will rise.

Option A is correct. The strong acid results in a salt component which is neutral. The weak base results in the salt component which is

a weak acid and will lower the pH.

Test Taking Skills Comment

This is a Dichotomy of Options (**SB A.2.3**) question which is a double dichotomy. One dichotomy is for strong versus weak acid. For any salt, you have to consider both the acid and base parts. For a weak acid, you will get a weak base which will move the pH in the wrong direction, so this dichotomy cannot be correct. Because the conjugate base of a strong acid is neutral, the conjugate acid from the base part can affect the pH as desired. So, the dichotomy of strong acid (A and B) would contain the correct answer.

A similar argument holds for the weak base versus strong base. The strong base conjugate has no effect, but the conjugate acid of the weak base will lower the pH as desired depending on the other half of the salt. So, this means options A or C (the weak base half) will be correct. As in any double dichotomy chosen correctly, since A is in both, it must be the correct option.

This is also a Three or More Step Analysis (**SB A.1.4**) which can make it more difficult: 1) you have to determine the effect of each of parts of the option, 2) you have to determine the overall effect of the two parts, 3) you have to determine if the option is True or False (**SB A.1.2**), and 4) you have to determine if the option is Correct or Incorrect (**SB A.1.2**).

CHAPTER 4

Q17 — Pre-Study Suggestions

Review the following if needed:
1) Fluid Pressure **PHY 6.1.2**
2) Density **PHY 6.1.1**
3) Equation Interpretation
4) Simultaneous Equations **PHY 10.3.1**
5) Camouflage and Distractions **SB A.1.3**
6) Three Out of Four Type Question **SB A.2.8**
7) Solve the problem.

Solution Discussion

The Fluid Pressure (**PHY 6.1.2**) (P in N/m^2) in a static fluid at given distance (h in meters) under the surface is given by:

$$P = P_e + \rho g h$$

P_e = external pressure in N/m^2

ρ = density (**PHY 6.1.1**) of fluid in kg/m^3

g = acceleration due to gravity (**PHY 1.3**).

It can be seen from the table given that the P_e would be found as follows:

$$250 = P_e + \rho (10)(0.05)$$
$$= P_e + 0.50 \rho$$
$$450 = P_e + \rho (10)(0.10)$$
$$= P_e + \rho$$

then,

$$\rho = 450 - P_e$$

and substituting for Simultaneous Equations (**PHY 10.3.1**),

$$250 = P_e + 0.5 (450 - P_e)$$
$$= P_e + 225 - (0.5)P_e$$
$$= (0.5)P_e + 225$$

$$(0.5)P_e = 250 - 225 = 25$$

$$P_e = 50 \ N/m^2.$$

Then for the 10 cm depth, the P is composed of:

$$P_{10cm} = P_e + \rho (10)(0.05)$$
$$= 50 + 400.$$

So, the contribution from the density and depth is the 400.

If the density is doubled, then this value will be doubled to 800 and the new pressure with the new density would be equal to 50 + 800 = 850.

Options A, B and D are incorrect. *See* the previous discussion.

Option C is correct. *See* the previous discussion.

Test Taking Skills Comment

An Alternative Solution (**SB A.1.3**), a type of Camouflage and Distractions (**SB A.1.3**), to this problem is to eliminate options. You should eliminate options A and B because they cannot be correct based on the formula and the table. You should be confident that the pressure at 10 cm in the new fluid is at least 450 or more.

When you look at the formula, you know the effect of the density is to increase the pressure at a certain depth. The effect would be:

$$P_{10x1} = \text{pressure of density one } (\rho_1) \text{ at 10cm}$$
$$= P_e + \rho_1 (10)(10)$$
$$= 450$$

$$P_{10x2} = \text{press. of density two } (2\rho_1) \text{ at 10 cm}$$
$$= P_e + 2\rho_1 (10)(10)$$
$$= P_{10x2}$$

Then by ratio and proportion, these can be divided:

$$\frac{P_{10x2}}{450} = \frac{1P_e + 2\rho_1(10)(10)}{1P_e + 1\rho_1(10)(10)}$$

CHAPTER 4

The ones (1) are put in to make the point that the P_{10x2} will be less than double the value of the 450. The amount less will be $1P_e$. If it was double the value, it would be $2P_e + 2_{\rho_1}(10)(10)$ and not $1P_e + 2_{\rho_1}(10)(10)$. So, you don't have to figure it out because of the answers. You know the correct answer will be less than 900 but more than 450. Since

there is only one option that fits this, it must be the answer.

This is also a weak Three Out of Four Type Question (**SB A.2.8**) because only numbers are involved. You can be bold and choose A, B and C because they are less than 1000. This means D is the outlier and outliers are usually incorrect.

Q18 — Pre-Study Suggestions

Review the following if needed:
1) Density **PHY 6.1.1**
2) Specific Gravity **PHY 6.1.1**
3) Buoyancy **PHY 6.1.2**
4) Equation Interpretation
5) Camouflage and Distractions **SB A.1.3**
6) Solve the problem.

Solution Discussion

To get the specific gravity (**PHY 6.1.1**) of an object, you must compare its density (**PHY 6.1.1**) to the density of water at the same temperature and pressure. Since all measurements are assumed to be at the same conditions and the density of water is 1000 kg/m^3 at most of the usual conditions,

the specific gravity of a substance is essentially its density. So, if you can determine the density, you have, in effect, determined the specific gravity. To determine the density of a substance you need its mass and the volume occupied by that mass.

In this problem, you have the mass but not the volume. How can you determine the volume with the information you are given? Since the mass is placed in benzene, the volume of benzene displaced is the volume of the mass. Since the mass displaces 5 g of benzene, and the specific gravity of the benzene is 0.7, it is reasonable to take its density as 0.7 g/ml (assume the units and just make them consistent), and the volume displaced will be (this is a skill of Equation Interpretation):

$$density = mass/volume$$

volume = mass/density
= 5/(0.7) ml.

This will be the volume of the mass. Then the density and, effectively, the specific gravity of the mass will then be:

Density = mass/volume
= 15 g/(5/0.7) ml
= (15)(0.7)/5
= (3)(0.7)
= 2.1 g/ml,

and the specific gravity is 2.1.

Options A, B and D are incorrect. See previous discussion.

Option C is correct. See previous discussion.

Test Taking Skills Comment

This shows how even basic concepts can be difficult. You have to pause and not panic and realize what you know from your Basic Knowledge (study, passage, general) (**SB A.2.2**) and then apply it. Everyone will say they understand density, yet only 55% got this question correct and probably fewer truly understood it as the guess rate can be as high as 25%. This is a Camouflage and Distractions (**SB A.1.3**) because you have to sort out the relationships as discussed previously.

CHAPTER 4

Q19 — Pre-Study Suggestions

Review the following if needed:
1) Melting Points **CHM 4.3.2**
2) Phases **CHM 4.3.1**
3) Energy of Phase Transitions **CHM 4.3.3, PHY 8.1**
4) Dichotomy of Options **SB A.2.3**
5) Solve the problem.

Solution Discussion

Option B is incorrect. A fraction of a second is not long enough to turn all of the solid metal into liquid metal. Even though the temperature is at the Melting Points (**CHM 4.3.2**), enough heat will still have to be transferred from the heat source to the metal to melt it. You have to appreciate Energy of Phase Transitions (**CHM 4.3.3, PHY 8.1**). The amount of heat is determined by the Heat of Fusion (ΔH_f = joules/mol or cal/mol) (**CHM 4.3.3**). The greater this value, the more heat has to be transferred for the melting of the solid.

Option C is incorrect. There will be no increase in temperature of the solid metal until all of the metal has been converted to liquid metal. So, the temperature of the solid and liquid metal will all remain the same until the phase change is complete.

Option D is incorrect. See the explanation in option C.

only a small amount of heat can be transferred. This will be just enough to melt a small amount of the solid metal closest to the heat source. Since the phase change will not be complete, the temperature will stay the same.

Option A is correct. Since the exposure to the flame is very short,

Q: What happens when electrons lose their energy?

A: They get Bohr'ed.

Q: What is a cation afraid of?

A: A dogion.

Test Taking Skills Comment

This problem is just testing your understanding of phase changes and this is not explicitly stated. This makes it a Camouflage and Distractions (**SB A.1.3**). You have to determine this question is about Phases (**PHY 4.3.1**) and Phase Interconversions (**PHY 4.3.1**). It is also a Dichotomy of Options (**SB A.2.3**). Remember to properly do a dichotomy, you must use your Basic Knowledge (study, passage, general) (**SB A.2.2**). The dichotomy options are 'temp stays same' (options A and B) and 'temp increases slightly' (options C and D). Basic knowledge should tell you that the temperature should not change given the short duration of heat application making options A or B correct.

CHAPTER 4

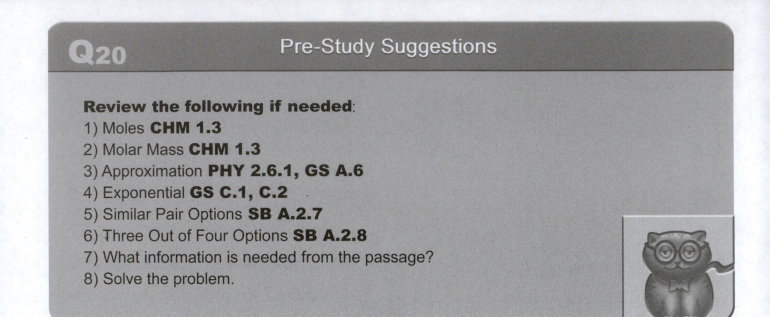

Q20 — Pre-Study Suggestions

Review the following if needed:
1) Moles **CHM 1.3**
2) Molar Mass **CHM 1.3**
3) Approximation **PHY 2.6.1, GS A.6**
4) Exponential **GS C.1, C.2**
5) Similar Pair Options **SB A.2.7**
6) Three Out of Four Options **SB A.2.8**
7) What information is needed from the passage?
8) Solve the problem.

Solution Discussion

The information from the passage is the Molar Mass (Molecular Weight, Atomic Weight, Atomic Mass) (**CHM 1.3**) of KHP found in third paragraph:

molar mass of KHP = 204.2;

and the grams of KHP of Student A found in Table 2:

grams of KHP of student A = 0.5500 g.

The problem is solved by using the basic formula for Moles (**CHM 1.3**):

$$\text{Moles} = \text{grams/gram molar mass}$$
$$= 0.5500/204.2$$
$$= 5.5000 \times 10^{-1}/2.042 \times 10^{2}$$
$$= (5.5000/2.042) \times 10^{-3}.$$

There is no need to go any further.

Option A, B, D is incorrect. The correct exponent is –3, and all of these are incorrect.

Option C is correct. The correct exponent is –3, so this must be the correct answer.

Test Taking Skills Comment

Notice you do not have to always complete the calculation. Also, delay actual divisions/additions/etc until you are forced to do them. Many times an approximation (**PHY 2.6.1**, **GS A.6**) is all that is required. This is also a Three Out of Four Options (**SB A.2.8**) problem. Options A, B and C are similar with negative exponents. Option D is an outlier with a positive exponent. Outliers tend to incorrect and can often be ignored.

This is also a Similar Pair Options (**SB A.2.7**) as options B and C are similar in having the same decimal (2.693). Since there are no other similar pairs present and since this similar pair is part of the three out of four, it is reasonable to guess B or C if you are in a true guess mode.

Q21 — Pre-Study Suggestions

Review the following if needed:
1) Thermodynamics **CHM 7.1-7.6**
2) Enthalpy (ΔH) **CHM 7.5, 7.6**
3) Entropy (ΔS) **CHM 8.9**
4) Free Energy (ΔG) **CHM 8.10**
5) Multiple Choice Question **SB A.1.2**
6) What information is needed from the passage?
7) Solve the problem.

CHAPTER 4

Solution Discussion

The information from the passage is found in the second paragraph:

"The instructor prepared a solution of NaOH(aq) by dissolving 8 g of NaOH(s) (MM = 40.00) in 2 L of H_2O … mixing process."

Option A is incorrect. It doesn't contain Item III.

Item I is true. The fact that the temperature of the solution increased is a sign that energy as heat was released by the reaction. This means the Enthalpy (ΔH) (**CHM 7.5, 7.6**) was negative (< 0).

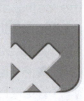

Option B is incorrect. It contains Item II.

Item II is false. Since there was spontaneous dissolution of the substance in water, this means the Free Energy (ΔG) (**CHM 8.10**) must have been negative, G < 0.

Option D is incorrect. It contains Item II.

Item III is true. The process involves solute molecules being dispersed in solvent molecules. This is a process of going from a more restricted state of each alone, to a state of the solution with many more possibilities. When the possible microstates increase, there is a positive Entropy (ΔS) (**CHM 8.9**).

Option C is correct. *See the previous discussion.*

Test Taking Skills Comment

This is a Multiple Choice Question (**SB A.1.2**) problem. If you are sure Item II is incorrect, as it is, then you can eliminate options B and D immediately. You are only left with option C. Since Item I must be correct, as it is in Options A and C, you only have to assess Item III for truth. If you only know that I is definitely correct, then you make your guesses, if needed, from options A and C. If you only know that Item III is correct, then you make your guess from options C or D. This is the value of a Multiple Choice Question (**SB A.1.2**).

Q22 — Pre-Study Suggestions

Review the following if needed:
1) Concentration Units **CHM 5.3.1**
2) Molarity **CHM 5.3.1**
3) Approximation **PHY 2.6.1, GS A.6**
3) Three Out of Four Options **SB A.2.8**
4) What information is needed from the passage?
5) Solve the problem.

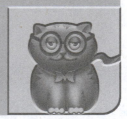

Solution Discussion

The key information from the passage is found in paragraph two:

"The instructor prepared a solution of NaOH(aq) by dissolving 8 g of NaOH(s) (MM= 40.00) in 2 L of H_2..."

The Molarity (**CHM 5.3.1**) is found as follows:

M = moles of solute/liters of solution
= (1/5)/2
= (1/5)(1/2)
= 1/10 = 0.1 M

Moles of solute = grams of solute / molar mass of solute
= 8/40 = 1/5.

Options B, C and D are incorrect. See the previous discussion.

Option A is correct. *See* the previous discussion.

Test Taking Skills Comment

This is also a Three Out of Four Options (**SB A.2.8**). Options A, B and C are all fractions or less than one. Option D is an outlier being greater than one. Outliers are usually incorrect and can be ignored. This means if you are not sure and you identify an outlier, eliminate it and take your guess from the other three options. They asked for an Approximation (**PHY 2.6.1, GS A.6**), but none was really required.

Q23   Pre-Study Suggestions

Review the following if needed:
1) Acid and Base Titrations **CHM 6.9, 6.9.1- 6.9.3**
2) pH **CHM 6.1, 6.2**
3) Salts **CHM 6.7**
4) Three Out of Four Options **SB A.2.8**
5) Similar Pair Options **SB A.2.7**
6) What information is needed from the passage?
7) Solve the problem.

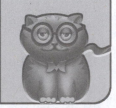

Solution Discussion

The information needed from the passage is Equation 3:

$$HC_7H_5O_2(aq) + NaOH\ (aq) \rightarrow NaC_7H_5O_2(aq) + H_2O(l).$$

At the neutralization (*see* Acid and Base Titrations **CHM 6.9, 6.9.1- 6.9.3**) point of the titration, the NaOH has completely neutralized the benzoic acid in solution. The only species present, other than water, is $NaC_7H_5O_2$. This is the Salts (**CHM 6.7**) of a weak acid and is the Conjugate Base (**CHM 6.3**) of the benzoic acid. The salt of a weak acid is a weak base. This will hydrolyze water as follows:

$$NaC_7H_5O_2 + H_2O \rightleftharpoons Na^+ + OH^- + HC_7H_5O_2.$$

Since the OH^- is produced, the solution is basic and should have a pH > 7.

Option B is incorrect. This would have been the situation if a weak base was titrated by a strong acid and the end product was a weakly acidic salt. The weakly acidic salt would hydrolyze the water to produce an acidic solution.

Option C is incorrect. A neutral solution with pH = 7 would result from the titration of a strong acid and a strong base.

Option A is incorrect. Since the acid was neutralized, the solution will not be acidic.

Option D is correct. *See* the previous discussion.

CHAPTER 4

Test Taking Skills Comment

This is a rare triple Three Out of Four Options (**SB A.2.8**) question. In the situation of triple Three Out of Four, the potentially correct answer is the remaining option when all of the Three Out of Fours are evaluated. Options B, C and D all contain the number 7. Option A is an outlier with no 7. Options A, B and D all have inequality relationships. Option C has an equal relationship and is the outlier. Options A, C and D all contain one relationship. Option B contains two relationships and is an outlier. Outliers tend to be incorrect and can often be ignored. Since option D is the only one that is not the outlier, it may correct. This is a possible Similar Pair Options (**SB A.2.7**), but it should not be used because there is more than one similar pair present (options A and B, options A and D).

Q24 — Pre-Study Suggestions

Review the following if needed:
1) Bronsted - Lowry Acids and Bases **CHM 6.1**
2) Conjugate Base **CHM 6.3**
3) Dichotomy of Options **SB A.2.3**
4) Internally Inconsistent **SB A.2.5**
5) Similar Pair Options **SB A.2.7**
6) What information is needed from the passage?
7) Solve the problem.

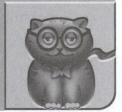

Solution Discussion

Chlorobenzoic acid has the following structure:

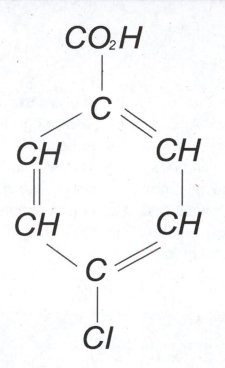

The Cl could be in other locations (where the H's are on the ring).

The conjugate base of Chlorobenzoic acid would be minus the H attached to the carboxylic acid group.

Option A is incorrect. This is the conjugate base of water, H_2O. This is Internally Inconsistent (**SB A.2.5**) because the Chlorobenzoic molecule will be part of the conjugate.

Option B is incorrect. This is the conjugate base of the hydronium ion, H_3O^+. This is Internally Inconsistent (**SB A.2.5**) like option A.

Option C is incorrect. This is a molecule with the wrong formula for Chlorobenzoic acid. It could be the conjugate base of a phenol. This is Internally Inconsistent (**SB A.2.5**).

Option D is correct. *See* the previous discussion. Remember, the only difference between the acid and its conjugate base is that the conjugate base has the acidic hydrogen removed.

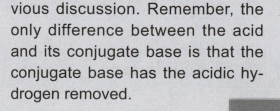

CHAPTER 4

Test Taking Skills Comment

This is a Dichotomy of Options (**SB A.2.3**). You should easily know options A and B cannot be correct because they do not have the proper atoms for Chlorobenzoic acid - they should be eliminated. So, options C and D would be the correct dichotomy to pick. Also, option C does not have enough oxygens to be a Carboxylic Acid (**ORG 8**) and should be eliminated. This is also a Three Out of Four Options (**SB A.2.8**). Options A, C and D are all negative ions. Option B is a neutral molecule and is the outlier. Outliers are generally incorrect and can be eliminated. This is also a Similar Pair Options (**SB A.2.7**) with options C and D being a good similar pair and part of the three out of four.

Q25 — Pre-Study Suggestions

Review the following if needed:
1) Acids and Bases **CHM 6.1- 6.6**
2) Concentration Units **CHM 5.3.1**
3) Acid and Base Titrations **CHM 6.9, 6.9.1- 6.9.3**
4) Carboxylic Acid **ORG 8**
5) Dichotomy of Options **SB A.2.3**
6) Internally Inconsistent **SB A.2.5**
7) What information is needed from the passage?
8) Solve the problem.

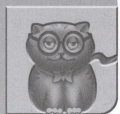

Solution Discussion

From Table 1, the formula for Succinic acid is: $H_2C_4H_4O_4$.

From Table 2, the equivalent weight of Succinic acid is 59.1.

Since the Molar (Molecular) Mass (Weight, MM, MW) (**CHM 1.3**) of Succinic acid is: $6H + 4C + 4O = 6(1) + 4(12) + 4(16) = 6 + 48 + 64 = 118$. Since the Equivalent Weight (see Normality **CHM 5.3.1**) is 59.1, the number of equivalents per mole is found as follows:

n = number of equivalents per mole
 = molar mass/equivalent weight
 = 118/59.1 = 2.

This means Succinic acid has two acidic hydrogens per molecule.

Option A is incorrect. This is Internally Inconsistent (**SB A.2.5**). If the acid is diprotic, it would require twice, not one - half, as many equivalents of base to neutralize it.

Option C is incorrect. This Internally Inconsistent (**SB A.2.5**) as for option A.

Option D is incorrect. This is consistent, but the molecule only has two acidic hydrogens as discussed previously.

Option B is correct. See the previous discussion.

Test Taking Skills Comment

This is a Dichotomy of Options (**SB A.2.3**) question. The dichotomy is the diprotic (options A and B) versus triprotic (options C and D). The analysis demonstrates the Succinic acid is diprotic, so, the triprotic options should be eliminated. If you didn't do this, then the Internally Inconsistency (**SB A.2.5**) of options A and C should cause them to be eliminated.

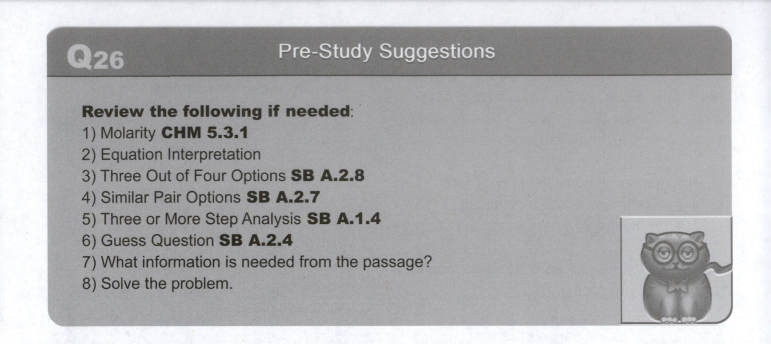

Q26 — Pre-Study Suggestions

Review the following if needed:
1) Molarity **CHM 5.3.1**
2) Equation Interpretation
3) Three Out of Four Options **SB A.2.8**
4) Similar Pair Options **SB A.2.7**
5) Three or More Step Analysis **SB A.1.4**
6) Guess Question **SB A.2.4**
7) What information is needed from the passage?
8) Solve the problem.

Solution Discussion

The information from the passage is as follows:

Table 2 - mass of KHP = 0.5500 g

Paragraph three:

   "NaOH(aq) was standardized by each student by titration against a pure sample of KHP (MM=204.2) …"

Equation 2:

KHP(aq) + NaOH(aq) $\rightleftharpoons$ KNaP(aq) + H_2O(l).

The Moles (**CHM 1.3**) of KHP is determined as follows:

Moles of KHP = mass KHP/molar mass (**CHM 1.3**)

KHP = 0.5500/204.2

The 0.5500 is expected to be pure KHP.

If the KHP is actually KHP, H_2O (contaminated with water), then some of the 0.5500 is water and not KHP. This means the moles of KHP is overestimated.

Since Molarity = moles/volume (**CHM 5.3.1**), the molarity of KHP will also be overestimated.

During the titration to determine the molarity of NaOH, the equation 2 would be used and the following relationship:

$$M_{KHP}V_{KHP} = M_{NaOH}V_{NaOH}$$

And,

$$M_{NaOH} = (M_{KHP}V_{KHP})/V_{NaOH}.$$

So, if M_{KHP} is overestimated, this means the M_{NaOH} will be overestimated. Notice the V_{KHP} required to titrate the NaOH will also be increased because the true amount of acid is less than expected.

Option B is incorrect. The number of moles of KHP used in the calculation is greater than the actual number used. So, this is a true statement. But, because this makes the molarity of KHP calculated greater than it should be, this causes the number of moles and molarity of NaOH to be greater than they should be.

Option C is incorrect. The number of moles of KHP in the calculation is greater not smaller than the actual number. This statement is incorrect.

Option D is incorrect. Since the number of moles of KHP is increased, the calculation and titration of NaOH will be distorted. The KHP was weighed before it was placed in water.

Option A is correct. This was discussed previously.

Test Taking Skills Comment

This is a Three Out of Four Options (**SB A.2.8**) question. Options A, B and C are change questions. Option D is an outlier and is a no – change option. Generally, outliers are incorrect, but you must be careful with change questions. This is also a Similar Pair Options (**SB A.2.7**) with options B and C being similar. These options would be a good guess if you're in the guessing mode even though neither is correct - remember these techniques increase your average guess and not every guess. This is a Guess Question (**SB A.2.4**) because the options are so complex and because it is also a Negative Question (**SB A.1.2**) which makes it more difficult.

This is a Three or More Step Analysis (**SB A.1.4**) which makes it more difficult: 1) you have to determine if it is high or low or unaffected, 2) then you have to determine if the explanation is consistent with these, 3) then you have to determine if the option is True or False (**SB A.1.2**), 4) finally, you have to determine if the option is Correct or Incorrect (**SB A.1.2**).

Q27 — Pre-Study Suggestions

Review the following if needed:
1) Mole Fraction **CHM 5.3.1**
2) Moles **CHM 1.3**
3) Dichotomy of Options **SB A.2.3**
4) Internally Inconsistent **SB A.2.5**
5) What information is needed from the passage?
6) Solve the problem.

Solution Discussion

The information from the passage:

In paragraph one:

Molar Mass (**CHM 1.3**) of potassium nitrate = 101.1 g/mol.

In Table 1: solute conc.

(KNO_3) = 226.5 g/L and water conc.

= 906.1 g/L.

The molar mass of H_2O is = 2(1) + 16 = 18.

The Mole Fraction, X, (**CHM 5.3.1**) (X_{KNO3}) of the KNO_3 is:

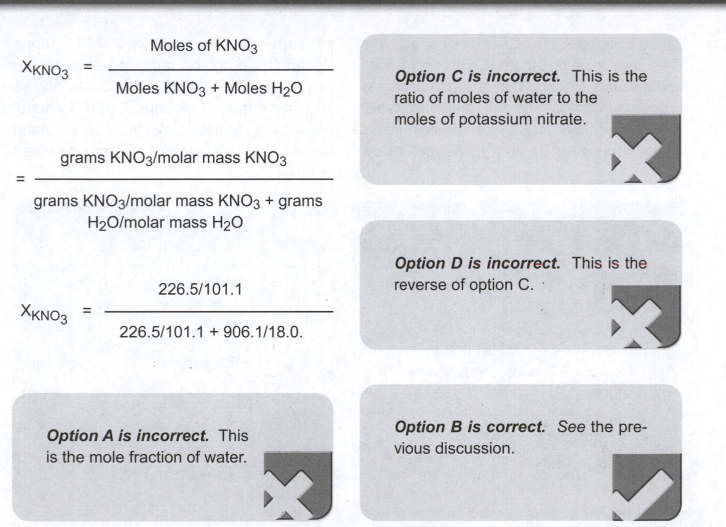

$$X_{KNO_3} = \frac{\text{Moles of } KNO_3}{\text{Moles } KNO_3 + \text{Moles } H_2O}$$

$$= \frac{\text{grams } KNO_3/\text{molar mass } KNO_3}{\text{grams } KNO_3/\text{molar mass } KNO_3 + \text{grams } H_2O/\text{molar mass } H_2O}$$

$$X_{KNO_3} = \frac{226.5/101.1}{226.5/101.1 + 906.1/18.0}$$

Option C is incorrect. This is the ratio of moles of water to the moles of potassium nitrate.

Option D is incorrect. This is the reverse of option C.

Option A is incorrect. This is the mole fraction of water.

Option B is correct. *See* the previous discussion.

Test Taking Skills Comment

This is a Dichotomy of Options (**SB A.2.3**) type question. If you are secure, Basic Knowledge (study, passage, general) (**SB A.2.2**), knowing that the mole fraction must have the total moles in the denominator, then you know there must be a term in the denominator for each component of the solution - this example requires two terms for the two components. Since options C and D only have one term, they cannot be correct and are immediately eliminated. Also, if you knew that for the mole fraction, the numerator must contain the moles of the substance of concern, the numerator must contain the term of 226.5/101.1.

CHAPTER 4

Since options A and C do not contain this term, they must be incorrect. This only leaves options B as correct. This question becomes a double dichotomy type. It is also Internally Inconsistent (**SB A.2.5**) for similar reasons if you apply your Basic Knowledge (study, passage, general) (**SB A.2.2**) - options C and D cannot be correct because you need the moles of all substances in the denominator. Also, options A and C cannot be correct, because the numerator must contain the substance of concern as noted previously.

Q28 — Pre-Study Suggestions

Review the following if needed:
1) Solubility **CHM 5.3**
2) Le Chatelier's Principle **CHM 9.9**
3) Solubility Factors **CHM 5.3**
4) Similar Pair Options **SB A.2.7**
5) Negative Question **SB A.1.2**
6) What information is needed from the passage?
7) Solve the problem.

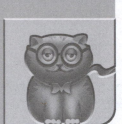

Solution Discussion

A saturated solution of KNO_3 will be:

$$KNO_3(s) + H_2O \rightleftharpoons K^+(aq) + NO_3^-(aq).$$

Option A is incorrect. The effect of adding $NH_4NO_3(s)$, which dissolves in water, will be to add NO_3^- ions to the solution as the NO_3^- will be added to the right side of the equation and will cause the equilibrium to shift to the left causing the KNO_3 to precipitate - this is Le Chatelier's Principle (**CHM 9.9**).

Option B is incorrect. The $Ca(NO_3)_2$ will dissolve in water, and the NO_3^- ions released will shift the equilibrium to the left causing more KNO_3 to precipitate.

will add to the right side of the equation and shift the equilibrium to the left. This will cause more of the KNO_3 to precipitate.

Option D is incorrect. The KCl will dissolve completely in the water and will release the K^+ ion which

Option C is correct. The NH_4Cl will dissolve completely in water, but neither of the ions released will affect the previous equilibrium.

Test Taking Skills Comment

This is the common ion effect (see Solubility Factors **CHM 5.3**) on solubility. It can be understood in terms of the Le Chatelier's Principle (**CHM 9.9**). This is why it is a Camouflage and Distractions (**SB A.1.3**) question. If a common ion, as in options A, B and D are added to solution with one of those ions, the effect is to decrease the solubility of the ions in solution. You might think this is a Similar Pair Options (**SB A.2.7**) as options A and C and options A and B are similar pairs. But, remember when there is more than one similar pair, do not use this technique.

CHAPTER 4

Q29 — Pre-Study Suggestions

Review the following if needed:
1) Graphs and Charts **GS A.3**
2) Dichotomy of Options **SB A.2.3**
3) Internally Inconsistent **SB A.2.5**
4) What information is needed from the passage?
5) Solve the problem.

Solution Discussion

The key information is found in the last paragraph:

"The condosity of a solution … specific conductance (electrical) as the solution."

And in Table 1:

The Molarity (**CHM 5.3.1**) of the solution is 2.241 mol/L.

The chart, Graphs and Charts (**GS A.3**), shows that the conductance is increasing as go up the vertical axis. It also shows that the molarity is increasing as go from left to right on the horizontal axis.

Option A is incorrect. This states the molarity of the student solution is the same as the NaCl. The student solution has a lower molarity that the NaCl. Also, the conductance should the same as the NaCl and this conductance is much higher. This is Internally Inconsistent (**SB A.2.5**) because the definition states condosity has the same conductance, not the same molarity, as is true for A and C, as the NaCl.

Option B is incorrect. This has the student solution's molarity much higher than the NaCl. The conductance is the same and this is appropriate, but the molarity of the student's solution is less than the NaCl.

Option C is incorrect. This is incorrect for the same reasons given in option A. This is Internally Inconsistent (**SB A.2.5**).

Option D is correct. The molarity of the student's solution is less than the molarity of the NaCl which is appropriate. Also, the conductance of both solutions is the same as required by the definition of condosity.

Test Taking Skills Comment

You have to properly interpret the Graphs and Charts (**GS A.3**) and know the definition as presented in the passage. Since the total conductance must be equal, the student's solution and the NaCl should be on the same horizontal line. This means options A and C cannot be correct; they are Internally Inconsistent (**SB A.2.5**), because they have a different conductance than the NaCl. Also, from the Table, it is clear that the molarity of the student's solution must be less than the NaCl. This means the student's molarity has to appear to the left of the NaCl. The only option that satisfies this, is option D. There is a Dichotomy of Options (**SB A.2.3**) based on the Passage Knowledge (**SB A.2.2**) in excerpt previously. Since the conductance has to be the same as the NaCl, the correct options must be B or D. You can eliminate A and C.

Q30 — Pre-Study Suggestions

Review the following if needed:
1) Concentration Units **CHM 5.3.1**
2) Ratio and Proportion
3) Moles **CHM 1.3**
4) Graphs and Charts **GS A.3**
5) Approximation **PHY 2.6.1, GS A.6**
6) Three Out of Four Options **SB A.2.8**
7) Camouflage and Distractions **SB A.1.3**
8) Similar Pair Options **SB A.2.7**
9) What information is needed from the passage?
10) Solve the problem.

Solution Discussion

From Table 1 - the solute concentration is 226.5 g L and Molarity = 2.241 mol/L (**CHM 5.3.1**). (*See* Graphs and Charts **GS A.3**).

From the first paragraph, the Molar Mass = 101.1 g/mol (**CHM 1.3**)

Solution using the solute concentration:
   Use Ratio and Proportion:

$$\frac{\text{Grams in 100 ml}}{100\ ml} = \frac{226.5\ g}{1000\ ml}$$

grams in 100 ml = (226.5)(100/1000)

= (226.5)(1/10)
= 22.65 g.

Solution using Moles (**CHM 1.3**):

First find moles of KNO_3 in 100 ml (= 0.10 L)
   Moles = MV
      = (2.241)(0.10 L)
      = 0.2241 mol

Then find grams of KNO_3:

   Moles = mass/molar mass
   Mass = moles x molar mass
      = 0.2241 x 101.1 = 22.66 g.

Options A, B and D are incorrect. *See* the previous discussion.

Option C is correct. *See* the previous discussion.

Test Taking Skills Comment

If one solution, the mole method, appears to be difficult, then quickly survey for an Alternative Solution (**SB A.1.3**), (*see* Camouflage and Distractions **SB A.1.3**). In general, you will not be expected to do complicated calculations as in the mole method. In the mole method, you can approximate (**PHY 2.6.1, GS A.6**) the calculation as the correct answer will be slightly greater than 22.41 (because the molar mass is 101.1). This means option C cannot be correct, option A is much too low and option D is much too high.

This is also a very subtle Three Out of Four Options (**SB A.2.8**) as options A, C and D are all multiples of option A. Option B is not a multiple and is an outlier. Outliers tend to be incorrect. You could also state this is a Similar Pair Options (**SB A.2.7**) as options B and C both have 22.x as the whole number part. You could guess from the B or C and would have correct guess in this instance. But, if you saw the three out of four previously, then the similar pair is not part of it and would not be used. The three out of four is a difficult read, but the similar pair is more obvious.

CHAPTER 4

Q31 — Pre-Study Suggestions

Review the following if needed:
1) Molarity **CHM 5.3.1**
2) Moles **CHM 1.3**

3) Avogadro's Number **CHM 1.3**
4) Ratio and Proportion
5) Approximation **PHY 2.6.1, GS A.6**
6) Three Out of Four Options **SB A.2.8**
7) Similar Pair Options **SB A.2.7**
8) Camouflage and Distractions **SB A.1.3**
9) What information is needed from the passage?
10) Solve the problem.

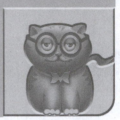

Solution Discussion

The key pieces of information:

From paragraph 2 - the volume of the solution is 1 L.

From Table 1- Molarity (**CHM 5.3.1**) of solution is 2.241 mol/L

To get the number of atoms, you have to determine the number of Moles (**CHM 1.3**):
Moles KNO_3 = MV = (2.241)(1) = 2.241 moles.

Then use Avogadro's number (**CHM 1.3**) to get the number of atoms using Ratio and Proportion:

$$\frac{\text{Number of atoms}}{\text{Moles of } KNO_3} = \frac{6.023 \times 10^{23}}{1 \text{ mole}}$$

Number of atoms = $(6.023 \times 10^{23}) (2.241)/(1)$
$\approx 6 \times 10^{23} \times 2.5 \approx 15 \times 10^{23}$
$\approx 1.5 \times 10^{24}$.

This is good example to use approximation (**PHY 2.6.1, GS A.6**).

Options A, B and C are incorrect. See the previous discussion.

Option D is correct. See the previous discussion.

Test Taking Skills Comment

Notice this calculation calls for an approximate answer as opposed to the prior one. This is also a Three Out of Four Options (**SB A.2.8**). Options B, C and D are similar in having double digit exponents (or even numbers which is less important). Option A has single digit exponents and is the outlier. In general, outliers are incorrect and can be ignored. Also, this is a soft Similar Pair Options (**SB A.2.7**) with options C and D both having exponents in the 20's. Since the similar pair is within the three out of four, you can reasonably guess it. In this instance, by guessing C or D, the similar pair, you would do better than the 45% correct the test group achieved.

It is disconcerting to reflect on the number of students we have flunked in chemistry for not knowing what we later found to be untrue.

– Quoted from Robert L. Weber, Science With a Smile (1992)

Q32 — Pre-Study Suggestions

Review the following if needed:
1) Chemical Reactions **CHM 1.5**
2) Ideal Gas Law **CHM 4.1.6**
3) Partial Pressure **CHM 4.1.7**
4) Mole Fraction, X, **CHM 5.3.1**
5) Equation Interpretation
6) Three Out of Four Options **SB A.2.8**
7) Camouflage and Distractions **SB A.1.3**
8) Solve the problem.

Solution Discussion

The reaction would be:

$$CH_4(g) + 2O_2(g) \rightleftharpoons CO_2(g) + 2H_2O(g).$$

The partial pressure of a gas is given by Dalton's Law of Partial Pressure (**CHM 4.1.7**):

$P_{H_2O} = X_{H_2O}P_T$ = partial pressure of water

P_T = total pressure = 1.2 torr

X_{H_2O} = Mole Fraction, X, (**CHM 5.3.1**) of water

= moles of water/total moles
= (2)/(1+2)
= 2/3 = 2/3.

These numbers are from the balanced equation - since the methane and oxygen reacts completely, they are no longer present

then,

$$P_{H_2O} = X_{H_2O}P_T$$
$$= (2/3)(1.2 \text{ torrs})$$
$$= (2)(0.4) \text{ torrs}$$
$$= 0.8 \text{ torrs}.$$

Options A, B and D are incorrect. You could select option B if you did not read the phrase reacts completely.

Option C is correct. See the previous question.

Test Taking Skills Comment

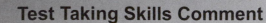

The MCAT does not try to trick you. But, you do have read the question carefully and interpret it directly. This question is a good example if you do not use the 'reacts completely' phrase. This is a Three Out of

Four Options (**SB A.2.8**) type question where options A, B and C are all less than one and option D is greater than one and is the outlier. Outliers will tend to be incorrect.

Q33 — Pre-Study Suggestions

Review the following if needed:
1) Molecular Formulas **CHM 1.2**
2) Empirical Formulas **CHM 1.2**
3) Internally Inconsistent **SB A.2.5**
4) Solve the problem.

Solution Discussion

Following the steps in the review (empirical formulas, **CHM 1.2**) for this problem:

Step 1:

moles of C = 12/12 = 1.0
moles of H = 2/1= 2.0
moles of O = 16/16 = 1.

Step 2/3:

this is already done and the empirical formula is $C_1H_2O_1$ or CH_2O.

Options B, C and D are incorrect.

Option A is correct. See the previous discussion.

CHAPTER 4

Test Taking Skills Comment

You should be able to eliminate options C and D because the formulas are not in the smallest ratio of atoms and this is Internally Inconsistent (**SB A.2.5**) with the definition of Empirical Formulas (**CHM 1.2**).

Q34 — Pre-Study Suggestions

Review the following if needed:
1) Standing Waves **PHY 7.1.5**
2) Wave Characteristics **PHY 7.1**
3) Equation Interpretation
4) Camouflage and Distractions **SB A.1.3**
5) Solve the problem.

Solution Discussion

The pipe described is equivalent to the string fixed at both ends (*see* Standing Waves **PHY 7.1.5**). The wavelengths associated with a string fixed at both ends are:

$$\lambda = 2L/n \quad \text{where } n = 1, 2, 3 \ldots$$

Then for $n = 1$ and $L = 1$ m,

$$\lambda = 2\,L/n$$
$$= 2(1)/1$$
$$= 2 \text{ m.}$$

The pipe open at both ends must have an antinode at the open end. This means one must be a crest, an antinode, and the other end must be a trough, or an antinode - this is the smallest portion of the wave that will fit into the constraints. The distance from a crest to a trough is ½ of a wavelength. If ½ of a wavelength is 1 m, then a full wavelength is twice this and is 2 m. This would be the fundamental wavelength which is the longest.

Options A, B and C are incorrect. *See* the previous discussion.

Option D is correct. *See* the previous discussion.

Test Taking Skills Comment

This is also a Camouflage and Distractions (**SB A.1.3**) question. Notice that you do not need the diameter of the pipe to solve the problem. Data is often presented that you do not need. The more confident you are, the better you have prepared, and the less you will be distracted by this type of data. You do have to recognize this as a Standing Waves (**PHY 7.1.5**) problem.

Q35 — Pre-Study Suggestions

Review the following if needed:
1) Waves **PHY 7.1**
2) Energy of Waves **PHY 7.1, 9.2.4**
3) Internally Inconsistent **SB A.2.5**
4) Solve the problem.

Solution Discussion

Option A is incorrect. Waves do not transport matter. They transport momentum and energy. Matter, in mechanical waves, would only oscillate about a point and not be transported through space. This is Internally Inconsistent (**SB A.2.5**) with your Basic Knowledge (study, passage, general) (**SB A.2.2**) of waves. All other options with matter would be incorrect as well.

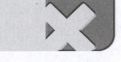

CHAPTER 4

Option C is incorrect. Matter is not transported. See option A. This is Internally Inconsistent (**SB A.2.5**).

Option D is incorrect. Energy is transported in waves.

"D DUV"

For **D**iverging mirrors and lenses, the image is always **D**iminished, **U**pright, and **V**irtual, regardless of the distance of the object from the mirror or lens.

Option B is correct. Energy as well as momentum is transported.

Test Taking Skills Comment

This is fundamental knowledge; you know it or not. You could try a Three Out of Four Options (**SB A.2.8**) or a Similar Pair Options (**SB A.2.7**) but the use of Internally Inconsistent (**SB A.2.5**) is better and is based on Basic Knowledge (study, passage, general) (**SB A.2.2**) which is very important.

Q36 — Pre-Study Suggestions

Review the following if needed:
1) Momentum **PHY 4.3**
2) Conservation of Momentum **PHY 4.3**
3) Collisions **PHY 4.4, 4.4.1**
4) Kinetic Energy **PHY 5.3**

5) Potential Energy **PHY 5.4**
6) Conservation of Energy **PHY 5.5**
7) What information is needed from the passage?
8) Solve the problem.

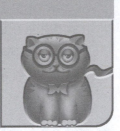

Solution Discussion

Information needed: In the first and third paragraphs, the passage describes a collision of the continents.

"The collision was brief on the time scale of geological ... and the Mauritanian Mountains."

"Consider a simplified model of this collision in which the ... "

Option C is incorrect. Potential Energy (**PHY 5.4**) is not a factor in the collision as the energy comes from the movement of the objects. Briefly during the collision there is the presence of potential energy that is converted back to kinetic or other energy.

Option B is incorrect. Kinetic Energy (**PHY 5.3**) is conserved in elastic Collisions (**PHY 4.4, 4.4.1**). This is not an elastic collision because the formation of the mountains represents a deformation of the colliding objects. This would have to been an inelastic collision.

Option D is incorrect. The impulse is similar to the momentum, but is viewed as the average force acting over the time of the collision. This can be confusing and could be a Mutually Excluding Options (**SB A.2.6**) if you understand the

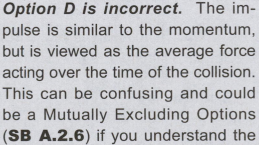

CHAPTER 4

relationship between the impulse and the momentum. Ultimately, you have to select the Best Option (**SB A.1.2**) which is option C.

Option C is correct. Momentum (**PHY 4.3**) is conserved in all collisions.

Test Taking Skills Comment

This is primarily knowledge, but review the previous comments in option D.

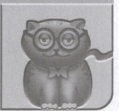

Teacher: What is the formula for water?

Premed student: H, I, J, K, L, M, N, O

Teacher: That's not what I taught you.

Premed student: But you said the formula for water was ... H to O.

Q37	Pre-Study Suggestions

Review the following if needed:
1) Radioactive Dating **PHY 12.4**
2) Similar Pair Options **SB A.2.7**
3) Complex Sounding Option(s) **SB A.2.2**
4) What information is needed from the passage?
5) Solve the problem.

Solution Discussion

The key information from the passage is from the first and second paragraphs:

First:

"and radioactive dating of rocks brought to the surface during the collision."

Second:

"In radioactive dating, the age of a rock ... the rock and the amount of its decay product, argon gas (^{40}Ar), in the sample."

Option B is incorrect. Gases in the rock before formation are not important as they only relate to pre - collision events.

Option D is incorrect. The passage states rocks brought to the surface are used for the dating.

Option A is incorrect. What is a role for organic material? The potassium's form is not noted. Potassium is an inorganic material. There is nothing in the passage nor in your prior study that can assess this option. This is a Complex Sounding Option(s) (**SB A.2.2**).

Option C is correct. Since the dating is comparing the potassium and the argon isotopes present, both should remain in the rock from its formation to get accurate dating.

CHAPTER 4

Test Taking Skills Comment

This only requires passage interpretation. You can eliminate option A because it is Complex Sounding Option(s) (**SB A.2.2**). Options B and C constitute a Similar Pair Options (**SB A.2.7**) because both relate to gases and there are no other obvious similar pairs in the question.

Q38 — Pre-Study Suggestions

Review the following if needed:
1) Momentum **PHY 4.3**
2) Conservation of Momentum **PHY 4.3**
3) Dimensional Analysis **GS Part II 2.3 # 16**
4) Collisions **PHY 4.4, 4.4.1**
5) Three Out of Four Options **SB A.2.8**
6) Similar Pair Options **SB A.2.7**
7) Camouflage and Distractions **SB A.1.3**
8) What information is needed from the passage?
9) Solve the problem.

Solution Discussion

Nothing is required from the passage.

Since the collision is a perfectly inelastic Collision (**PHY 4.3**), Kinetic Energy (**PHY 5.3**) is not conserved, but Momentum (**PHY 4.3**) is conserved:

initial momentum = final momentum

$$m_1 v_1 + m_2 v_2 = v_f (m_1 + m_2)$$

then,

$$v_f = (m_1v_1 + m_2v_2)/(m_1 + m_2)$$
$$= \text{final velocity.}$$

Option A is correct. See the previous discussion.

Option B, C and D are incorrect. See the previous discussion.

Test Taking Skills Comment

This is a basic application of the Conservation of Momentum (**PHY 4.3**) and it must be recognized (*see* Camouflage and Distractions **SB A.1.3**). Nothing is required from the passage. This could be a Three Out of Four Options (**SB A.2.8**) as options A, C and D do not contain exponents and option B, the outlier does. This could also be a

Similar Pair Options (**SB A.2.7**) as options A and D both contain fractions and are part of the three out of four. You should check Dimensional Analysis (**GS Part II 2.3 # 16**) but all the options has the appropriate dimensions for velocity and it does not help in this problem.

CHAPTER 4

Q39 — Pre-Study Suggestions

Review the following if needed:
1) Nuclear Particles **PHY 12.1, 12.2**
2) Nuclear Reactions **PHY 12.4**
3) Periodic Table **CHM 2.3**
4) What information is needed from the passage?
5) Solve the problem.

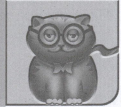

Solution Discussion

The information needed is from paragraph 2:

"In radioactive dating, the age of a rock … amount of its decay product, argon gas (^{40}Ar), in the sample."

The Nuclear Reactions (**PHY 12.4**) is then (get the Atomic Number **PHY 12.2**, or number of protons from the Periodic Table **CHM 2.3**):

$$_{19}K^{40} \rightarrow {}_{18}Ar^{40} + {}_{x}Z^{y}.$$

Then,

$$x = 19 - 18 = +1$$

$$y = 40 - 40 = 0.$$

The Z particle is then,

$_{+1}Z^{0}$ and this is a Positron, $_{1}\beta^{0}$ or $_{1}e^{0} = {}_{+1}e^{0}$
(**PHY 12.1, 12.2**).

Options A, B and C are incorrect. *See* the previous discussion.

Option D is correct. *See* the previous discussion.

Test Taking Skills Comment

Minimal information about the decay product is needed from the passage. You solve this problem by knowing the Basic Knowledge (study, passage, general) (**SB A.2.2**).

Q40 — Pre-Study Suggestions

Review the following if needed:
1) Newton's Laws of Motion **PHY 2.2, 2.3, 4.2**
2) Three Out of Four Options **SB A.2.8**
3) Similar Pair Options **SB A.2.7**
4) Camouflage and Distractions **SB A.1.3**
5) What information is needed from the passage?
6) Solve the problem.

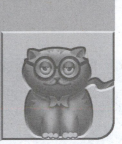

Solution Discussion

This is a direct application of Newton's Third Law of Motion (**PHY 2.2, 2.3, 4.2**) of equal and opposite forces.

Options A, C and D are incorrect. See the previous discussion.

Option B is correct. Per Newton's Third Law of Motion.

Test Taking Skills Comment

Everyone knows Newton's Laws of Motion (**PHY 2.2, 2.3, 4.2**). Only 45% got this question correct. This is also a Three Out of Four Options (**SB A.2.8**) question. Options A, B and C are non-zero options. Option D is zero and is the outlier. Outliers tend to be incorrect. An exception is change questions or question with none or zero as an option;

but generally zero/no change options are incorrect. Also, this is a Similar Pair Options (**SB A.2.7**) question as options B and C are non fractions. But, you could also say that options A and C are a similar pair because both have the factor 2 involved. If you see more than one similar pair, it is best not to use this technique. This is also a problem of recognizing the concept, Camouflage and Distractions (**SB A.1.3**), because the concept is well camouflaged by all the superfluous information.

Q41 — Pre-Study Suggestions

Review the following if needed:
1) Electric Field, E, **PHY 9.1.3**
2) Resistance, R, **PHY 10.2**
3) Relationships of Variables **GS A.3.1**
4) Dichotomy of Options **SB A.2.3**
5) What information is needed from the passage?
6) Solve the problem.

Solution Discussion

The key information from the passage is found in paragraph two:

"The electric field at all points between the electrodes is equal to the electrode voltage difference divided by L."

Inversely Related (Proportional) (**GS A.3.1**) to L as described previously:

$$E = V/L$$

where

V = electrode voltage difference.

Option B is incorrect. The Electric Field (**PHY 9.1.3**) (E) is

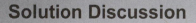

This means as L decreases, the E will increase. Notice that this equation is nothing more than the relationship you are supposed to know about Electric Field (**PHY 9.1.3**) and electric Potential, V (**PHY 9.1.4**).

So, the E is usually a Direct Relationship (**GS A.3.1**) to the resistance. But, the layout shows that the outside R of the loop affecting the field of the electrodes.

Options C and D are incorrect. Usually, the voltage (V) and then the electric field (E) will be related as follows and will be related to the resistance (R):

$V = IR$ where I = current
$V = Ed$ where d = distance between charges
$Ed = IR$
$E = IR/d$
$= V/d = V/L$

Option A is correct. Since E and L are inversely related, any increase in L will cause a decrease in E:

$$E \propto 1/L.$$

Test Taking Skills Comment

Sometimes you are given specific relationships that are different from the Basic Knowledge (study, passage, general) (**SB A.2.2**) you have. You are expected to use this information to solve problems even if it is in conflict with your basic knowledge.

This does not mean your basic knowledge is incorrect, it just means you are given advanced information and must apply it. In this case, there is actually no conflict. This is also a Dichotomy of Options (**SB A.2.3**) question.

CHAPTER 4

Since you have a specific relationship with L in the passage, you always use Basic Knowledge (study, passage, general) (**SB A.2.2**) to pick your dichotomy, you must use it and should eliminate any relationship with the R in this particular problem. Options C and D would have been considered if the R was part of the loop of the photodiode. Note that the voltage (V) across the diode is not affected by R.

Q42 — Pre-Study Suggestions

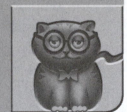

Review the following if needed:
1) Kinetic Energy **PHY 5.3**
2) Potential Energy **PHY 5.4**
3) Conservation of Energy **PHY 5.5**
4) Three Out of Four Options **SB A.2.8**
5) Similar Pair Options **SB A.2.7**
6) Camouflage and Distractions **SB A.1.3**
7) What information is needed from the passage?
8) Solve the problem.

Solution Discussion

From the first paragraph:

"The ejected electron will have a kinetic energy equal to the photon's energy minus the work function."

From the second paragraph:

"The potential energy of an electron immediately after it is released from the cathode is equal to qV ..."

Option A is incorrect. The total energy is as follows:

Photon energy = work function
+ excess energy.

The excess energy is initially

potential energy of the electron as noted previously. As the electron begins to move, the potential energy is converted into kinetic energy. By Conservation of Energy (**PHY 5.5**), these two energies must be equal and not more or less.

Option D is incorrect. *See* discussion of option A.

Option C is incorrect. *See* discussion of option A.

Option B is correct. Since there is a Conservation of Energy (**PHY 5.5**), the excess energy from the photon will be converted to other forms of energy. The majority of this energy will be kinetic energy and will be a 1:1 relationship.

Test Taking Skills Comment

This question is a Camouflage and Distractions (**SB A.1.3**) type question. The concept is of Conservation of Energy (**PHY 5.5**). This is also a Three Out of Four Options (**SB A.2.8**) question but may be a difficult one to see. Options A, B and C all have a comparison to the potential energy. Option D is an outlier being zero and is not a comparison. Outliers tend to be incorrect. But, also no change/zero options tend to be incorrect, but there are two here - so, this makes it more confusing. Anytime there appears to be confusion about these techniques, don't use them.

Q43 — Pre-Study Suggestions

Review the following if needed:
1) Three Out of Four Options **SB A.2.8**
2) Mutually Excluding Options **SB A.2.6**
3) What information is needed from the passage?
4) Solve the problem.

Solution Discussion

From the first paragraph:

"To free an electron, the energy of a photon ... energy equal to the photon's energy minus the work function."

From the second paragraph:

"The potential energy of an electron immediately after it is released from the cathode is equal to qV"

"The electric field at all points between the electrodes is equal to the electrode voltage difference divided by L."

Option B is incorrect. The Potential Energy (**PHY 5.4**) of each electron is given by qV and is nearly the same for all ejected electrons.

Option C is incorrect. The Electric Field (**PHY 9.1.3**) is not dependent on the photons, it is dependent upon V and L as defined previously.

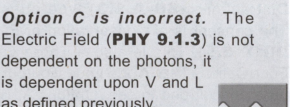

Option D is incorrect. If the potential energy is nearly the same, the speed at the Anode (**CHM 10.4**) depends on the conversion of the potential to Kinetic Energy (**PHY 5.3, 9.1**) and would be nearly the same. This is an option similar to option B and is a Mutually Excluding Options (**SB A.2.6**) based on the information in the passage.

Option A is correct. Each photon above the work function can result in one electron being ejected. As more photons with energy above the work function strike the metal, more electrons will be ejected. Notice it is the number of photons that increases not the energy per photon (then options B and D would be correct).

Test Taking Skills Comment

This problem requires careful reading of the passage. It is also a Mutually Excluding Options (**SB A.2.6**) for options B and D as discussed. Remember you use mutually excluding options when the effect of the option is the same. If potential energy increases, then kinetic energy increases and the speed increase - this makes options B and D the same. This is also a Three Out of Four Options (**SB A.2.8**) question with options A, B and D all relating to electrons. Option D does not relate to electrons and is an outlier - outliers are usually incorrect.

CHAPTER 4

Q44 — Pre-Study Suggestions

Review the following if needed:
1) Coulomb's Law **PHY 9.1.2**
2) Electric Field **PHY 9.1.3**

3) Acceleration **PHY 1.3**
4) Camouflage and Distractions **SB A.1.3**
5) Complex Sounding Option(s) **SB A.2.2**
6) Three Out of Four Options **SB A.2.8**
7) Similar Pair Options **SB A.2.7**
8) What information is needed from the passage?
9) Solve the problem.

Solution Discussion

From the second paragraph:

  "The cathode is made of a photoelectric metal and is connected to the negative terminal of the battery."

  "The electric field at all points between the electrodes …"

The Figure 1:
This shows the anode being connected to the positive terminal and would be positive; it also shows the direction of motion of the electron from the cathode to the anode.

  Option A is incorrect. A charge in an Electric Field (**PHY 9.1.3**) will move in the direction based on its charge and the direction of the field. Positive charges move in the direction of the field. Negative charges move in the direction opposite to the field. Coulomb's Law (**PHY 9.1.2**) gives the forces acting on the charge and also gives the direction of movement. There is an electric field present and forces present as described in the passage. This is also a Complex Sounding Option(s) (**SB A.2.2**) as how do you invoke the collisions as a factor. This is beyond your Basic Knowledge (study, passage, general) (**SB A.2.2**).

Option B is incorrect. There is a Force (**PHY 5.6**) on the charge given by Coulomb's Law (**PHY 9.1.2**). Since a force is acting, there is acceleration (**PHY 1.3**) and the speed (**PHY 1.3**) will not be constant.

Option D is incorrect. Where did this come from? You have nothing in the passage to suggest this. There is nothing in your study to assess this. This is a Complex Sounding Option(s) (**SB A.2.2**)

well beyond your Basic Knowledge (study, passage, general) (**SB A.2.2**).

Option C is correct. The anode (**CHM 10.4**) is positively charged and the electric Field (**PHY 9.1.3**) would emanate from it to the cathode (**CHM 10.4**). The electron moves opposite to the electric field or toward positive charges under a force given by Coulomb's Law (**PHY 9.1.3**).

Test Taking Skills Comment

There is a Complex Sounding Option(s) (**SB A.2.2**) as discussed for options A and D previously. This is also a Three Out of Four Options (**SB A.2.8**) question with options A, B and C all relating to the motion of the electron and deal with the anode. Option D is an outlier that deals with neither of these. This is also a Similar Pair Options (**SB A.2.7**) as options B and D relate directly to

the motion of the electron directly. But, the similar pair conflicts with the three out of four … when this occurs, you should not use the similar pair unless you have some compelling reason. Also, Camouflage and Distractions (**SB A.1.3**) is used because the question really deals with your understanding of the effect of forces on the motion of particles, electrons in this instance.

CHAPTER 4

Q45 — Pre-Study Suggestions

Review the following if needed:
1) Electrical Power, W, **PHY 10.2**
2) Current, I (amperes, A), **PHY 10.1**
3) What information is needed from the passage?
4) Solve the problem.

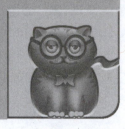

Solution Discussion

From the second paragraph:

The Resistance, R (ohms), (**PHY 10.2**) of the resistor is 100 .

The Voltage, V (volts), (**PHY 10.1, 10.3**) of the battery is 50 V.

Electrical Power, P (watts), (**PHY 10.2**) (P) is given as:

P = IV and this gives the power through the battery,

and Ohm's Law (**PHY 10.1**) is:

$$\boxed{V = IR}$$

Then to get the power loss through the resistor:

$$P = (I)(IR) = I^2R$$
$$= (1 \times 10^{-3})^2(100)$$
$$= (1 \times 10^{-6})(10^2)$$
$$= 10^{-4} \text{ W.}$$

Options A, C and D are incorrect. See the previous discussion.

Option B is correct. See the previous discussion.

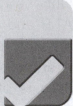

Test Taking Skills Comment

This was an application of basic knowledge.

Q46 — Pre-Study Suggestions

Review the following if needed:
1) Voltage, V (volts), **PHY 10.1, 10.3**
2) Current, I (amperes), **PHY 10.1**
3) Resistance, R (ohms), **PHY 10.2**
4) Similar Pair Options **SB A.2.7**
5) What information is needed from the passage?
6) Solve the problem.

Solution Discussion

From the second paragraph:

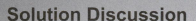

"The potential difference between the cathode and anode is approximately equal to the battery voltage, V = 50 V."

cathode to the anode because that is the direction opposite to the electric field. The expected motion of the electron is to the positive pole of the battery as shown in Figure 1.

Option A is incorrect. The electron responds to the electric field and potential and not vice-versa. The electron moves from the

CHAPTER 4

Option B is incorrect. The voltage difference is maintained by the battery. If the circuit was not maintained by a battery, the voltage would eventually decline to zero.

Option C is correct. When electrons move, this is current flow. By convention, in an electrical circuit, the current flow is the motion of positive charges. So the electrical current flow would be opposite to the direction of electron flow.

Option D is incorrect. Resistance is the effect of slowing the electrons down and is not caused by the electrons.

Longitudinal waves move parallel to the source. Think of the the two l's in the word 'longitudinal' as the symbol for parallel lines. Transverse waves move perpendicular to the source. Think of the capital 'T' in 'Transverse' as being an upside down perpendicular symbol.

Test Taking Skills Comment

This is an application of basic knowledge. There is a Similar Pair Options (**SB A.2.7**) as options A and B are similar and you could guess them - you would be wrong. None of the techniques are 100%, but on the average, you would be better off using them.

Q47 — Pre-Study Suggestions

Review the following if needed:
1) Energy of Waves **PHY 7.1, 9.2.4**
2) Dichotomy of Options **SB A.2.3**
3) Camouflage and Distractions **SB A.1.3**
4) Internally Inconsistent **SB A.2.5**
5) What information is needed from the passage?
6) Solve the problem.

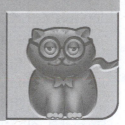

Solution Discussion

The key information from the passage:
From the first paragraph:

"To free an electron, the energy of a photon … minus the work function."

"The energy of the photon is given by the equation $E = hf$, where $h = 6.6 \times 10^{-34}$ Js (Planck's constant), and f = frequency of the photon."

If the number of photons that strike the cathode above the work function increases, then the number of ejected electrons will increase. If the energy of the photons that strike the cathode above the work function increases, then the energy of the ejected electrons will increase.

Options A and B are incorrect. Photons are not ejected. They impinge on the metal and cause electrons to be ejected. These options are a dichotomy and should be rejected immediately. These are also Internally Inconsistent (**SB A.2.5**) based on passage information.

Option C is incorrect. As the frequency of the photon increases, so does its energy. This one and option D are Camouflage and Distractions (**SB A.1.3**) because the test-maker is using frequency (**PHY 7.1**) as a proxy for Energy of Waves (**PHY 7.1, 9.2.4**). This means more excess energy is available to increase the Kinetic Energy (**PHY 5.3**) of the electrons. If the electrons have more kinetic energy, they should speed (**PHY 1.3**) up and not slow down.

Option D is correct. Higher frequency of photons means more excess energy to increase the kinetic energy ($mv^{2n}/2$) of the ejected electron and increase its speed. See the discussion in option C.

Test Taking Skills Comment

Careful reading solves this problem. This is a Camouflage and Distractions (**SB A.1.3**) question as discussed in option C. It also has Internally Inconsistent (**SB A.2.5**) options as discussed in options A and B. It is also a Dichotomy of Options (**SB A.2.3**) as options A and B relate to number of photons and options C and D relate to the speed of the ejected electrons. Based on passage knowledge, part of your Basic Knowledge (study, passage, general) (**SB A.2.2**), you should select options C and D and not even consider A or B.

Q48 — Pre-Study Suggestions

Review the following if needed:
1) Bohr Atom **CHM 2.1, PHY 12.1, 12.5**
2) Electron Transitions **CHM 2.2, 2.3, PHY 12.5**
3) Three Out of Four Options **SB A.2.8**
4) Similar Pair Options **SB A.2.7**
5) Complex Sounding Option(s) **SB A.2.2**
6) Solve the problem.

Solution Discussion

Option A is incorrect. This is a true statement. If there was not a better answer, it would be correct. The problem is lack of specificity about how the orbit is changed.

evaluate it with Basic Knowledge (study, passage, general) (**SB A.2.2**).

Option B is incorrect. This option is a Complex Sounding Option(s) (**SB A.2.2**). It sounds as if it would make sense, but there is no way to

Option D is incorrect. When electrons move to orbits of larger radius, they gain or absorb energy and emit energy - *see* Electron Transitions (**CHM 2.2, 2.3**, **PHY 12.5**).

CHAPTER 4

Option C is correct. When electrons move to orbits of lower energy, energy is emitted as radiation, e.g. - *see* Electron Transitions (**CHM 2.2, 2.3, PHY 12.5**).

Test Taking Skills Comment

This is a Three Out of Four Options (**SB A.2.8**) question. Options A, C and D all deal with orbits. Option B is an outlier not dealing with orbits. Outliers tend to be incorrect and may be ignored. There is a Complex Sounding Option(s) (**SB A.2.2**) in option B.

Q49 — Pre-Study Suggestions

Review the following if needed:
1) Phases **PHY 4.3.1**
2) Phase Interconversions **PHY 4.3.1**
3) Phase Energy Changes **CHM 4.3.3**
4) Similar Pair Options **SB A.2.7**
5) Mutually Excluding Options **SB A.2.6**
6) Solve the problem.

Solution Discussion

Option B is incorrect. The Sublimation (**PHY 4.3.1**) of a solid is the conversion to a gas, and the energy would be the Heat of Sublimation (ΔH_{sub} = joules/mol or cal/mol) (**CHM 4.3.3**).

Option C is incorrect. The Boiling (**CHM 5.1.2**), similar to evaporation, of a liquid would be the change of liquid to gas and would involve the Heat of Vaporization (ΔH_v = joules/ mol or cal/mol) (**CHM 4.3.3**).

Option D is incorrect. The Condensation (**PHY 4.3.1**) of a liquid is the process of going from a gas to a liquid. This is the reverse of liquid to gas. The energy associated is the given by the negative of the Heat of Vaporization (ΔH_v = joules/mol or cal/mol) (**CHM 4.3.3**). This option is essentially the same as option C. This makes options C and D Mutually Excluding Options (**SB A.2.6**) because both involve the same phase transition, just in opposite directions, and would measure the same energy change other than the sign of it.

Option A is correct. The Melting (**PHY 4.3.2**) of a solid, from solid to liquid, or the freezing of a liquid (liquid to solid) are complementary processes and both are reflected by the Heat of Fusion (ΔH_f = joules/mol or cal/mol) (**CHM 4.3.3**) with only opposite signs.

Test Taking Skills Comment

There is Mutually Excluding Options (**SB A.2.6**) as discussed in option D previously. There is also a Similar Pair Options (**SB A.2.7**) for options A and B. Since there are no other similar options present, this is a good guess opportunity. So, you have options C and D eliminated twice by the previous techniques and this gives a high probability of your answer coming from A or B.

Q50 — Pre-Study Suggestions

Review the following if needed:
1) Parallel Circuits **PHY 10.2.1**
2) Series Circuits **PHY 10.2.1**
3) Resistance **PHY 10.2**
4) Current **PHY 10.1**
5) Solve the problem.

Solution Discussion

The circuit is as follows:

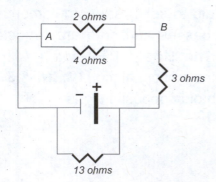

The two resistors (2 and 4 ohms) in the top portion of the circuit are in Parallel (**PHY 10.2.1**). The Current, I (ampere, **PHY 10.1**, I_T) entering at junction A is split (I_2 and I_4) between the two resistors inversely related to their Resistance, R (ohms), (**PHY 10.2**) (R_2 and R_4):

Since,

$$I_2 \propto 1/R_2$$

$$I_4 \propto 1/R_4$$

Making a Ratio and Proportion by dividing these:

$$\frac{I_2}{I_4} = \frac{1/R_2}{1/R_4}$$

$$= \frac{1/2}{1/4} = (1/2)(4/1) = 2$$

$$I_4 = I_2/2$$
$$= 2/2$$
$$= 1\ A.$$

Then,

$$I_T = I_2 + I_4$$
$$= 2 + 1$$
$$= 3\ A.$$

The 3 A of current exists at junction B and is the same at the 3 ohm resistor which is in Series (**PHY 10.2.1**) with the 2 and 4 ohm resistors.

Options A, C and D are incorrect. *See* the previous discussion.

Option B is correct. *See* the previous discussion.

Test Taking Skills Comment

If you were confident, you could have quickly determined that the current through the four ohm resistor must be ½ (2/4) of the current through the 2 ohm resistor and is 1 A.

Q51 — Pre-Study Suggestions

Review the following if needed:
1) Plane Mirrors **PHY 11.3**
2) Three Out of Four Type Question **SB A.2.8**
3) Solve the problem.

Solution Discussion

An image is formed in a plane Mirrors (**PHY 11.3**) at a perpendicular distance behind the mirror that the object is in front of the mirror. If the distance between the object, the Near-Sighted (**BIO 6.2.4; PHY 11.5, 11.5.1**) person, and the image is 300 cm, the maximum distance for clear vision, then the person must be one half of this from the mirror, or 150 cm.

Remember the image is not at the mirror, the image is a Real Image (**PHY 11.3**) and is a distance behind the mirror.

Options A, C and D are incorrect. See the previous discussion.

Option B is correct. See the previous discussion.

Test Taking Skills Comment

This is a very hard question. It illustrates the importance of thinking carefully about Basic Knowledge (study, passage, general) (**SB A.2.2**) and not giving in to panic and thinking there is something else that you should have studied. The concept is very basic. The application appears to have got 60% of the students. This is a soft Three Out of Four Type Question (**SB A.2.8**) with options B, C and D all being over 100. Option A is the outlier being less than 100. Outliers tend to be incorrect.

Q52 — Pre-Study Suggestions

Review the following if needed:
1) pH **CHM 6.1, 6.2, 6.5.1**
2) Logarithms **GS A.4**
3) Exponential **GS A.4**
4) Three Out of Four Options **SB A.2.8**
5) Similar Pair Options **SB A.2.7**
6) Solve the problem.

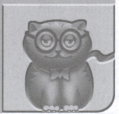

Solution Discussion

If the pH = 6.0, the Logarithms (**GS A.4**) form, then it must be converted back to the Exponential (**GS A.4**) form as follows:

$$[H^+] = 10^{-6}.$$

This is a direct conversion from a 'p' function to the exponential form. The value of the 'p' function becomes the negative exponent of 10.

Options A, B and C are incorrect. *See* the previous discussion.

Option D is correct. *See* the previous discussion.

Test Taking Skills Comment

This is also a Three Out of Four Options (**SB A.2.8**). Options B, C and D are all negative exponents. Option A is a positive exponent and is an outlier. Outliers tend to be incorrect and may be ignored. You may see a second three out of four, with options A, C and D all having 6 as an exponent and option B as an outlier with a 7, neglecting signs. The option B would be the outlier and probably incorrect in this grouping. So, you can eliminate options A and B by applying both of these three out of fours. Finally, Options C and D are a reasonable Similar Pair Options (**SB A.2.7**) as well.

Q. What do you do when you find a dead chemist?

A. Barium.

Q. What is the purpose of a doctor?

A. Helium.

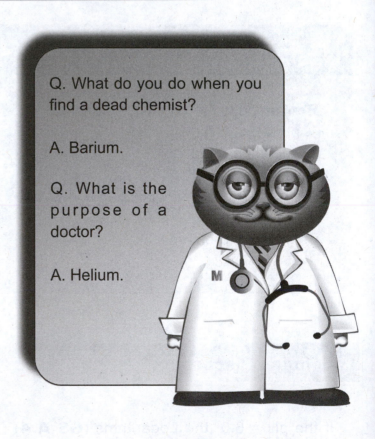

Chapter 5
VERBAL REASONING

Chapter 5

AAMC MCAT PRACTICE TEST 4

Verbal Reasoning Workbook
with Analysis Online

MCAT-Prep.com

Passage I - Questions 53-58

For 4CBT Verbal Reasoning Solutions, do the following:

1. Take the AAMC 4CBT Verbal Reasoning Test.
2. Apply the skills and techniques demonstrated in the review of 3CBT VR Solutions.
3. Then review each passage and complete the following skeleton (do this before you use the online solutions to 4CBT). You will benefit by using additional lined paper to complete your analysis.
4. Then compare your analysis to our analysis as found online. You have

free access to the 4CBT VR analysis at DrFlowersMCAT.com.

Good Luck.

We present three different ways to approach the Verbal Reasoning subtest. You should determine which works the best for you. We recommend the "Highlighting for Holistic and Central Thesis Analysis":

1) Highlighting for Holistic and Central Thesis Analysis
2) Standard Highlighting Analysis
3) Option Elimination Analysis

Highlighting For Holistic and Central Thesis Analysis

A Note on the Highlighting
See SB Chapter 2.

Putting It All Together: The Critical Path
See SB Chapter 2.

Passage I - Questions 53-58

Holistic Highlighting
You should attempt to go through the passage in 3 minutes or less highlighting the following (or simply read the passage and try to focus on/remember the following).

Look for the new concept keys and the author opinion keys. You should write in the following spaces what you considered to be the key highlighting and which relate to the author's opinion (do for each paragraph):

Paragraph 1:_____
_____

Paragraph 2:_____
_____

Paragraph 3:_____
_____

Paragraph 4:_____
_____

Headlining or Signposting the Passage

In this section, you should summarize the paragraph in one sentence.

Paragraph 1:_____
_____

Paragraph 3:_____
_____

Paragraph 2:_____
_____

Paragraph 4:_____
_____

The Central Thesis

Next, provide a summary of the Central Thesis and why.

_____
_____
_____
_____

Passage at a Glance

• Can you describe the key descriptors of the passage? _____
• Genre: _____
• Passage difficulty level: _____
• Abstract/concrete: _____
• Subject: _____
• Author's attitude to subject: _____
• Question types: _____

Passage I - Questions 53-58

Standard Passage Highlighting

Passage Highlighting
This is done as if skimming during an actual test and is not meant to be a "perfect" highlighting - learn from the following discussion: see Highlighting (SB B.6, B.7).

Use the standard approach to highlighting as discussed in the concepts about Highlighting. Note the key words or phrases for each paragraph.

Paragraph 1:_____
_____

Paragraph 3:_____
_____

Paragraph 2:_____
_____

Paragraph 4:_____
_____

The Questions and Solutions by the Different Techniques

Using the Holistic Approach

Question Discussion

Discuss the solution to the question; how you arrive at it, how the highlighting, central thesis or inferences play a part in the solution. Try to discuss each option as to its correct/incorrect status.

_____

_____

_____

_____

The Critical Path
How would you quickly summarize and arrive at the answer to this question?

_____

_____

Using the Standard Approach

Highlighting (HL) Analysis
Using the highlighting you have done previously, solve each question. You have about 1 minute (on the real test, but you may take longer here as you're learning) for each question. Try to discuss each option. You will need extra paper.

_____

_____

_____

_____

Using Option Elimination Analysis

Concepts to Review
Which of the Option Elimination Analysis skills are applicable in this question?

_____

Solution Discussion
Please review the AAMC solution for this problem.

Test Taking Skills Comment
Use the Test Taking Skills to explain how to eliminate options.

_____

_____

CHAPTER 5

Holistic Highlighting
You should attempt to go through the passage in 3 minutes or less highlighting the following (or simply read the passage and try to focus on/remember the following).

Look for the new concept keys and the author opinion keys. You should write in the following spaces what you considered to be the key highlighting and which relate to the author's opinion (do for each paragraph):

Paragraph 1:_____

Paragraph 2:_____

Paragraph 3:_____

Paragraph 4:_____

Paragraph 5:_____

Paragraph 6:_____

Headlining or Signposting the Passage
In this section, you should summarize the paragraph in one sentence.

Paragraph 1:_____

Paragraph 2:_____

Paragraph 3:_____

Paragraph 4:_____

Paragraph 5:_____

Paragraph 6:_____

The Central Thesis
Next, provide a summary of the Central Thesis and why.

_____

_____

_____

_____

Passage at a Glance

• Can you describe the key descriptors of the passage? _____
• Genre: _____
• Passage difficulty level: _____
• Abstract/concrete: _____
• Subject: _____
• Author's attitude to subject: _____
• Question types: _____

Standard Passage Highlighting

Passage Highlighting
This is done as if skimming during an actual test and is not meant to be a "perfect" highlighting - learn from the following discussion: see Highlighting **(SB B.6, B.7)**.

Use the standard approach to highlighting as discussed in the concepts about Highlighting. Note the key words or phrases for each paragraph.

Paragraph 1:_____
_____

Paragraph 4:_____
_____

Paragraph 2:_____
_____

Paragraph 5:_____
_____

Paragraph 3:_____
_____

Paragraph 6:_____
_____

The Questions and Solutions by the Different Techniques

Using the Holistic Approach

Question Discussion
Discuss the solution to the question; how you arrive at it, how the highlighting, central thesis or inferences play a part in the solution. Try to discuss each option as to its correct/incorrect status.

_____
_____
_____
_____

The Critical Path
How would you quickly summarize and arrive at the answer to this question?

_____
_____

Using the Standard Approach

Highlighting (HL) Analysis
Using the highlighting you have done previously, solve each question. You have about 1 minute (on the real test, but you may take longer here as you're learning) for each question. Try to discuss each option. You will need extra paper.

_____
_____
_____
_____

Using Option Elimination Analysis

Concepts to Review
Which of the Option Elimination Analysis skills are applicable in this question?

_____

Solution Discussion
Please review the AAMC solution for this problem.

Test Taking Skills Comment
Use the Test Taking Skills to explain how to eliminate options.

_____

Passage III - Questions 65-70

Holistic Highlighting
You should attempt to go through the passage in 3 minutes or less highlighting the following (or simply read the passage and try to focus on/remember the following).

Look for the new concept keys and the author opinion keys. You should write in the following spaces what you considered to be the key highlighting and which relate to the author's opinion (do for each paragraph):

Paragraph 1:_____

Paragraph 2:_____

Paragraph 3:_____

Paragraph 4:_____

Paragraph 5:_____

Paragraph 6:_____

CHAPTER 5

Headlining or Signposting the Passage

In this section, you should summarize the paragraph in one sentence.

Paragraph 1:_____

Paragraph 4:_____

Paragraph 2:_____

Paragraph 5:_____

Paragraph 3:_____

Paragraph 6:_____

The Central Thesis

Next, provide a summary of the Central Thesis and why.

_____
_____
_____
_____

Passage at a Glance

• Can you describe the key descriptors of the passage? _____
• Genre: _____
• Passage difficulty level: _____
• Abstract/concrete: _____
• Subject: _____
• Author's attitude to subject: _____
• Question types: _____

Standard Passage Highlighting

Passage Highlighting
This is done as if skimming during an actual test and is not meant to be a "perfect" highlighting - learn from the following discussion: see Highlighting **(SB B.6, B.7)**.

Use the standard approach to highlighting as discussed in the concepts about Highlighting. Note the key words or phrases for each paragraph.

Paragraph 1:_____
_____

Paragraph 4:_____
_____

Paragraph 2:_____
_____

Paragraph 5:_____
_____

Paragraph 3:_____
_____

Paragraph 6:_____
_____

The Questions and Solutions by the Different Techniques

Using the Holistic Approach

Question Discussion
Discuss the solution to the question; how you arrive at it, how the highlighting, central thesis or inferences play a part in the solution. Try to discuss each option as to its correct/incorrect status.

_____
_____
_____
_____

CHAPTER 5

The Critical Path

How would you quickly summarize and arrive at the answer to this question?

_____

_____

Using the Standard Approach

Highlighting (HL) Analysis

Using the highlighting you have done previously, solve each question. You have about 1 minute (on the real test, but you may take longer here as you're learning) for each question. Try to discuss each option. You will need extra paper.

_____

_____

_____

_____

Using Option Elimination Analysis

Concepts to Review

Which of the Option Elimination Analysis skills are applicable in this question?

_____

Solution Discussion

Please review the AAMC solution for this problem.

Test Taking Skills Comment

Use the Test Taking Skills to explain how to eliminate options.

_____

_____

Passage IV - Questions 71-77

Holistic Highlighting

You should attempt to go through the passage in 3 minutes or less highlighting the following (or simply read the passage and try to focus on/remember the following).

Look for the new concept keys and the author opinion keys. You should write in the following spaces what you considered to be the key highlighting and which relate to the author's opinion (do for each paragraph):

Paragraph 1:_____
_____

Paragraph 4:_____
_____

Paragraph 2:_____
_____

Paragraph 5:_____
_____

Paragraph 3:_____
_____

Headlining or Signposting the Passage

In this section, you should summarize the paragraph in one sentence.

Paragraph 1:_____
_____

Paragraph 4:_____
_____

Paragraph 2:_____
_____

Paragraph 5:_____
_____

Paragraph 3:_____
_____

CHAPTER 5

The Central Thesis
Next, provide a summary of the Central Thesis and why.

_____
_____
_____
_____

Passage at a Glance

• Can you describe the key descriptors of the passage? _____
• Genre: _____
• Passage difficulty level: _____
• Abstract/concrete: _____
• Subject: _____
• Author's attitude to subject: _____
• Question types: _____

Standard Passage Highlighting

Passage Highlighting
This is done as if skimming during an actual test and is not meant to be a "perfect" highlighting - learn from the following discussion: see Highlighting (SB B.6, B.7).

Use the standard approach to highlighting as discussed in the concepts about Highlighting. Note the key words or phrases for each paragraph.

Paragraph 1:_____
_____

Paragraph 2:_____
_____

Paragraph 3:_____
_____

Paragraph 4:_____
_____

Paragraph 5:_____
_____

The Questions and Solutions by the Different Techniques

Using the Holistic Approach

Question Discussion
Discuss the solution to the question; how you arrive at it, how the highlighting, central thesis or inferences play a part in the solution. Try to discuss each option as to its correct/incorrect status.

_____
_____
_____
_____

The Critical Path
How would you quickly summarize and arrive at the answer to this question?

_____
_____

Using the Standard Approach

Highlighting (HL) Analysis
Using the highlighting you have done previously, solve each question. You have about 1 minute (on the real test, but you may take longer here as you're learning) for each question. Try to discuss each option. You will need extra paper.

_____
_____
_____
_____

Using Option Elimination Analysis

Concepts to Review
Which of the Option Elimination Analysis skills are applicable in this question?

_____

Solution Discussion
Please review the AAMC solution for this problem.

Test Taking Skills Comment
Use the Test Taking Skills to explain how to eliminate options.

_____

_____

Passage V - Questions 78-82

Holistic Highlighting
You should attempt to go through the passage in 3 minutes or less highlighting the following (or simply read the passage and try to focus on/remember the following).

Look for the new concept keys and the author opinion keys. You should write in the following spaces what you considered to be the key highlighting and which relate to the author's opinion (do for each paragraph):

Paragraph 1:_____
_____

Paragraph 4:_____
_____

Paragraph 2:_____
_____

Paragraph 5:_____
_____

Paragraph 3:_____
_____

Paragraph 6:_____
_____

Headlining or Signposting the Passage
In this section, you should summarize the paragraph in one sentence.

Paragraph 1:_____
_____

Paragraph 4:_____
_____

Paragraph 2:_____
_____

Paragraph 5:_____
_____

Paragraph 3:_____
_____

Paragraph 6:_____
_____

The Central Thesis
Next, provide a summary of the Central Thesis and why.
_____
_____
_____
_____

Passage at a Glance

• Can you describe the key descriptors of the passage? _____
• Genre: _____
• Passage difficulty level: _____
• Abstract/concrete: _____
• Subject: _____
• Author's attitude to subject: _____
• Question types: _____

Standard Passage Highlighting

Passage Highlighting
This is done as if skimming during an actual test and is not meant to be a "perfect" highlighting - learn from the following discussion: see Highlighting **(SB B.6, B.7)**.

Use the standard approach to highlighting as discussed in the concepts about Highlighting. Note the key words or phrases for each paragraph.

Paragraph 1:_____

Paragraph 4:_____

Paragraph 2:_____

Paragraph 5:_____

Paragraph 3:_____

Paragraph 6:_____

The Questions and Solutions by the Different Techniques

Using the Holistic Approach

Question Discussion
Discuss the solution to the question; how you arrive at it, how the highlighting, central thesis or inferences play a part in the solution. Try to discuss each option as to its correct/incorrect status.

_____
_____
_____
_____

The Critical Path
How would you quickly summarize and arrive at the answer to this question?

_____

_____

Using the Standard Approach

Highlighting (HL) Analysis
Using the highlighting you have done previously, solve each question. You have about 1 minute (on the real test, but you may take longer here as you're learning) for each question. Try to discuss each option. You will need extra paper.

_____

_____

_____

_____

Using Option Elimination Analysis

Concepts to Review
Which of the Option Elimination Analysis skills are applicable in this question?

_____

Solution Discussion
Please review the AAMC solution for this problem.

Test Taking Skills Comment
Use the Test Taking Skills to explain how to eliminate options.

_____

_____

Holistic Highlighting

You should attempt to go through the passage in 3 minutes or less highlighting the following (or simply read the passage and try to focus on/remember the following).

Look for the new concept keys and the author opinion keys. You should write in the following spaces what you considered to be the key highlighting and which relate to the author's opinion (do for each paragraph):

Paragraph 1:_____

Paragraph 4:_____

Paragraph 2:_____

Paragraph 5:_____

Paragraph 3:_____

Paragraph 6:_____

Headlining or Signposting the Passage

In this section, you should summarize the paragraph in one sentence.

Paragraph 1:_____

Paragraph 4:_____

Paragraph 2:_____

Paragraph 5:_____

Paragraph 3:_____

Paragraph 6:_____

The Central Thesis

Next, provide a summary of the Central Thesis and why.

_____
_____
_____
_____

Passage at a Glance

• Can you describe the key descriptors of the passage? _____
• Genre: _____
• Passage difficulty level: _____
• Abstract/concrete: _____
• Subject: _____
• Author's attitude to subject: _____
• Question types: _____

Standard Passage Highlighting

Passage Highlighting

This is done as if skimming during an actual test and is not meant to be a "perfect" highlighting - learn from the following discussion: see Highlighting **(SB B.6, B.7)**.

Use the standard approach to highlighting as discussed in the concepts about Highlighting. Note the key words or phrases for each paragraph.

Paragraph 1:_____
_____

Paragraph 4:_____
_____

Paragraph 2:_____
_____

Paragraph 5:_____
_____

Paragraph 3:_____
_____

Paragraph 6:_____
_____

CHAPTER 5

The Questions and Solutions by the Different Techniques

Using the Holistic Approach

Question Discussion

Discuss the solution to the question; how you arrive at it, how the highlighting, central thesis or inferences play a part in the solution. Try to discuss each option as to its correct/incorrect status.

_____
_____
_____
_____

The Critical Path

How would you quickly summarize and arrive at the answer to this question?

_____
_____

Using the Standard Approach

Highlighting (HL) Analysis

Using the highlighting you have done previously, solve each question. You have about 1 minute (on the real test, but you may take longer here as you're learning) for each question. Try to discuss each option. You will need extra paper.

_____
_____
_____
_____

Using Option Elimination Analysis

Concepts to Review
Which of the Option Elimination Analysis skills are applicable in this question?

_____

Solution Discussion
Please review the AAMC solution for this problem.

Test Taking Skills Comment
Use the Test Taking Skills to explain how to eliminate options.

_____

_____

Passage VII - Questions 88-92

Holistic Highlighting
You should attempt to go through the passage in 3 minutes or less highlighting the following (or simply read the passage and try to focus on/remember the following).

Look for the new concept keys and the author opinion keys. You should write in the following spaces what you considered to be the key highlighting and which relate to the author's opinion (do for each paragraph):

Paragraph 1:_____

_____

Paragraph 2:_____

_____

Paragraph 3:_____

_____

Paragraph 4:_____

_____

Paragraph 5:_____

_____

CHAPTER 5

Headlining or Signposting the Passage
In this section, you should summarize the paragraph in one sentence.

Paragraph 1:_____
_____

Paragraph 4:_____
_____

Paragraph 2:_____
_____

Paragraph 5:_____
_____

Paragraph 3:_____
_____

The Central Thesis
Next, provide a summary of the Central Thesis and why.

_____
_____
_____
_____

Passage at a Glance

• Can you describe the key descriptors of the passage? _____
• Genre: _____
• Passage difficulty level: _____
• Abstract/concrete: _____
• Subject: _____
• Author's attitude to subject: _____
• Question types: _____

Standard Passage Highlighting

<u>Passage Highlighting</u>
This is done as if skimming during an actual test and is not meant to be a "perfect" highlighting - learn from the following discussion: see Highlighting **(SB B.6, B.7)**.

Use the standard approach to highlighting as discussed in the concepts about Highlighting. Note the key words or phrases for each paragraph.

Paragraph 1:_____
_____

Paragraph 4:_____
_____

Paragraph 2:_____
_____

Paragraph 5:_____
_____

Paragraph 3:_____
_____

The Questions and Solutions by the Different Techniques

Using the Holistic Approach

Question Discussion
Discuss the solution to the question; how you arrive at it, how the highlighting, central thesis or inferences play a part in the solution. Try to discuss each option as to its correct/incorrect status.

_____
_____
_____
_____

The Critical Path

How would you quickly summarize and arrive at the answer to this question?

_____

_____

Using the Standard Approach

Highlighting (HL) Analysis

Using the highlighting you have done previously, solve each question. You have about 1 minute (on the real test, but you may take longer here as you're learning) for each question. Try to discuss each option. You will need extra paper.

_____

_____

_____

_____

Using Option Elimination Analysis

Concepts to Review

Which of the Option Elimination Analysis skills are applicable in this question?

_____

Solution Discussion

Please review the AAMC solution for this problem.

Test Taking Skills Comment

Use the Test Taking Skills to explain how to eliminate options.

_____

_____

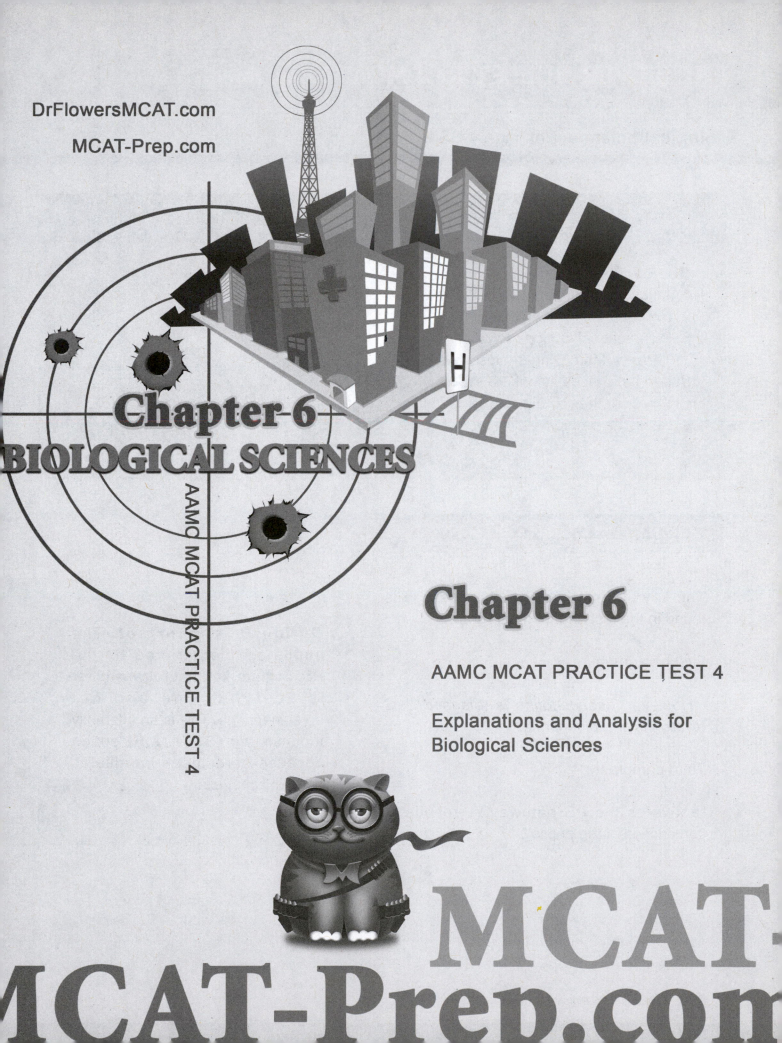

DrFlowersMCAT.com

MCAT-Prep.com

Chapter 6
BIOLOGICAL SCIENCES

AAMC MCAT PRACTICE TEST 4

Chapter 6

AAMC MCAT PRACTICE TEST 4

Explanations and Analysis for
Biological Sciences

MCAT-Prep.com

Q95   Pre-Study Suggestions

Review the following if needed:
1) Autonomic Nervous System **BIO 6.1.4**
2) Neurotransmitters **BIO 5.1**
3) Dichotomy of Options **SB A.2.3**
4) Three or More Step Analysis **SB A.1.4**
5) Internally Inconsistent **SB A.2.5**
6) What are the key pieces of information from the passage?
7) Solve the problem.

Solution Discussion

The key information from the passage is found in the first and third paragraphs:

First paragraph:

"However, acetylcholine is released ... S division is norepinephrine."

Third paragraph:

"activates the PS pathway ... results in constriction of the pupils."

Option B is incorrect. The pupils are constricted by the PS, but the key neurotransmitter is acetylcholine and not norepinephrine. This is an Internally Inconsistent **(SB A.2.5)** option because norepinephrine dilates and not constricts.

Option C is incorrect. The pupils are not dilated because the PS system is activated. This is an Internally Inconsistent **(SB A.2.5)** option because the acetylcholine will result in constriction and not dilation.

pupils would be dilated, so the option is internally consistent.

Option A is correct. The PS system results in constriction and the acetylcholine is the end-organ neurotransmitter released.

Option D is incorrect. The pupils are not dilated because the PS system is activated. If the norepinephrine was released, the

Test Taking Skills Comment

You should solve this problem by information in the passage. Although you are supposed to understand the general structure and function of the autonomic nervous system **(BIO 6.1.4)**, you are not required to know all the details. This is why you are given some specific details of the function of the ANS. This is a double Dichotomy of Options **(SB A.2.3)**. The first dichotomy is dilation or constriction. Based on paragraph three, you should determine it has to be constriction and eliminated options C and D. The other dichotomy is norepinephrine vs. acetylcholine. The question states the PS system is activated and based on paragraph one, you should eliminate norepinephrine. This will eliminate options B and D. As is typical in double dichotomy questions, if you correctly eliminate both dichotomies, there is only one, the correct, option remaining - option A.

This is also an Internally Inconsistent **(SB A.2.5)** question as discussed in options B and C. For both internally inconsistent questions and dichotomy questions, you can use your Basic Knowledge (study, passage, general knowledge) **(SB A.2.2)** to eliminate certain options.

Finally, this is a Three or More Step Analysis **(SB A.1.4)** question. Usually, this type of question will be more difficult, and if not more difficult, they are more time consuming. The steps involved are:

1) to determine if constricted/dilated;
2) to determine if this is True or False **(SB A.1.2)** based on acetylcholine or norepinephrine;
3) to determine if the option is True or False **(SB A.1.2)**; and,
4) to determine if the option is Correct or Incorrect **(SB A.1.2)**.

You should be aware of the basic neurotransmitters **(BIO 5.1)** which encompass both acetylcholine and norepinephrine. Study the section if you are not familiar with the other common neurotransmitters.

Q96   Pre-Study Suggestions

Review the following if needed:
1) Neurotransmitters **BIO 5.1**
2) Dichotomy of Options **SB A.2.3**
3) Internally Inconsistent **SB A.2.5**
4) Three or More Step Analysis **SB A.1.4**
5) What information is needed from the passage?
6) Solve the problem.

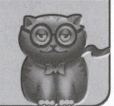

Solution Discussion

The key information from the passage is found in paragraph one:

"However, acetylcholine is released ... S division is norepinephrine."

You could answer the question without this information because you are given so much information in the Stem **(SB A.1.1)**.

Option B is incorrect. The mechanism is passive because the atropine does not mimic acetylcholine but prevents it from attaching to the receptor. But blocking acetylcholine does not block the sympathetic system. This is Internally Inconsistent **(SB A.2.5)** because you should know that since acetylcholine is involved, you are dealing

Option C is incorrect. Any active mechanism is Internally Inconsistent **(SB A.2.5)** with the blocking effect of atropine as defined in the stem.

Option D is incorrect. The mechanism is not active because the atropine blocks and does not mimic. Also, it is the PS system and not the S system which is affected by acetylcholine. So, this option is Internally Inconsistent **(SB A.2.5)** for two reasons.

Option A is correct. Because the atropine blocks the action of acetylcholine, it is a passive mechanism. The system blocked is the parasympathetic system; the system that will exert more of its effects is the sympathetic.

Test Taking Skills Comment

with the parasympathetic system. This is a Dichotomy of Options **(SB A.2.3)** question.

Based on the definition provided and the description of the action of atropine, the mechanism must be passive and options C and D are eliminated - this is using your Passage Knowledge **(SB A.2.2)** from your Basic Knowledge (study, passage, general knowledge) **(SB A.2.2)**.

There were a number of Internally Inconsistent **(SB A.2.5)** options as discussed previously. Also, this was a Three or More Step Analysis **(SB A.1.4)** question as follows:

1) you had to determine if passive or active was True or False **(SB A.1.2)**;

2) you had to determine if blocked/mimicked was consistent with passive/active;

3) you had to determine if the option was True or False **(SB A.1.2)**;

4) you had to determine if the Options **(SB A.1.1)** were Correct or Incorrect **(SB A.1.2)**.

Usually these are harder options because of the number of steps involved - this one was relatively easy. Part of this reason is that the information was included in the Stem **(SB A.1.1)** and not in the passage itself.

Q97 Pre-Study Suggestions

Review the following if needed:
1) Autonomic Nervous System **BIO 6.1.4**
2) Negative Question **SB A.1.2**
3) Similar Pair Options **SB A.2.7**
4) What information is needed from the passage?
5) Solve the problem.

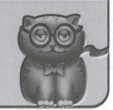

Solution Discussion

The key information from the passage is found in paragraph one:

"However, acetylcholine is released … S division is norepinephrine."

Options A, B and C are incorrect. All of these are sympathetic functions and would depend on the presence of norepinephrine.

Option D is correct. This is a parasympathetic (PS) function. Acetylcholine relates to PS functions.

Test Taking Skills Comment

Some information is required from the passage regarding acetylcholine and PS; but this should be basic knowledge about the PS and the autonomic nervous system **(BIO 6.1.4)**. The general rule is that the sympathetic system moves the organism away from homeostasis **(BIO 6.1)** and the parasympathetic system moves toward homeostasis and maintains it. Pupil dilation, blood vessel dilation and rise in blood pressure would all be moves away from homeostasis that would prepare the organism for 'fight or flight'.

This is also a Negative Question **(SB A.1.2)** which is a bit different from the usual type. The negative part is caused by the phrase 'rapidly inactivated'. This means you have to determine which is negated by the description; which is the parasympathetic system in this instance.

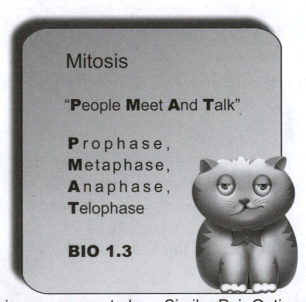

Mitosis

"**P**eople **M**eet **A**nd **T**alk"

Prophase,
Metaphase,
Anaphase,
Telophase

BIO 1.3

This may appear to be a Similar Pair Options **(SB A.2.7)** question but you should not apply the technique because, reasonably, more than one similar pair is present. Options A and B are a similar pair due to 'dilation', options B and C are a similar pair due to references to 'blood'.

Q98 — Pre-Study Suggestions

Review the following if needed:

1) Autonomic Nervous System **BIO 6.1.4**
2) Nervous System Concepts **BIO 6.1**
3) Dichotomy of Options **SB A.2.3**
4) Internally Inconsistent **SB A.2.5**
5) What are the key pieces of information from the passage?
6) Solve the problem.

Solution Discussion

No information is needed from the passage.

Option A is incorrect. The motor fibers are correct because an action, efferent, results instead of a sensation. Sympathetic fibers cause the heart rate to increase.

Sympathetic efferent fibers cause a speeding up of the heart. This option is Internally Inconsistent **(SB A.2.5)** because an action/effect is not consistent with sensory.

Option B is incorrect. The sensory fibers are incorrect as they detect sensations and are afferent.

Option D is incorrect. Sensory fibers are afferent and detect sensations and do not cause actions. Parasympathetic efferent fibers do slow the heart down. This is Internally Inconsistent **(SB A.2.5)** as in option B.

Option C is correct. The parasympathetic fibers do slow the heart and are motor, efferent, fibers.

Test Taking Skills Comment

This is a double Dichotomy of Options **(SB A.2.3)** problem. One dichotomy is the sensory vs. motor. Sensory fibers are afferent going from the periphery to the central nervous system (CNS) (*see* nervous system concepts; **BIO 6.1**). They carry the sensations to the brain and spinal cord. Motor fibers are efferent going from the CNS to the periphery. They result in some action of some type such as muscle contractions. Since cardiac slowing is an action, the fibers must be motor and efferent. This means options B and D must be incorrect and are

Internally Inconsistent **(SB A.2.5)** based on your Basic Knowledge (study, passage, general knowledge) **(SB A.2.2)**. The other dichotomy is between the PS and S systems. Remember the sympathetic moves away from homeostasis or prepares for fight or flight actions. Increasing the heartbeat would be a preparation for fight or flight and would be sympathetic (S). Slowing the heartbeat would be parasympathetic (PS). Then options A and B would be eliminated and the correct option would be C.

Biological Science Passage 4.BS.I

Q99   Pre-Study Suggestions

Review the following if needed:
1) Autonomic Nervous System **BIO 6.1.4**
2) Dichotomy of Options **SB A.2.3**
3) What information is needed from the passage?
4) Solve the problem.

Solution Discussion

From the first paragraph:

"the S ganglia appear near the spinal … do not connect with each other."

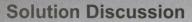

Option C is incorrect. The PS division is incorrect. It is true the ganglia are not connected and this is the reason it cannot generate a rapid whole body response.

Option B is incorrect. Norepinephrine is not the reason the S can produce a more rapid whole body response. Why would a neurotransmitter from any given nerve ending generate an immediate whole body response in and of itself from a specific nerve or ganglia? There is no evidence in the passage to support this claim.

Option D is incorrect. See options B and C.

Option A is correct. This interconnection of ganglia is the key reason the S system can pull off the fight or flight response as a total body response.

Test Taking Skills Comment

This is another double Dichotomy of Options **(SB A.2.3)**. If you know the S is the correct response, then you can eliminate options C and D. From the required study, this could be known. If you know, from the passage that the interconnection of the ganglia is the key and not the neurotransmitters, then you eliminate options B and D. This leaves option A as the correct option. But, this is a difficult dichotomy to choose correctly, and it is very reasonable that you could not use this technique here. It relies on your logic to determine if the explanation given can explain the effect as previously discussed.

Q100 — Pre-Study Suggestions

Review the following if needed:
1) Neurotransmitters **BIO 5.1**
2) Dichotomy of Options **SB A.2.3**
3) Negative Question **SB A.1.2**
4) Internally Inconsistent **SB A.2.5**
5) Three or More Step Analysis **SB A.1.4**
6) What are the key pieces of information from the passage?
7) Solve the problem.

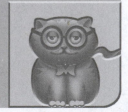

Solution Discussion

The key information from the passage is found in the first and third paragraphs:

First Paragraph:

"However, acetylcholine is released … S division is norepinephrine."

Third Paragraph:

"activates the PS pathway leading … in constriction of the pupils."

Option A is incorrect. If acetylcholine (ACh) was decreased, the pupils would dilate due to unopposed sympathetic activity. But, the ACh levels will increase because the enzyme, acetylcholinesterase, that breaks it down is blocked by the physostigmine.

Option B is incorrect. This is incorrect because if ACh levels were increased, the pupils should con-

strict. This is an Internally Inconsistent **(SB A.2.5)** option based on your Basic Knowledge (study, passage, general knowledge) **(SB A.2.2)** as presented in the passage.

Option C is incorrect. If the ACh was decreased, the unopposed sympathetic system would dilate the pupils. This is also an Internally Inconsistent **(SB A.2.5)** option based on your Passage Knowledge **(SB A.2.2)** that increased ACh is PS and constricts the pupils.

Option D is correct. The physostigmine blocks the acetylcholinesterase that would normally degrade the ACh. Since the ACh is not being degraded, it will build up making it more available to stimulate

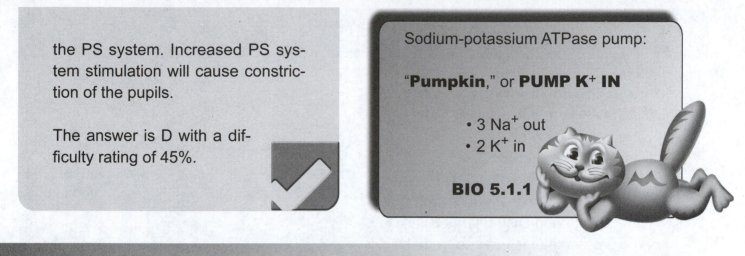

the PS system. Increased PS system stimulation will cause constriction of the pupils.

The answer is D with a difficulty rating of 45%.

Sodium-potassium ATPase pump:

"Pumpkin," or **PUMP K$^+$ IN**

- 3 Na$^+$ out
- 2 K$^+$ in

BIO 5.1.1

Test Taking Skills Comment

This is another double Dichotomy of Options **(SB A.2.3)** question. If you determine the pupils will constrict, then you eliminate options A and B. Or, if you determine the acetylcholine will increase, then you eliminate options A and C. A double dichotomy elimination results in the correct answer which is D. There are also Internally Inconsistent **(SB A.2.5)** answer choices as discussed in options B and C. An acetylcholine increase will cause more constriction and vice versa. This means options B and C are inconsistent.

This is also a subtle/tricky Negative Question **(SB A.1.2)**. Usually you have 'NOT' or 'EXCEPT' or similar key words for negative questions. But, many will have a phrase or a description that negates the positive. In this question, it is the 'inhibits' which performs this function. In fact, this is a double negative

because of the enzyme used. You focus on ACh which would give a PS response and be positive. But you are given the enzyme which breaks down the ACh and decreases it (like a negative effect). But, then you are given something that inhibits the enzyme and this reverses the inhibition - this is a double negative in effect.

This is also a Three or More Step Analysis **(SB A.1.4)** which makes it more difficult:

1) you must determine whether 'dilate' or 'constrict' is correct;
2) then you have to determine if the reason given correlates with the dilate or constrict;
3) then you have to determine if the option is True or False **(SB A.1.2)**; and finally,
4) you have to determine if the option is Correct or Incorrect **(SB A.1.2)**.

Q101 — Pre-Study Suggestions

Review the following if needed:

1) Colligative Properties **CHM 5.1**
2) Osmosis **BIO 1.1.1**
3) Energy Metabolism **BIO 4**
4) Membrane Transport **BIO 1.1**
5) Complex Sounding Option(s) **SB A.2.2**
6) Camouflage and Distractions **SB A.1.3**
7) What information is needed from the passage?
8) Solve the problem.

Solution Discussion

The key information from the passage is found in the second paragraph:

"accelerated glucose release from hepatic … dehydration of cells and other"

> ***Option A is incorrect.*** Glucose is an energy source, but where in the review or in the passage does it discuss glucose accelerating the osmotic work performed by plasma membranes. This is one of the 'scientifically sounding' options

that cannot be assessed. This is beyond Basic Knowledge (study, passage, general knowledge) **(SB A.2.2)** and that makes this a Complex Sounding Option(s) **(SB A.2.2)**. Your study knowledge and passage knowledge do not allow you to answer this question.

Option B is incorrect. Same as option A. Where did you learn this or get this information? The only way you fall for this is if you have not adequately prepared in the basics. This is also a Complex Sounding Option(s) **(SB A.2.2)**.

is not the process of osmosis **(BIO 1.1.1)**. It is not in the passage; it cannot be correct.

Option D is incorrect. Again, same as options A and B. This is not what you learned about with membrane transport **(BIO 1.1)** and it is not Basic Knowledge (study, passage, general knowledge) **(SB A.2.2)**. This certainly

Option C is correct. This is a question about understanding osmosis. Hyperglycemia means there is an increase in the number of glucose molecules on one side of a membrane; in this situation, it is on the outside of the cell membrane. Water, by osmosis, will move from the inside of the cell to the outside to balance its concentration across the membrane.

Test Taking Skills Comment

This is a somewhat Camouflage and Distractions **(SB A.1.3)** type question, but you have to recognize it. All you're being asked about is osmosis. The stem does not give you a clue, but the options do give you clues and you have to pick up on them. This is also a subtle dichotomy type question. If you recognize the key concept is osmosis,

then you eliminate the 'energy' dichotomy of options A and B. As noted, there are also Complex Sounding Option(s) **(SB A.2.2)** that should be recognized and eliminated as previously discussed.

Q102 — Pre-Study Suggestions

Review the following if needed:

1) Blood Sugar (Glucose) Metabolism **BIO 4, 6.3.4**
2) Pancreatic Hormones **BIO 6.3.4**
3) Similar Pair Options **SB A.2.7**
4) Complex Sounding Option(s) **SB A.2.2**
5) What information is needed from the passage?
6) Solve the problem.

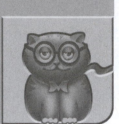

Solution Discussion

The key information from the passage is found in the second paragraph:

"strategy involves accelerated … the glucose concentration of body fluids."

Option B is incorrect. Since glucagon **(BIO 6.3.4)** raises blood sugar levels, the suppression of it would result in a lowering of the blood sugar and not the extreme hyperglycemia noted. Also, in the second paragraph, it is noted the glycogen is released from the liver which is an action of glucagon.

Option C is incorrect. Since glycogen is a storage product for glucose (blood sugar), if the breakdown (anabolism; **BIO 4**) of glycogen was slowed, the amount of glucose in the blood should decrease and not increase. Also, a key to the process is the breakdown of glycogen as in the passage.

Option D is incorrect. What is this about? "Scientifically sounding" non-sense! You have no way of assessing this statement. What does increased 'sensitivity' do? What happens? 'All pancreatic endocrine response' means what? Some pancreatic **(BIO 6.3.4)** hormone functions will increase insulin and others will decrease it - which way will it go? All of this is not basic knowledge. It is not discussed in the passage. It is a Complex Sounding Option(s) **(SB A.2.2)** that cannot be answered with your Basic Knowledge (study, passage, general knowledge) **(SB A.2.2)**.

Option A is correct. This makes sense based on your 'basic knowledge'. You know that the effect of insulin **(BIO 6.3.4)** is to lower blood sugar when it is elevated. So, if insulin was functioning properly, and if the blood sugar was elevated, then the insulin would lower the blood sugar. Since the blood sugar remains elevated, one plausible reason is that something is suppressing insulin. All of this fits. You don't have to know why it happens, but if it does happen, it makes sense.

Test Taking Skills Comment

Notice that for options A, B and C, based on your knowledge and the passage, you could assess whether they made sense or not. Option D is not assessable based on your knowledge base or the passage and is a Complex Sounding Option(s) **(SB A.2.2)** as previously discussed. Again, the only way you can come to these conclusions is to have studied well.

This is also a Similar Pair Options **(SB A.2.7)** as options A and B are a similar pair with both dealing the suppression of a hormone during freezing. Because this is the only obvious similar pair, it is a good guess to choose one of them.

Q103 — Pre-Study Suggestions

Review the following if needed:
1) Graphs and Charts **GS A.3**
2) Dichotomy of Options **SB A.2.3**
3) What information is needed from the passage?
4) Solve the problem?

Solution Discussion

The Figure 1 is needed - please refer to it.

The key information from the passage is found in the second paragraph:

"strategy involves accelerated glucose ... the freezing point of body fluids"

this equilibration relate to the cryoprotective effect? It is not clear from the passage.

Option B is incorrect. You have to focus on the question. The question asks why the transiently persistent heartbeat is important to the cryoprotective effect of glucose. Circulating blood may equilibrate the temperature throughout the body - so the statement is probably true. But, how does

Option C is incorrect. See option B. While it may be true that a beating heart, by circulating blood, can warm body tissues and slow ice production, how does this directly affect the cryoprotective effect of glucose? There is no answer from the passage.

Option D is incorrect. The heart eventually stops or nearly stops beating as shown in Figure 1. This occurs when the glucose is at its highest. So, even with glucose, the heart stops beating, so this cannot be a correct statement in this situation. Generally, a beating heart will require glucose, but may use other nutrients for energy as well.

Option A is correct. The glucose is released from the liver at the onset of the process; it takes time for it to be distributed throughout the body. If the heart beat stopped right away, this redistribution would not take place and the effectiveness of the cryoprotective effect would diminish.

Test Taking Skills Comment

This is a Dichotomy of Options **(SB A.2.3)** of options questions with A/B being one option with 'circulating' and options C/D being the other set with 'beating heart'. For a dichotomy, you must use Basic Knowledge (study, passage, general knowledge) **(SB A.2.2)** to determine which half of the dichotomy is correct. This may not be an easy decision in this case. If you cannot use some info to make the decision, it is best not to use the technique. The previous excerpt suggests the circulation is what is important - this eliminates options C/D.

Meso Compounds

"**Me**s**o** compounds have a **M**irror of **S**ymmetry"

Thus even though they may have stereogenic centers, they are achiral and so do not have enantiomers.

ORG 2.3.3

Biological Science Passage 4.BS.II

Q104 — Pre-Study Suggestions

Review the following if needed:
1) Cell Structure and Function **BIO 1**
2) Cardiovascular System **BIO 7**
3) Lymphatic Vessels **BIO 7.6**
4) Blood Vessels **BIO 7.3**
5) Fluid Homeostasis **BIO 6.1**
6) Multiple Choice Question **SB A.1.2**
7) Three Out of Four Type Question **SB A.2.8**
8) What information is needed from the passage?
9) Solve the problem.

Solution Discussion

The key information from the passage is found in the first paragraph:

"slow cooling permits redistribution … only extracellular water freezes."

Option II is correct. The blood plasma **(BIO 7.5)** is extracellular.

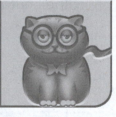

Option I is incorrect. The cytoplasm **(BIO 1.2)** is inside the cell and not extracellular.

Option III is correct. The lymph **(BIO 7.6)** is extracellular.

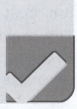

Options A, B and C are incorrect.

Option D is correct. Only extracellular **(BIO 1.2)** tissues freeze.

Test Taking Skills Comment

This is a Multiple Choice Question **(SB A.1.2)**. The first set of choices are the I, II and III options. If you can determine which of these are Correct or Incorrect **(SB A.1.2)**, then you can eliminate certain of the A, B, C or D options. In this question, since the key is 'extracellular', you may be able to determine that option I, cytoplasm, cannot be correct since it is clearly intracellular **(BIO 1.2)**. Just by knowing this, you know option C cannot be correct. Then if you know that blood plasma **(BIO 7.5)** is extracellular, you know that option II has to be correct; then you can eliminate option B and know the answer must be C or D. Then you have to

determine if option III is Correct or Incorrect **(SB A.1.2)** to pick the correct letter option. Sometimes, multiple choice questions will provide a variety of opportunities for elimination of options. These will have to be evaluated on an individual basis.

This is also a Three Out of Four Type Question **(SB A.2.8)** with options A, C and D all containing Choice II. Usually two or more choice will be correct, so you could guess that C or D must be correct (this is generally, but not always true).

Q105 Pre-Study Suggestions

Review the following if needed:
1) Energy Metabolism **BIO 4**
2) Anaerobic Respiration **BIO 4**
3) Three Out of Four Type Question **SB A.2.8**
4) Similar Pair Options **SB A.2.7**
5) What information is needed from the passage?
6) Solve the problem.

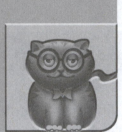

Solution Discussion

The information needed is the data found in Figure 1.

Options A, B and C are incorrect. *See* the discussion of option D.

that will be related directly to the presence of oxygen is the heart rate. When the heart stops or slows significantly, there will not be delivery of oxygen to the tissue and anaerobic conditions will prevail. The heart rate stops at about 12 hours and continues to about 26 hours.

Option D is correct. Anaerobic metabolism will ensue when there is no longer oxygen being provided to the tissues. The only variable

Test Taking Skills Comment

This is a Three Out of Four Type Question **(SB A.2.8)**. Options B, C and D are similar because they are all 'between' with option A being the outlier. Outliers are usually incorrect. This is also a Similar Pair Options **(SB A.2.7)** as options B and C are similar in starting with a zero. In this situation, you would guess wrong but this is the hazard of guessing. On the average, you will do better with the technique if properly applied.

Q106 — Pre-Study Suggestions

Review the following if needed:
1) Blood **BIO 7.5**
2) Graphs and Charts **GS A.3**
3) Dichotomy of Options **SB A.2.3**
4) Three or More Step Analysis **SB A.1.4**
5) Best Option **SB A.1.2**
6) Complex Sounding Option(s) **SB A.2.2**
7) What information is needed from the passage to solve the problem?
8) Solve the problem.

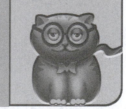

Solution Discussion

The information needed is found in Figure 2.

The Figure 2 shows that as the glucose concentration injected increases, the survival increases but the plasma hemoglobin will decrease. Plasma hemoglobin is related to the extent of hemolysis. The greater the plasma hemoglobin, the greater the hemolysis of red blood cells. Hemoglobin should not be present in the plasma - it should be in the red blood cells. Survival is lowest and plasma hemoglobin is highest for saline only.

CHAPTER 6

Biological Science Passage 4.BS.II

Option B is incorrect. Death is directly related to the hemolysis, shown by the amount of plasma hemoglobin. As hemolysis decreases, the survival increases. Since the extent of hemolysis is inversely related to the concentration of exogenous glucose, this could support the hypothesis. This is a True **(SB A.1.2)** option but is not the Best Option **(SB A.1.2)**.

Option D is incorrect. Where is the connection made between hemolysis and circulatory collapse? There is no basic knowledge to support this, and there is nothing from the passage to support this. This is a Complex Sounding Option(s) **(SB A.2.2)** that goes beyond Basic Knowledge (study, passage, general knowledge) **(SB A.2.2)**.

Option C is incorrect. There is no data on the blood hemoglobin to make this assessment. Blood hemoglobin and plasma hemoglobin are not the same. Remember plasma **(BIO 7.5)** is the fraction that results from centrifuging and removing the cellular components of blood. Blood is made of the cellular portion and the plasma. The cellular portion of blood contains hemoglobin. The graph is showing the lowering of plasma hemoglobin. This would suggest that blood hemoglobin is at worst unaffected.

Option A is correct. The graphs clearly show these facts. This is the best option.

Test Taking Skills Comment

Note option B is plausible but it is not the best option. The Dichotomy of Options **(SB A.2.3)** should be done and you should eliminate options C and D because the graphs clearly show a survival advantage for injected glucose and would support the hypothesis. Remember, you use your Basic

Knowledge (study, passage, general knowledge) **(SB A.2.2)** to determine which part of the dichotomy is correct. This also requires the use of Best Option **(SB A.1.2)** and Complex Sounding Option(s) **(SB A.2.2)** as previously discussed.

Q107 — Pre-Study Suggestions

Review the following if needed:
1) Similar Pair Options **SB A.2.7**
2) Complex Sounding Option(s) **SB A.2.2**
3) What information is needed from the passage?
4) Solve the problem.

Solution Discussion

The key information from the passage is found in paragraphs 1 and 2:

From paragraph one:

"in these animals, slow cooling ... extracellular water freezes."

From the second paragraph:

"strategy involves accelerated glucose ... freezing point of body fluids"

Figures 1 and 2 are needed.

Option A is incorrect. The passage does not call for total body dehydration. The dehydration is selective for the cells only as previously described.

Option C is incorrect. Again, high blood hemoglobin concentrations are not shown or discussed in the passage. This is a Complex Sounding Option(s) **(SB A.2.2)** because this information is not in the passage and is not study knowledge.

Option D is incorrect. The high glucose concentrations are important for the tissues. So, this would be a survival benefit. But, how do the tissues get high glucose? They get it from the liver, option B. Notice also that high glucose tissue levels at times other than the freeze is not good.

Option B is correct. Having large supplies of glycogen present in the liver is the best preparation, of those listed, for the winter survival. Glycogen is broken down into glucose for distribution around the body.

Test Taking Skills Comment

This is a Complex Sounding Option(s) **(SB A.2.2)** as discussed for option C. It is also a subtle Similar Pair Options **(SB A.2.7)** because glycogen and glucose are very similar. You could guess from these two options.

Q108 — Pre-Study Suggestions

Review the following if needed:

1) Solubility of Organics **ORG 3.1.1, 6.1, 8.1, 9.4, 10.1, 11.1.2, 12.1.1**
2) Functional Group **ORG 1.6**
3) Three Out of Four Type Question **SB A.2.8**
4) Similar Pair Options **SB A.2.7**
5) Three or More Step Analysis **SB A.1.4**
6) What information is needed from the passage?
7) Solve the problem.

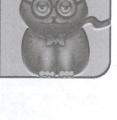

Solution Discussion

The key information is from paragraph three:

"Compound C was optically inactive and soluble in both dilute acid and base."

Camphoric acid, hippuric acid and 4-aminobenzoic acid all have acid groups.

Option A is incorrect. The carboxylic acid **(ORG 8)** component would be soluble **(ORG 8.1)** in base. The amide **(ORG 9.3)** is not acidic or basic and wouldn't necessarily be soluble in either acid or base. The only amide group is in hippuric acid.

Option B is incorrect. The amine **(ORG 11)** would be soluble **(ORG 11.1.2)** in acid. The only amine is 4-aminobenzoic acid. Amides are not soluble in either - *see* option A.

CHAPTER 6

Option C is incorrect. *See* option A for comments about amides. There is no nitro group **(ORG 1.6, 5.2.2)** on any of the compounds in Table 1.

Option D is correct. Acids are soluble in bases; bases are soluble in acids (*see* solubility of organics; **ORG 3.1.1, 6.1, 8.1, 9.4, 10.1, 11.1.2, 12.1.1**). The amine group is basic and would be soluble in acid. The carboxylic acid group is acidic and would be soluble in base. The 4-aminobenzoic acid fits both of these requirements.

Test Taking Skills Comment

It is important that you be familiar with the common organic functional groups **(ORG 1.6)** and their characteristics. This is a Three Out of Four Type Question **(SB A.2.8)**. Options A, B and C all contain amide. Option D is the outlier without amide. Generally, the outlier will be incorrect. This is a rare occasion where the outlier is the correct option - remember guessing is guessing, but using the techniques will, on the average, give you an advantage. This is also a Similar Pair Options **(SB A.2.7)** with options A and D both containing a carboxylic acid. Generally, you should not go for a similar pair that is not part of your three out of four, but in this question, you would have guessed correctly.

This is also a Three or More Step Analysis **(SB A.1.4)** which generally makes it more difficult:

1) first you have to determine the first compounds features;
2) then you have to determine the second compounds features;
3) then you have to determine if they are consistent with the description of Compound C;
4) then you have to determine if the option is True or False **(SB A.1.2)**; and
5) then you have to determine if the option is Correct or Incorrect **(SB A.1.2)**.

Q109 — Pre-Study Suggestions

Review the following if needed:
1) Infrared Spectroscopy **ORG 14.1**
2) Functional Group **ORG 1.6**
3) What information is needed from the passage?
4) Solve the problem.

Solution Discussion

The key information from the passage is from Table 1:

The functional groups **(ORG 1.6)** in each compound:

1) Camphoric acid: Carboxylic Acid **(ORG 8)**
                        Carbonyl **(ORG 7.1)**
                        Hydroxyl (Alcohols; **ORG 6**)
                        Aliphatic hydrogens (alkanes; **ORG 3**)

2) Hippuric Acid: Carboxylic acid
                       Carbonyl
                       Hydroxyl
                       Amides **(ORG 9.3)**
                       Benzene ring/hydrogens **(ORG 14.1)**

3) Diethlybarbituric Acid: Imide **(ORG 11.2)**
                               Carbonyl

4) Aminobenzoic Acid: Amine **(ORG 11)**
                          Carboxylic acid
                          Hydroxyl
                          Carbonyl
                          Benzene ring/hydrogens

Option A is incorrect. The range of greater than 3000 cm^{-1} is for aromatic hydrogens and hydrogens attached to multiple bonded carbons as in a benzene ring. Compounds 2 and 4 would have peaks in this range. If the peaks were at 2900 cm^{-1}, then the aliphatic hydrogens of compounds 1, 2 and 3 would have been likely.

Option B is incorrect. The only functional group near 2100 cm^{-1} is the acetylene or carbon triple bond **(ORG 1.3.1)**. No compound has a triple bond. Note nitrile, or cyano **(ORG 14.1)**, (triple bond carbon and nitrogen) is near 2250 cm^{-1}.

Option D is incorrect. This is close to the carbon-oxygen single bond as in a hydroxyl group. This value is usually closer to 1100 cm^{-1}, but these are approximations. Compounds 1, 2 and 4 all contain the C-O functional group.

Option C is correct. The functional group that absorbs at about 1700 cm^{-1} is the carbonyl functional group. All four compounds contain a carbonyl **(ORG 7.1)**.

Test Taking Skills Comment

Notice all the locations of absorption are approximate. You should know the approximate locations of the absorption of the major functional groups as discussed in infrared spectroscopy **(ORG 14.1)**. You should know the structure of all of the common functional groups **(ORG 1.6)**.

Q110

Pre-Study Suggestions

Review the following if needed:

1) Melting Points of Organic Compounds **ORG 3.1.1, 6.1, 8.1, 9.2, 10.1, 11.1.2**
2) Melting Points (Freezing Points) **ORG 3.1.1, 6.1, 8.1, 9.2, 10.1, 11.1.2**
3) Dichotomy of Options **SB A.2.3**
4) Three Out of Four Type Question **SB A.2.8**
5) Similar Pair Options **SB A.2.7**
6) Illogical Sequence of Options **SB A.2.9**
7) What information is needed from the passage?
8) Solve the problem.

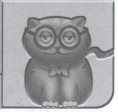

Solution Discussion

From Table 1, the MP of the compounds are given:

Camphoric acid = 183-186 °C
4-Aminobenzoic acid = 188-189 °C.

Option A is incorrect. Impurities lower the melting point (MP), or freezing point **(ORG 3.1.1, 6.1, 8.1, 9.2, 10.1, 11.1.2)**, of the substance. Since the main component is 4-aminobenzoic acid, the MP must be lower than 189 °C when an impurity is present.

Option C is incorrect. It is difficult to state the exact MP without knowing the concentration. It will not be sharp because of the presence of the impurity. The MP should be less than the 188 °C of the 4-aminobenzoic acid, but you cannot determine the exact MP without more details such as the molality (m = moles/kg of solvent; **CHM 5.1.2**) and concentration of the mixture. Another key reason this is incorrect is because of the sharp MP - any

CHAPTER 6

impurity will broaden the MP range.

Option D is incorrect. This is incorrect for two reasons. First, the MP of the solution will be depressed below the 189 °C because of freezing point depression (**ORG 3.1.1, 6.1, 8.1, 9.2, 10.1, 11.1.2**). Second, the MP will not be sharp, but will be over a range because of the impurity.

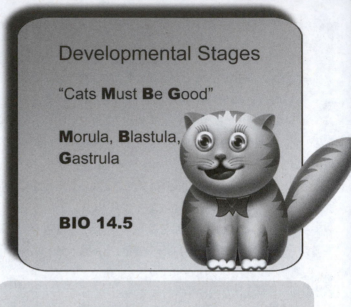

Developmental Stages

"Cats **M**ust **B**e **G**ood"

Morula, **B**lastula, **G**astrula

BIO 14.5

Option B is correct. The MP will be depressed below the 188 °C and the range will be broad because there is an impurity present.

Test Taking Skills Comment

This is a double Dichotomy of Options (**SB A.2.3**) type question. One dichotomy is sharp versus broad MP. If you know the MP will be broad, and you should based on your Study Knowledge (**SB A.2.2**) as in melting points (freezing points) (**ORG 3.1.1, 6.1, 8.1, 9.2, 10.1, 11.1.2**) and melting points of organic compounds (**ORG 3.1.1, 6.1, 8.1, 9.2, 10.1, 11.1.2**), you should eliminate options C and D. The second dichotomy is whether the MP will be depressed below

that of 4-aminobenzoic acid. The MP will be depressed by an impurity and will be lower than the lowest number of the 4-aminobenzoic acid which is 188 °C. This means options A and D would be incorrect. As usual, for double dichotomy questions, if you correctly identify both, the correct answer remains which is B in this question.

This is also a Three Out of Four Type Question (**SB A.2.8**) as options A, B and D all relate to the MP of 4-aminobenzoic acid (4-ABA). This means option C is an outlier because it does not relate to 4-ABA. Outliers are usually incorrect.

Options A and D could be called a Similar Pair Options **(SB A.2.7)** as both relate to 189 degrees. But, caution should be used, and really you should not use this option, when the similar pair is not part of the three out of four, or when there are more than one similar pair present. Note any dichotomy is automatically a set of similar pairs.

There is also an Illogical Sequence of Options **(SB A.2.9)** which is a rare occurrence.

Options A and B are reversed; B should be before A logically as 188 °C is smaller than 189 °C. So, one of these was moved to fit a random option being correct. You really cannot tell which was moved. So, you still can only guess from A or B. But, there are other skills available to narrow down the guess as previously discussed.

Q111 — Pre-Study Suggestions

Review the following if needed:
1) Functional Group **ORG 1.6**
2) Ethers **ORG 1.6, 10.1, 7.2.2**
3) Ketone **ORG 7**
4) Aldehydes **ORG 7**
5) Esters **ORG 9.4**
6) Three Out of Four Type Question **SB A.2.8**
7) Similar Pair Options **SB A.2.7**
8) Camouflage and Distractions **SB A.1.3**
9) What are the key pieces of information from the passage?
10) Solve the problem.

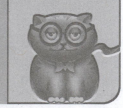

Solution Discussion

The following information is found in the passage:

First Paragraph:

"It was also observed that Compound A … formation of two new compounds."

Second Paragraph:

"The first compound (Compound B) was a water-soluble alcohol"

Third Paragraph:

"The second compound (Compound C) … soluble in both dilute acid and base."

Option C is incorrect. Ketones **(ORG 7)** do not break down into alcohols by refluxing NaOH. ketones may be converted to alcohols by reduction or by an aldol condensation **(ORG 7.2.4)**.

Option D is incorrect. Aldehydes **(ORG 7)** are similar to ketones.

Option A is incorrect. The ethers **(ORG 1.6, 7.2.2, 10.1)** would not result in the two compounds with the refluxing NaOH.

Option B is correct. This is an ester **(ORG 9.4)**. The alcohol would result from the refluxing NaOH. The carboxylic acid **(ORG 8)** portion would be formed by the acidification of the NaOH. Also, the acid part would be soluble in base.

Test Taking Skills Comment

This is Three Out of Four Type Question **(SB A.2.8)** as options B, C and D all have a carbonyl group **(ORG 7.1)**. Option A is an outlier, and outliers are usually incorrect. There is also a reasonable Similar Pair Options **(SB A.2.7)** present for A and D as they are carbonyls. In this question, you would guess wrong using these but this is the risk of guessing. On the average, you would be better off by doing the guessing, if you have to guess.

This is a type of Camouflage and Distractions **(SB A.1.3)** as the issue here is whether you understand the reactions of esters **(ORG 9.4)** and the products formed from hydrolysis.

Q112 — Pre-Study Suggestions

Review the following if needed:
1) Solubility of Organics **ORG 3.1.1, 6.1, 8.1, 9.4, 10.1, 11.1.2, 12.1.1**
2) Melting Points of Organic Compounds **ORG 3.1.1, 6.1, 8.1, 9.2, 10.1, 11.1.2**
3) Alcohols **ORG 6**
4) Molar Mass (MM = g per mole) **CHM 1.3**
5) Graphs and Charts **GS A.3**
6) Three Out of Four Type Question **SB A.2.8**
7) What information is required from the passage?
8) Solve the problem.

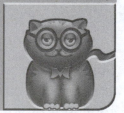

Solution Discussion

The information is found in Table 1.

Option A is incorrect. The compounds have many of the same functional groups **(ORG 1.6)**. This means they will have similar solubility **(ORG 3.1.1, 6.1, 8.1, 9.4, 10.1, 11.1.2, 12.1.1)** and solubility of organics **(ORG 3.1.1, 6.1, 8.1, 9.4, 10.1, 11.1.2, 12.1.1)**.

Option C is incorrect. The melting points **(ORG 3.1.1, 6.1, 8.1, 9.2, 10.1, 11.1.2)** are very close together and actually overlap. So, they cannot be distinguished on this basis.

Option B is incorrect. Most of the compounds contain a carboxylic acid **(ORG 8)** group. The acid group will react with alcohols **(ORG 6)** to form esters **(ORG 9.4)**.

Option D is correct. I wouldn't determine the molecular weight of each of the compounds. I reach this conclusion by being certain of my elimination of the other options.

Test Taking Skills Comment

Sometimes you can only eliminate options to reach the correct answer. If you were not confident of your elimination of options, you could determine the molar mass (MM = g per mole) **(CHM 1.3)** of each one. This is very time consuming. This is a Three Out of Four Type Question **(SB A.2.8)** as options A, C and D deal with physical properties. This means option B is an outlier, it is a chemical property, and is probably incorrect.

Q113 — Pre-Study Suggestions

Review the following if needed:
1) Bacterial Reproduction **BIO 2.2**
2) Similar Pair Options **SB A.2.7**
3) Complex Sounding Option(s) **SB A.2.2**
4) Internally Inconsistent **SB A.2.5**
5) What information is needed from the passage?
6) Solve the problem.

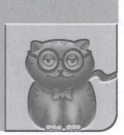

Solution Discussion

The key information from the passage is from:

Paragraph One:

"Because plasmids are not ... distributed among daughter cells."

Paragraph two:

"Conjugation occurs when ... and a bacterium lacking such genes."

Option A is incorrect. You would have to be given specific information to make this assessment. Since the MCAT is not out to trick you, you assume that the normal processes you learned will occur unless you are given specific information to the contrary. This would be a Complex Sounding Option(s) **(SB A.2.2)**. Notice the difference between this option in this question and the same option if the question was different. In some persuasive type problems or new information problems, the question might ask you the effect on something given this observation, as in option A.

In questions like this, you are to assume the option, statement, is true and determine its impact on the question being asked. In this particular question, you are not instructed to assume the option, statement, is true. So, you must first determine if it is True or False **(SB A.1.2)** before you can determine if it is Correct or Incorrect **(SB A.1.2)**. Option A now must be true for it to be a possible correct option. But, your Study Knowledge **(SB A.2.2)** or Passage Knowledge **(SB A.2.2)** does not allow you to make that determination. Therefore, the option is indeterminate as to True or False **(SB A.1.2)** and cannot be the Correct **(SB A.1.2)** answer. Try to understand this distinction and how to apply it.

Option B is incorrect. This is the same as option A. You have to determine if 'the cell membrane failed

to move the replicated chromosomes apart' is a true statement or not. But, there is no way for you to determine this based on your Basic Knowledge (study, passage, general knowledge) **(SB A.2.2)**. Therefore, this is a Complex Sounding Option(s) **(SB A.2.2)** and cannot be the correct option.

Option D is incorrect. This is the same as options A and B. *See* previously. This is even more 'out there' than A or B and is a Complex Sounding Option(s) **(SB A.2.2)** - how are you going to determine if something ate something else? You cannot unless it is in the passage which it is not. But even more to the point, it is an Internally Inconsistent **(SB A.2.5)** option because bacteria do not have lysosomes **(BIO 1.2.1)** because they are prokaryotic **(BIO 2.2)** and do not have membrane **(BIO 1.2.1)** bound cell organelles **(BIO 1.2.1)**.

Option C is correct. You are given specific information in the passage that this occurs - this is Passage Knowledge **(SB A.2.2)**. You should also be familiar with this from your Study Knowledge **(SB A.2.2)**. Contrast this option with the options in A, B and D - the better you understand why this option is correct and the others are not given Basic Knowledge (study, passage, general knowledge) **(SB A.2.2)** will help you immensely.

Test Taking Skills Comment

There are Complex Sounding Option(s) **(SB A.2.2)** and Internally Inconsistent **(SB A.2.5)** options in this question - these are previously discussed.

This is also a Similar Pair Options **(SB A.2.7)** with options C and D being similar with both dealing with 'plasmids'. Since this is the only reasonable similar pair present and there are no other confounders present, this would be a good guess.

Q114   Pre-Study Suggestions

Review the following if needed:
1) Mutations **BIO 3, 15.5**
2) Immune Response **BIO 8**
3) Complex Sounding Option(s) **SB A.2.2**
4) Internally Inconsistent **SB A.2.5**
5) Similar Pair Options **SB A.2.7**
6) Three Out of Four Type Question **SB A.2.8**
7) What information is needed from the passage?
8) Solve the problem.

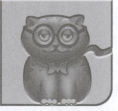

Solution Discussion

The key information from the passage is from the first paragraph:

"Plasmids (small, circular … resistance to specific antibiotics."

Option A is incorrect. You have no information to assess if this option is correct or not - it is a Complex Sounding Option(s) **(SB A.2.2)** based on Basic Knowledge (study, passage, general knowledge) **(SB A.2.2)**. Your prior Study Knowledge **(SB A.2.2)** did not require you to know this and it is not contained within the Passage Knowledge **(SB A.2.2)**.

Option B is incorrect. This is just like option A and is a Complex Sounding Option(s) **(SB A.2.2)**. This is even more out in left field than option A. It is also incompatible with your

Study Knowledge **(SB A.2.2)** of bacteria. A bacterium does not generate immune responses **(BIO 8)**, which makes this Internally Inconsistent **(SB A.2.5)** as well.

Option C is incorrect. This is like option A and is a Complex Sounding Option(s) **(SB A.2.2)** because this information is beyond your Basic Knowledge (study, passage, general knowledge) **(SB A.2.2)**. Also, this is Internally Inconsistent **(SB A.2.5)** because antibiotics are directed at bacteria and not the cells of the human body.

Option D is correct. You can assess this. It only calls for chance mutations **(BIO 3, 15.5)** that may occur. It does not state the antibiotics caused the mutations as in option A. You also know from the passage that plasmids may contain genes that are antibiotic resistant. Of all the options, this one has

statements that you can evaluate based on your study and the passage; your Basic Knowledge (study, passage, general knowledge) **(SB A.2.2)**.

Test Taking Skills Comment

There are Complex Sounding Option(s) **(SB A.2.2)** and Internally Inconsistent **(SB A.2.5)** options as previously discussed.

This is also a Three Out of Four Type Question **(SB A.2.8)** as options A, C and D all deal with 'resistance' of some type. Option B deals with 'immune response' and is an

outlier - outliers are usually incorrect. This is also a reasonable Similar Pair Options **(SB A.2.7)** as options A and D both deal with mutations and are part of the three out of four set. Options A or D would be a good guess.

Q115 — Pre-Study Suggestions

Review the following if needed:
1) Bacterial Reproduction **BIO 2.2**
2) Complex Sounding Option(s) **SB A.2.2**
3) What information is needed from the passage?
4) Solve the problem.

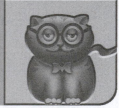

Solution Discussion

The key information is from:

Paragraph One:

"Plasmids (small, circular … resistance to specific antibiotics."

Paragraph Two:

"Conjugation occurs when … a bacterium lacking such genes."

"Conjugation may occur between of the same, or different, bacterial species."

Option C is incorrect. Same as option B and is a Complex Sounding Option(s) **(SB A.2.2)**. How would you assess this? You have no basis for doing so. Since you cannot determine if it is True or False **(SB A.1.2)** based on your Basic Knowledge (study, passage, general knowledge) **(SB A.2.2)**, it cannot be correct.

Option B is incorrect. Where do you get the information to assess this is correct or not? There is none; none from your study nor from the passage. Therefore, this is a Complex Sounding Option(s) **(SB A.2.2)** not assessable using Basic Knowledge (study, passage, general knowledge) **(SB A.2.2)** and is not correct.

Option D is incorrect. Same as option B. This may be plausible, but where and how can you determine its veracity based on Basic Knowledge (study, passage, general knowledge) **(SB A.2.2)**? You can't.

Option A is correct. This is assessable. You are told in the passage that plasmids have resistance genes, that plasmids direct conjugation, and that conjugation can occur between unrelated species - all of this is Passage Knowledge **(SB A.2.2)**. Since the E. coli were exposed to ampicillin and kana- mycin, they could have become resistant to them and then could have shared the genes with the TB bacterium. Notice the difference between this option and the previous options.

Test Taking Skills Comment

There are Complex Sounding Option(s) **(SB A.2.2)** as previously discussed.

Q116   Pre-Study Suggestions

Review the following if needed:
1) Gastrointestinal System **BIO 9**
2) Bacteria **BIO 2.2**
3) Three Out of Four Type Question **SB A.2.8**
4) Similar Pair Options **SB A.2.7**
5) What information is needed from the passage?
6) Solve the problem.

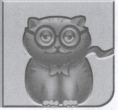

Solution Discussion

The information is from the third paragraph:

"A man was hospitalized with a ruptured appendix"

"Shortly after leaving the hospital, he … from a coworker."

and would have similar colonization.

Option A is incorrect. The M. tuberculosis was not acquired until after the patient left the hospital and the appendix had been treated.

Option D is incorrect. Same as option B.

Option B is incorrect. The colon and appendix are continuous

Option C is correct. The ruptured appendix allows the contents of the colon/appendix to spill into the abdominal cavity leading to peritonitis (not necessary for MCAT).

Test Taking Skills Comment

This is a Three Out of Four Type Question **(SB A.2.8)**. Options B, C and D are similar because each deals with E. coli. Option A is an outlier and deals with M. tuberculosis. Outliers tend to be incorrect. This is also a reasonable Similar Pair Options **(SB A.2.7)** question even though you would get the wrong answer - again, this is the risk of guessing. Options B and D are very similar and would be a reasonable guess. You are guessing to increase your overall average percent correct, which the techniques will do.

Q117 — Pre-Study Suggestions

Review the following if needed:
1) Bacteria **BIO 2.2**
2) Complex Sounding Option(s) **SB A.2.2**
3) Similar Pair Options **SB A.2.7**
4) Three Out of Four Type Question **SB A.2.8**
5) What information is needed from the passage?
6) Solve the problem.

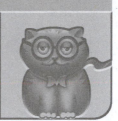

Solution Discussion

The key information from the passage is from paragraph 1:

"Escherichia coli, a bacterial … producing vitamins such as B_{12} and K."

Option B is incorrect. There is no information in the passage regarding this, and you did not have to prepare for this. Vitamin B_{12} production is mentioned in the passage as beforehand, but the passage does not address whether or not this feature makes E. coli more successful than other bacteria - this is what the question is asking. Therefore, this is a Complex Sounding Option(s) **(SB A.2.2)** which is beyond your Basic Knowledge (study, passage, general knowledge) **(SB A.2.2)**. *See* option A discussion.

Option C is incorrect. You are given no information on the metabolism of glucose. Furthermore, you are not given any indication of the relative survival value of metabolizing glucose even if the statement is true. This is a Complex Sounding Option(s) **(SB A.2.2)** which is beyond your Basic Knowledge (study, passage, general knowledge) **(SB A.2.2)**. *See* option A

(study, passage, general knowledge) **(SB A.2.2)**. *See* discussion in option A.

Option D is incorrect. This is even more extreme and in 'left field' than options B or C. You not only have to know if this is true, you again have to know whether it results in a better survival if it is true. There is no way of knowing this and this is a Complex Sounding Option(s) **(SB A.2.2)** which is beyond your Basic Knowledge

Option A is correct. This is also a Complex Sounding Option(s) **(SB A.2.2)**. But, this makes sense and can be evaluated. The difference between this option and options A, B and C is that it is logical, without any other information, and that if more viable offspring are produced than other bacteria, then E. coli will survive better. It seems kind of obvious, which it is. The other options cannot be assessed because they make a statement whose effect cannot be assessed in terms of survival which is the question being asked.

Test Taking Skills Comment

There are Complex Sounding Option(s) **(SB A.2.2)** in this question as previously discussed. But, this is different from some other questions of this type. Because of the manner in which the Stem **(SB A.1.1)** is phrased, you are to assume the statement is True **(SB A.1.2)**, and you have to determine if it answers the questions being asked without questioning its veracity. Notice that for options B, C or D, even if the statement is true, how do you determine that it translates into better survival for E. coli. This is where the Complex Sounding Option(s) **(SB A.2.2)** comes in - you cannot assess any of the statements in options B, C or D as relates to survival.

Option A is a statement of survival itself, 'more viable descendants', so there is nothing else to assess. For all of these except option B, which is stated in the passage, you don't really know if the statement is True or False **(SB A.1.2)**, but because of the manner of stating the question, you are to assume each is true and then assess it in relation to survival, the question being asked.

This could also be a Similar Pair Options **(SB A.2.7)** question as options A and B both discuss 'produce' of some type. This is soft, but a guess is a guess.

Q118 — Pre-Study Suggestions

Review the following if needed:
1) Complex Sounding Option(s) **SB A.2.2**
2) Similar Pair Options **SB A.2.7**
3) What information is needed from the passage?
4) Solve the problem.

Solution Discussion

The key information from the passage is from paragraph one:

"Escherichia coli, a bacterial … producing vitamins such as B_{12} and K."

Option A is incorrect. There is nothing in the passage about digestive enzymes. This is a Complex Sounding Option(s) **(SB A.2.2)** because the determination if it is True or False **(SB A.1.2)** is beyond your Basic Knowledge (study, passage, general knowledge) **(SB A.2.2)**.

Option D is incorrect. This is the same as options A and C. Nothing at all is stated about absorption in the passage. It is a Complex Sounding Option(s) **(SB A.2.2)** and is beyond your Basic Knowledge (study, passage, general knowledge) **(SB A.2.2)**.

Option C is incorrect. Again there is nothing in the passage about increases in intestinal tract infections if E. coli is decreased. This is a Complex Sounding Option(s) **(SB A.2.2)** because the assessment is beyond your Basic Knowledge (study, passage, general knowledge) **(SB**

Option B is correct. This is assessable as the information is found in the passage as is discussed beforehand. Notice this is not Study Knowledge **(SB A.2.2)**. The only you can determine if it is True or False **(SB A.1.2)** and Correct or Incorrect **(SB A.1.2)** is the Passage Knowledge **(SB A.2.2)** from paragraph one.

Test Taking Skills Comment

This is a Complex Sounding Option(s) **(SB A.2.2)** as previously discussed. Please notice how this Complex Sounding Option(s) **(SB A.2.2)** is different from the complex sounding option as discussed in Q 117.

This is also a possible soft Similar Pair Options **(SB A.2.7)** question. Options A and B both relate to 'deficiencies' and would be a reasonable guess.

Q119 — Pre-Study Suggestions

Review the following if needed:
1) Meiosis **BIO 14.2**
2) Bacterial Reproduction **BIO 2.2**
3) Recombination **BIO 15.3**
4) Similar Pair Options **SB A.2.7**
5) What are the key pieces of information from the passage?
6) Solve the problem.

Solution Discussion

The key information from the passage is from paragraph 2; the whole paragraph describes conjugation.

The process of sexual reproduction in eukaryotic **(BIO 1)** organisms is by the process of meiosis **(BIO 14.2)**. Meiosis results in haploid **(BIO 14.2)** gametes **(BIO 14.2)** which then combine in fertilization **(BIO 14.5)** to form diploid **(BIO 14.2)** gametes.

Option B is incorrect. The combining of the two sets of chromosomes **(BIO 14.2)** is the process of fertilization **(BIO 14.5)** during sexual reproduction. This is not what is occurring during bacterial conjugation (*see* paragraph 2).

Option C is incorrect. All reproduction has the potential to increase organisms in the population whether sexual or asexual.

Biological Science Non-Passage 4R.NPI

Option D is incorrect. Sexual reproduction in eukaryotic cells **(BIO 1)** is generally only effective between members of the same species. As noted in the 2nd paragraph, conjugation is not restricted to the same species.

Option A is correct. The key feature of both conjugation and sexual reproduction in eukaryotes is the recombination of genes which produces genetic variability **(BIO 15.5)**.

Test Taking Skills Comment

This is a reasonable Similar Pair Options **(SB A.2.7)** as options A and B are dealing with genes/chromosomes/combinations. A guess is a guess but these techniques enhance your correct guess percentage.

Q120 — Pre-Study Suggestions

Review the following if needed:
1) Formal Charge **CHM 2.2, 2.3**
2) Three Out of Four Type Question **SB A.2.8**
3) Solve the problem.

Solution Discussion

The structure is:

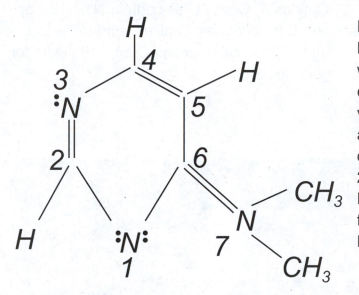

From the periodic chart **(CHM 2.3)**, N has an atomic number **(CHM 1.3)** of 7 which means it has 7 electrons. Its electron configuration **(CHM 2.2)** is $1s^2\ 2s^2\ 2p^3$. The valence electrons **(CHM 2.2)** are the 2s and the 2p giving it 5 valence electrons. In determining its formal charge **(CHM 2.2, 2.3)**, these must be taken into account. Each bond counts as one electron and each free pair of electrons count as two electrons. For each of the nitrogens:

Nitrogen	Valence Electrons	-bonds	-2 x electron pairs	= formal charge
1	5	-2	-2 (2)	= 5-2-4 = -1
3	5	-3	-2 (1)	= 5-3-2 = 0
7	5	-4	-2 (0)	= 5-4-0 = 1

Option A, B and D are incorrect.

Option C is correct. See the previous discussion.

CHAPTER 6

Test Taking Skills Comment

If you knew for sure one or the other was correct: you could eliminate options. E.g. if you knew for sure that N7 was positive, then you could eliminate options A and D.

This is also a double Three Out of Four Type Question **(SB A.2.8)**. Options B, C and D all contain N7. Then option A is an outlier. Options A, C and D all contain N1. Then option B is an outlier. Outliers tend to be incorrect. This leaves options C or D to select for your guess.

Q121 — Pre-Study Suggestions

Review the following if needed:
1) Nervous System Concepts **BIO 6.1**
2) Three Out of Four Type Question **SB A.2.8**
3) Illogical Sequence of Options **SB A.2.9**
4) Solve the problem.

Solution Discussion

At site I is the peripheral receptor. This is the transducer that converts the stimulus, e.g. pain, into electrical impulses. There will be no other connections at this point. Site IV is the peripheral effecter site. This is where the action will be carried out. No other connections will exist here. At sites II and III, which are in the spinal cord **(BIO 6.1)** or central nervous system **(BIO 6.1)**, there may be many other connections.

Options B, C and D are incorrect.

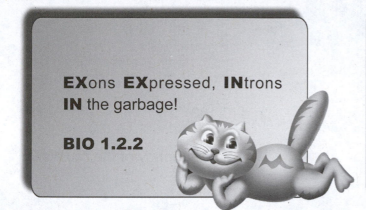

EXons EXpressed, INtrons IN the garbage!

BIO 1.2.2

Option A is correct. The middle neuron is an interneuron. Interneurons **(BIO 6)** have connections to multiple other neurons in the nervous system.

Test Taking Skills Comment

You should be able to eliminate sites I and IV as these are peripheral end sites - one is the receptor and the other is the effecter. If you do this, then the only option left is A. This is also a Three Out of Four Type Question **(SB A.2.8)**. But, in this case, as occasionally occurs, the outlier, option A that does not have site IV as a choice, is correct. On the average, Three Out of Four Type Question **(SB A.2.8)** is a very effective technique and will give you most guesses correctly. But,

guessing is guessing and it is not 100%.

This is a potential Illogical Sequence of Options **(SB A.2.9)**, but there are more than one possible logical sequences interrupted and whenever this occurs, it is best not to use the technique. Option D is out of sequence. It should either be A or B, but which one? Since this conflict exists, it is best not to use it.

Q122 — Pre-Study Suggestions

Review the following if needed:
1) Hardy-Weinberg Principle **BIO 15.4**
2) Camouflage and Distractions **SB A.1.3**
3) Solve the problem.

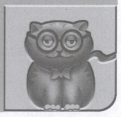

Solution Discussion

The two genes are the dominant **(BIO 15.1, 15.3)** gene with a frequency of p and the recessive **(BIO 15.1, 15.3)** gene with a frequency of q. Then,

p + q = 1.00
= the sum of the frequencies of the alleles **(BIO 15.3)** in the population.

The distribution of the genotype **(BIO 15)** is given by the binomial expansion of:

$$(p + q)^2 = p^2 + 2pq + q^2 = 1.00.$$

Where

p^2 = homozygous **(BIO 15.1, 15.3)** genotype
2pq = frequency of heterozygous **(BIO 15.1, 15.3)**
q^2 = frequency of homozygous recessive genotype

It is known that:

q^2 = 160/1000
= 0.160
= the frequency of the homozygous recessive genotype

Then,

$q = (0.160)^{1/2}$
= 0.40
= the frequency of the recessive allele.

Then,

p + 0.40 = 1.00
p = 0.60
= the frequency of the dominant allele.

Then, the frequency of heterozygotes in the population is:

2pq = 2 (0.60)(0.40)
= 2 (0.24)
= 0.48.

Then, the actual number of heterozygotes in the population is:

Number of heterozygotes	=	frequency of heterozygotes x total population
	=	0.480 x 1000
	=	480.

Options A, B and D are incorrect. *See* the previous discussion.

Option C is correct. *See* the previous discussion.

Test Taking Skills Comment

This is Passage Knowledge **(SB A.2.2)** and interpretation problem. There are Similar Pair Options **(SB A.2.7)** present. Options A and C are similar and would constitute a reasonable guess.

Q123   Pre-Study Suggestions

Review the following if needed:
1) Graphs and Charts **GS A.3**
2) Three Out of Four Type Question **SB A.2.8**
3) Similar Pair Options **SB A.2.7**
4) What information is required from the passage?
5) Solve the problem.

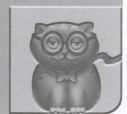

Solution Discussion

The key information is found in Figure 1 - refer to it in the chart.

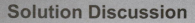

Biological Science Passage 4R.V

Option A is incorrect. The tension increases with or without endothelium (**BIO 7.4**) when the norepinephrine is added.

Option D is incorrect. The tension is expected to decrease when the ACh and NE are removed.

Option B is incorrect. The rate of decrease of tension appears to be the same by looking at the slopes of the curves. The reasons for the decrease are different in the two rings.

Option C is correct. When the pressure or tension reaches a certain level, endothelium produces the NO to result in a lowering of the tension in the blood vessels which will increase flow in them. This occurs when the ACh reaches 10^{-7} M in the endothelial lined ring, but does not occur in the other ring without endothelium even when the concentration of the ACh is continued to be increased.

Test Taking Skills Comment

This is Passage Knowledge (**SB A.2.2**) and Graphs and Charts (**GS A.3**) interpretation.

This is a Three Out of Four Type Question (**SB A.2.8**) as options B, C and D all relate to endothelium. Option A is an outlier and is incorrect. It is also a Similar Pair Options (**SB A.2.7**) as options B and D are 'without', and there is a similar pair with A and C as both deal with the neurotransmitters (**BIO 5.1**) chemicals used in the experiment. When there is more than one similar pair, it is best not to use the technique.

Q124 — Pre-Study Suggestions

Review the following if needed:
1) Graphs and Charts **GS A.3**
2) Dichotomy of Options **SB A.2.3**
3) Complex Sounding Option(s) **SB A.2.2**
4) What information is needed from the passage?
5) Solve the problem.

Solution Discussion

The Figure 1 is required and the following from paragraph two:

"Both rings were first contracted by adding norepinephrine to the baths."

Option A is incorrect. There is no graph to compare the presence and absence of NE for ACh. This is a Complex Sounding Option(s) **(SB A.2.2)** because there is no Passage Knowledge **(SB A.2.2)** to answer the question.

Option B is incorrect. There is no graph comparing the presence and absence of NE for ACh. This is a Complex Sounding Option(s) **(SB A.2.2)** as is option A.

Biological Science Passage 4R.V

Option D is incorrect. The 10^{-8} M concentration of ACh is to the left of the peak tensions. All of these peak tensions have greater ACh concentrations than 10^{-8} M.

Option C is correct. With the endothelium, the peak tension is reached at ACh of 10^{-7} M. Without the endothelium, the peak tension is reached at 10^{-6} M. This is approximately a 10 fold increase in tension with the endothelium.

Test Taking Skills Comment

Passage interpretation needed. This is a Dichotomy of Options **(SB A.2.3)** question. You should assess you cannot evaluate the epinephrine options as they are written. This means you would eliminate options A and B and guess from options C or D giving you a 50% correct guess rate. This is as good as the whole group of students did on this question. Remember, you have to use Basic Knowledge (study, passage, general knowledge) **(SB A.2.2)** to select the correct half of the dichotomy.

Q125   Pre-Study Suggestions

Review the following if needed:
1) Graphs and Charts **GS A.3**
2) Slope **GS A.3**
3) Complex Sounding Option(s) **SB A.2.2**
4) What information is needed from the passage?
5) Solve the problem.

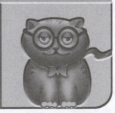

Solution Discussion

The most sensitive tension will be where the tension has the greatest value (rise) for a given concentration. The greatest tension occurs at about 10^{-7} M because the curves are highest at about this concentration. This is where the slope **(GS A.3)** is undergoing the greatest rate of change for a given change in concentration.

Option D is incorrect. The peak takes longer to develop and there is less slope increase in the ring without endothelium. This suggests less sensitivity to all concentrations. This is also a Complex Sounding Option(s) **(SB A.2.2)**.

Option A is incorrect. The curve is still rising, and not at its peak, as it goes from 10^{-8} M to 10^{-7} M.

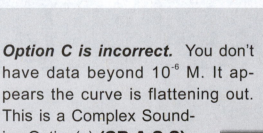

Option B is correct. The curves are near or at the peak at about 10^{-7} M.

Option C is incorrect. You don't have data beyond 10^{-6} M. It appears the curve is flattening out. This is a Complex Sounding Option(s) **(SB A.2.2)**.

Test Taking Skills Comment

This is a Three Out of Four Type Question **(SB A.2.8)**. Options A, B and C all deal with concentration. Option D does not deal with concentrations and is an outlier. Outliers tend to be incorrect.

There are Complex Sounding Option(s) **(SB A.2.2)** discussed previously. Option C is complex sounding because you do not have the Passage Knowledge **(SB A.2.2)** given to answer it. Option D is complex sounding because it is stated much more complexly than any of the other options. When you see an option that appears or is stated with more complexity than the other options, as is option D compared to the others, it is best to ignore it.

Q126 — Pre-Study Suggestions

Review the following if needed:
1) Blood Pressure **BIO 7.4**
2) Complex Sounding Option(s) **SB A.2.2**
3) What information is needed from the passage?
4) Solve the problem.

Solution Discussion

The information from the passage is in the third paragraph (but none of this is absolutely needed to answer the question):

"The relaxing substance ... from the amino acid L-arginine."

"competitive inhibitors of ... L-NMMA is one such inhibitor."

Option A is incorrect. L-NMMA is not normally in the body, so this is incorrect. NE could play a role in blood pressure **(BIO 7.4)** (BP). But, the question asked 'normally determine', and an exogenous substance like L-NMMA would not normally determine the BP.

Option C is incorrect. The blood volume and amount of L-arginine could potentially affect the blood pressure. But, this is a Complex Sounding Option(s) **(SB A.2.2)**, because your Basic Knowledge (study, passage, general knowledge) **(SB A.2.2)** does not provide L-arginine as being a substance that 'normally' affects the BP. Blood

volume certainly normally affects BP though.

Option D is incorrect. The heart rate and the stroke volume determine the cardiac output. Since cardiac output helps determine the blood pressure, this is a viable answer. *See* the following discussion in option B.

Option B is correct. Blood pressure **(BIO 7.4)** is determined by the cardiac output and the resistance in the blood vessels. This relationship is the same as Ohm's law **(PHY 10.1)**:

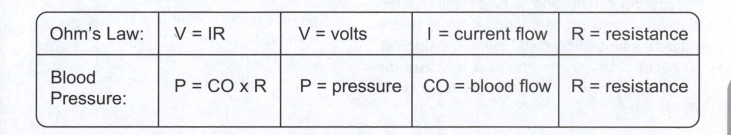

Ohm's Law:	$V = IR$	V = volts	I = current flow	R = resistance
Blood Pressure:	$P = CO \times R$	P = pressure	CO = blood flow	R = resistance

Test Taking Skills Comment

There is a Complex Sounding Option(s) **(SB A.2.2)** as discussed for option C. Similar Pair Options **(SB A.2.7)** is present but should not be used because there is more than one similar pair present - options A and C or B and D could be similar pairs.

Q127   Pre-Study Suggestions

Review the following if needed:
1) Blood Vessels **BIO 7.3**
2) What are the key pieces of information from the passage?
3) Solve the problem.

Solution Discussion

No specific information needed from the passage.

Vasoconstriction **(BIO 7.5, 11.2, 13.1)** means the constriction of blood vessels, the decrease in a cross-sectional area, and a decrease blood flow distal to the constriction. Vasoconstriction also increases resistance which will increase the blood pressure **(BIO 7.4)**.

Option A is incorrect. Vasodilation **(BIO 7.5, 11.2, 13.1)** causes the decrease in blood pressure associated with fainting.

Option B is incorrect. Vasodilation causes the increase in blood flow to muscles during exercise. Vasoconstriction decreases the flow.

Option D is correct. When blood vessels constrict, vasoconstriction, the blood pressure will increase and this is very important during hemorrhage.

Option C is incorrect. Vasodilation increases blood flow to the skin during blushing.

Test Taking Skills Comment

This is a Study Knowledge **(SB A.2.2)** question. You must know the previous concepts to answer the question.

Q128   Pre-Study Suggestions

Review the following if needed:
1) Similar Pair Options **SB A.2.7**
2) Three Out of Four Type Question **SB A.2.8**
3) What are the key pieces of information from the passage?
4) Solve the problem.

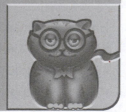

Solution Discussion

The information from the passage is found in the third paragraph:

"The relaxing substance was found ... the amino acid L-arginine."

"competitive inhibitors of ... L-NMMA is one such inhibitor."

should decrease the dilation of the vessel.

Option A is incorrect.

Option D is incorrect.

Option B is incorrect. The NO causes the vessel to dilate. The L-NMMA is an inhibitor of the enzyme which produces NO. This would mean NO would decrease and this

Option C is correct. Since L-NMMA blocks the enzyme producing NO, this would cause NO to decrease. This removes the stimulus for dilation, so the vessel should contract.

Test Taking Skills Comment

This is a Three Out of Four Type Question **(SB A.2.8)** with options B, C and D all relating to 'tension'. Option A is not related to tension and is an outlier - outliers are usually incorrect. This is also a reasonable Similar Pair Options **(SB A.2.7)** as options B and C both relate to a related effect (dilation/contraction).

Q129 — Pre-Study Suggestions

Review the following if needed:
1) Polarity **CHM 3.3**
2) Covalent Bonds **CHM 3.2**
3) Molecular Polarity **CHM 3.3**
4) Molecular Geometry **CHM 3.5**
5) Electronegative **CHM 3.3**
6) Vectors **PHY 1.1**
7) Three Out of Four Type Question **SB A.2.8**
8) Negative Question **SB A.1.2**
9) Solve the problem.

Solution Discussion

To determine whether a molecule is polar or not, you have to determine its hybrid orbitals **(ORG 1.2)** and then its molecular geometry **(CHM 3.5)**. Next you have to determine the polarity **(CHM 3.3)** of each bond and then use vectors **(PHY 1.1)** to determine the net polarity. All of the options shown are sp^3 hybridized (tetrahedral, 4 orbitals, 109.5 degrees) **(ORG 1.2)**.

Option B is incorrect. The hybridization on the carbon is sp^3, so the molecular geometry will be tetrahedral.

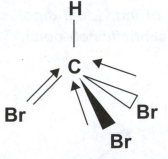

Directions of individual dipoles. The C-H bond is essentially non-polar.

The net dipole: this means this is a polar compound.

Option C is incorrect. The hybridization on the carbon is sp^3, so the molecular geometry will be tetrahedral.

Option D is incorrect. The hybridization on the carbon is sp^3, so the molecular geometry will be tetrahedral.

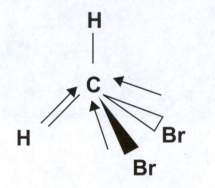

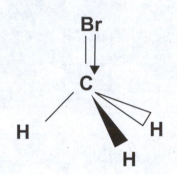

Directions of individual dipoles. The C-H bond is essentially non-polar.

Directions of individual dipoles. The C-H bond is essentially non-polar.

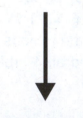

The net dipole: this means this is a polar compound.

The net dipole: this means this is a polar compound.

Option A is correct. The hybridization on the carbon is sp^3, so the molecular geometry will be tetrahedral.

$$Net = 0$$

There is no net dipole. This means this is a non-polar compound.

Br

C

Br   Br

Br

Directions of individual dipoles.

The polarity of the compound depends on the molecular geometry of the molecule and the vector summation of the vectors of the bonds. In this case, all of the bond dipole moments cancel out. The molecule has polar bonds, but is not a polar molecule. Note that you can show the dipoles from positive to negative - the result is the same.

Test Taking Skills Comment

This is a direct application of Study Knowledge **(SB A.2.2)**. Since all of a logical sequence is shown, it is not wise to try to apply various test taking skills e.g., if you tried to apply Three Out of Four Type Question **(SB A.2.8)** and select options B, C and D as the three because of the presence of H,

you would eliminate the correct answer. But, this is a Negative Question **(SB A.1.2)**. Remember that in negative questions, you have to be careful with the test skills. In particular, for three out of four and a negative question, the correct answer is often the outlier.

Q130   Pre-Study Suggestions

Review the following if needed:
1) Carbonyl Group **ORG 7.1**
2) Tautomerism **ORG 7.1**
3) Resonance in Organic Chemistry **ORG 1.4**
4) Oxidation Reduction Reactions **CHM 1.6, ORG 6.22, 8.2**
5) Mutarotation **BIO 12.3.2**
6) Solve the problem.

Solution Discussion

The compounds are:

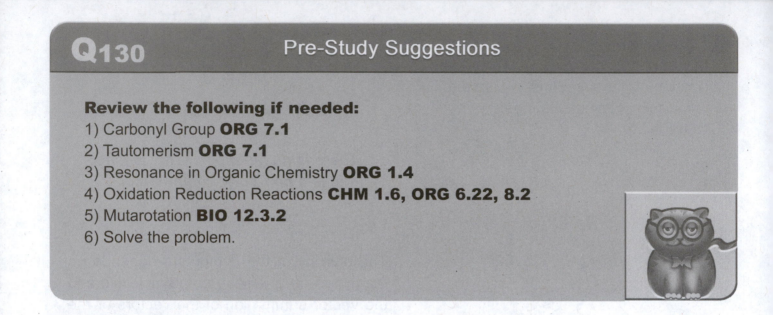

Compound 1   Compound 2

Option A is incorrect. In a reduction reaction **(CHM 1.6)**, there must be the gain of electrons by the molecule. This means the oxidation state **(CHM 1.6)** must become less positive or more negative or decrease. None of the atoms in these two compounds change their oxidation state. Then, this cannot be reduction. Also, if reduction occurs, oxidation must also occur.

Option B is incorrect. Resonance in organic chemistry **(ORG 1.4)** involves the attempt to correctly represent the electron distribution of a molecule with stick and dot methods. Only one molecule is involved. This means the same atoms are attached to the same atoms and have the same geometry. The H moves from the carbon to the oxygen between Compound 1 and Compound 2 - so this cannot be resonance as the two molecules are different. Also, since the MCAT is not trying to trick you, the equation shows an equilibrium and this is not how resonance is symbolized (resonance uses a double headed arrow).

Option D is incorrect. Mutarotation **(ORG 12.3.2)** is the conversion from one carbohydrate anomer **(ORG 12.3.2)** to another anomer.

Option C is correct. This is tautomerism **(ORG 7.1)**: the intramolecular shift of one atom between atoms in the same molecule. This is typical of aldehydes **(ORG 7)** and ketone **(ORG 7)**.

Test Taking Skills Comment

This is an application of Study Knowledge **(SB A.2.2)**.

Q131 — Pre-Study Suggestions

Review the following if needed:
1) Fungi **BIO 2.3**
2) Similar Pair Options **SB A.2.7**
3) Solve the problem.

Solution Discussion

Option A is incorrect. The spores are inactive and essentially gametes **(BIO 14.2)** and are haploid **(BIO 14.2)**.

Option D is incorrect. Part of the resistance to environmental conditions is the casing which is impermeable to the environment and is not the cell nucleus **(BIO 1.2)** membrane.

Option C is incorrect. The spores are very resistant to nearly all environmental conditions.

Option B is correct. The spores are essentially gametes, haploid, that are dormant until growth conditions are right.

Test Taking Skills Comment

This is Study Knowledge **(SB A.2.2)**. A Similar Pair Options **(SB A.2.7)** is present for options A and B which are very similar. Since there are no other similar pairs present, these would be a reasonable guess.

Q132   Pre-Study Suggestions

Review the following if needed:
1) Genetic Calculations **BIO 15.3**
2) Probability **BIO 15.3.1**
3) Similar Pair Options **SB A.2.7**
4) Solve the problem.

Solution Discussion

Assume H = normal gene (allele) and h = hemophilia allele.

The genotype of the father is h- since he is normal. He received the h, hemophilia gene, from his mother. His Y chromosome has no gene and is '-'. The mother must be Hh since she does not have hemophilia. She had to get the hemophilic h gene from her father

who was hemophilic (*see* X-linked traits; **BIO 15.3**). Since she does not have hemophilia, her mother's X chromosome gene was H, the normal gene. This means the gametes formed and their frequencies are:

Father (H-): H = ½   and   '-' = ½

but the son can only get the '-' and then the

probability of it is 1.0

Mother (Hh): H = ½ and   h = ½.

For a son to get hemophilia, he must get the '-', 1.0, from the father and the h, 0.5, from the mother with the following probability:

Probability of having one son with hemophilia: = ½ x 1.0 = ½.

The probability of three sons, since each are independent events **(BIO 15.3.1)** is:

½ x ½ x ½ = 1/8.

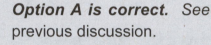

Options B, C and D are incorrect. *See* previous discussion.

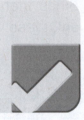

Option A is correct. See previous discussion.

Test Taking Skills Comment

Notice the little pitfalls if you do not think through the problem. Review the sections in genetic calculations **(BIO 15.3)** and probability **(BIO 15.3.1)** and especially independent events **(BIO 15.3.1)** carefully. This could be a soft Similar Pair Options **(SB A.2.7)** because options A and C both have fractions with 8 as the denominator - but this is risky but possible with number result options.

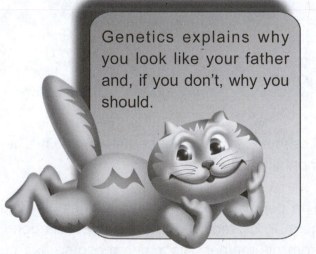

Genetics explains why you look like your father and, if you don't, why you should.

Q133 — Pre-Study Suggestions

Review the following if needed:
1) Immune Response **BIO 8**
2) Dichotomy of Options **SB A.2.3**
3) Complex Sounding Option(s) **SB A.2.2**
4) What information is needed from the passage?
5) Solve the problem.

Solution Discussion

The key information is:

Treatment 2:

"Administration of an antibody … protein complex on macrophages."

Figure 1:

This shows the endotoxin binding protein = 'endotoxin and binding protein complex' must attach to the macrophage to activate it for the shock cascade to occur.

tivation that leads to the problems. This should be blocked.

Option A is incorrect. It is the macrophage **(BIO 2.1, 5.4.1)** ac-

Option B is incorrect. There are no T cells, or T lymphocytes, **(BIO 8)** mentioned and since it is not in the passage nor does your Basic Knowledge (study, passage, general knowledge) **(SB A.2.2)** cover this aspect of T cells, there is no way to assess this option. Then

it is incorrect. This is a Complex Sounding Option(s) **(SB A.2.2)**.

Option C is incorrect. Same as option B for the T cells **(BIO 8)**. This is a Complex Sounding Option(s) **(SB A.2.2)**.

Option D is correct. This is directly from the Figure 1 and this will stop the cascade. It is the activation of the macrophage **(BIO 2.1, 5.4.1)** that lead to final pathway for the production of shock.

Test Taking Skills Comment

There are Complex Sounding Option(s) **(SB A.2.2)** as previously discussed. This is a Dichotomy of Options **(SB A.2.3)** question. You are given no information on T-cells and their role in shock in the passage and this is beyond basic knowledge. Therefore, they cannot be correct and you should eliminate options B and C. There is also the dichotomy of stimulate/inhibit. From the passage, you want to inhibit the pathway shown and should eliminate options A and B. As in all double dichotomies, when you select each one correctly, you have the correct answer which is D in this question.

Q134 — Pre-Study Suggestions

Review the following if needed:
1) Blood **BIO 7.5**
2) Blood Pressure **BIO 7.4**
3) Complex Sounding Option(s) **SB A.2.2**
4) What information is needed from the passage?
5) Solve the problem.

Solution Discussion

The information on treatment 1:

"Administration of a general anti-inflammatory ... infected with endotoxin."

The information in Figure 1 is also important.

Complex Sounding Option(s) **(SB A.2.2)** and is beyond your Basic Knowledge (study, passage, general knowledge) **(SB A.2.2)**.

Option B is incorrect. There is no information in the passage about the effect of anti-inflammatory drugs on the platelets **(BIO 7.5)** number; there is no basic information you are supposed to know about the effect of these drugs on platelets. So, there is no way for you to assess this option. This is a

Option C is incorrect. This is the same as option B but deals with red blood cells (RBC, erythrocytes) **(BIO 7.5)**. It is a Complex Sounding Option(s) **(SB A.2.2)** that cannot be answered with your Basic Knowledge (study, passage, general knowledge) **(SB A.2.2)**.

Option D is incorrect. This is the same as options B and C but deals with blood pressure **(BIO 7.4)**. It is a Complex Sounding Option(s) **(SB A.2.2)**.

Option A is correct. The Figure 1 shows that the white cells (WBC, leukocytes) **(BIO 8)**, are proliferated in the normal response. Although, some of this may add to the problems of septic shock, the white cells are also important in fighting the infection itself. So, if the drug knocks out the white cells (the inflammatory cell response) this could decrease the antibacterial activities, which can be dangerous.

Test Taking Skills Comment

There are several Complex Sounding Option(s) **(SB A.2.2)** options in this question. You must understand why option D is not a complex sounding option and why options A, B and C are. Review the previous discussions until you are certain about this point.

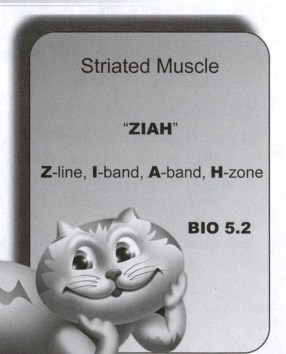

Striated Muscle

"**Z**IAH"

Z-line, **I**-band, **A**-band, **H**-zone

BIO 5.2

Q135 — Pre-Study Suggestions

Review the following if needed:
1) Temperature Regulation (Thermoregulation) **BIO 13.1**
2) Capillaries **BIO 7.5.2**
3) Muscle **BIO 5.2, 11.2**
4) Respiratory System (Pulmonary) **BIO 12**
5) Similar Pair Options **SB A.2.7**
6) Negative Question **SB A.1.2**
7) What are the key pieces of information from the passage?
8) Solve the problem.

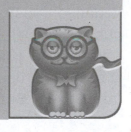

Solution Discussion

Option B is incorrect. Increased muscle activity, e.g. shivering, is a means to raise the body temperature. This would not be a mechanism to compensate for it.

Option D is incorrect. Fevers result in increased fluid losses not decreased fluid losses. Decreasing fluid loss would not lower the fever as for option C.

Option C is incorrect. Rapid breathing leads to loss of water as vapor and this would lower the temperature. So, slow breathing would result in the opposite effect desired.

Option A is correct. Vasodilation **(BIO 7.5, 11.2, 13.1)** of blood vessels results in increased loss of heat which would result in lowering of body temperature.

Test Taking Skills Comment

This is a Negative Question **(SB A.1.2)** which does not use 'NOT', 'EXCEPT', etc. The fever is the positive and the word 'compensation' is a negative of the fever. So, you would have to treat this question as a negative question when applying the various techniques. This is also a soft Similar Pair Options **(SB A.2.7)** as options C and D both have 'decrease' and you could guess from these. But, be careful with negative questions, because options A and B could also be considered, by stretching it, a similar pair (both are increasing something), and remember to never use similar pairs when more than one similar pair is evident. In this question, your guess would not be correct.

Q136 — Pre-Study Suggestions

Review the following if needed:
1) Cell Cycle **BIO 1.3**
2) DNA Duplication **BIO 1.2.2**
3) Three Out of Four Type Question **SB A.2.8**
4) What are the key pieces of information from the passage?
5) Solve the problem.

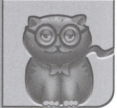

Solution Discussion

There is nothing from passage necessary to answer this question.

Option A is incorrect. The G_0 phase is a rest phase in which there is no cell division occurring.

Option D is incorrect. The G_2 is the short phase after duplication of DNA has occurred.

Option B is incorrect. The G_1 phase is the phase before duplication of the DNA occurs.

Option C is correct. The S phase is the phase of DNA duplication.

Test Taking Skills Comment

This is your Study Knowledge **(SB A.2.2)** at work. You could try to apply Three Out of Four Type Question **(SB A.2.8)** to this question, but remember when the options are a complete or logical sequence, it is best not to use it. All of the phases of the cell cycle **(BIO 1.3)** are listed. If you did not know better you would select options A, B and D as the 'three' because each has a 'G' and you would make your incorrect guess for this question from those three.

Q137 — Pre-Study Suggestions

Review the following if needed:
1) Acetoacetic Ester Synthesis **ORG 9.4**
2) Nomenclature **ORG 3.1, 6.1, 7.1, 8.1, 9.1-9.4, 11.1**
3) Similar Pair Options **SB A.2.7**
4) What information is needed from the passage?
5) Solve the problem.

Solution Discussion

The information needed is mainly the reaction sequence shown in Scheme 1 - refer to it if needed.

The acetoacetic ester synthesis **(ORG 9.4)** was specifically added in the 2003 revision of the MCAT. But, they still describe most of its features in the passage itself. You will probably be able to answer most of the questions about it from the passage information, but this will not always be a given. Yet, if you had studied the synthesis prior to the test, you would still be at an advantage.

The key here is that the reaction involves the addition of the alkyl halide **(ORG 3)** at the enol (enolate) **(ORG 7.1)** position of the acetoacetate molecule:

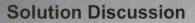

$$CH_3CO\text{-}CH_2\text{-}CO_2Et \rightarrow CH_3CO\text{-}CH^-\text{-}CO_2Et + H^+$$
Acetoacetate   Enolate ion

A base removes the hydrogen ion from the carbon shown resulting in an enolate **(ORG 7.1)** ion. The enol **(ORG 7.1)** is formed when the H shifts to one of the carbonyl **(ORG 7.1)** carbons, on the oxygen with a double bond to carbon (*see* the link for details), instead of being dissociated from the molecule.

The enol (enolate) **(ORG 7.1)** then displaces the halide from the alkyl group of the alkyl halide **(ORG 3)** substituting for it (an alkylation step). One or both of the hydrogens on the enolic carbon may be so substituted.

The compound desired (5) from Table 1 is 4-methyl-2-pentanone. Based on the rules of nomenclature (**ORG 3.1, 6.1, 7.1, 8.1, 9.1-9.4, 11.1**), this compound's structure is:

$$CH_3CH(CH_3)CH_2COCH_3$$

The #1 carbon is on the right side and #5 is on the far left. The O is bound to the #2 carbon and is a keto group. At carbon #4 is the methyl group. You should be able to go from the name of a compound to its structure and from its structure to its name.

The Scheme 1 shows the reaction of the malonic ester. The only difference for the aceto-acetate is that a ketone (**ORG 7**) group, instead of a carboxylic acid (**ORG 8**) group, remains (always one carboxylic acid group is lost as carbon dioxide). This means the R group of the added alkyl halide is everything except the methyl ketone and the enolic carbon of the acetoacetate:

$$CH_3CO-CH_2-CO_2Et \rightarrow CH_3CO-CH_2-R.$$

This means the alkyl halide must be the following from the structure of 5 from the table:

$$CH_3CH(CH_3)CH_2COCH_3 \rightarrow CH_3CH(CH_3) + {}^-CH_2COCH_3$$

Molecule #5 from Table 1   #A   #B

This is not a reaction; #5 is split apart for illustrative purposes. Molecule #A is the alkyl halide fragment. The angle line is where the halide was bonded and is where the bond forms with the enolate ion of acetoacetate. Fragment #B is the fragment that remains from the acetoacetate. The horizontal dashed line is where the enolate ion displaces the halide.

This means the original alkyl halide was:

$$CH_3CHX(CH_3).$$

From the sections on nomenclature (**ORG 3.1, 6.1, 7.1, 8.1, 9.1-9.4, 11.1**), specifically the section on branched alkyl groups (iso-, sec- and tertiary) (**ORG 3.1**), the alkyl halide would be an isopropyl halide.

Options A, B and C are incorrect. See the previous analysis.

CHAPTER 6

Option D is correct. See the previous analysis.

Test Taking Skills Comment

This is a Basic Knowledge (study, passage, general knowledge) **(SB A.2.2)** which can be determined using the passage but also from your study because you were required to know this reaction. Knowing the information from your study would make the question easier to do. This is not a good Similar Pair Options **(SB A.2.7)** because there is more than one set of similar options - C and D are similar and A and C are similar.

Q138 — Pre-Study Suggestions

Review the following if needed:
1) Carboxylic Acid **ORG 8**
2) Saponification **ORG 9.4.1**
3) Three Out of Four Type Question **SB A.2.8**
4) Similar Pair Options **SB A.2.7**
5) What are the key pieces of information from the passage?
6) Solve the problem.

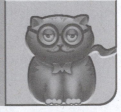

Solution Discussion

The information from the passage is not critical but is found in the first paragraph:

"The starting ester is alkylated, saponified, acidified, and pyrolyzed"

Saponification **(ORG 9.4.1)** is the process of treating an ester with a base and converting it to a salt of the acid. Acidification would then convert the salt to the acid form.

Option B is incorrect. An acid added to an acid will not result in a salt. Nothing may happen. To convert an acid to a salt **(CHM 6.7)**, a base is added to the acid.

Option D is incorrect. The reaction of an ester and acid results in the hydrolysis of the ester as discussed in option A.

Option A is incorrect. An ester is not the product of the saponification **(ORG 9.4.1)**. An ester **(ORG 9.4)** may be converted to a carboxylic acid **(ORG 8)** and an alcohol **(ORG 6)** by acid catalysis. So, the statement is True **(SB A.1.2)** but it is not Correct **(SB A.1.2)**.

Option C is correct. Saponification **(ORG 9.4.1)** and the subsequent acid hydrolysis are as previously discussed.

Biological Science Passage 4.BS.VII

Test Taking Skills Comment

This is a Three Out of Four Type Question **(SB A.2.8)** where options A, B and C all involve an acid. Option D is an outlier which does not involve an acid. Outliers are usually incorrect. Options B and C are a type of a Similar Pair Options **(SB A.2.7)** and would be an ok guess. But, remember when there is more than one similar pair, you have to be careful.

Q139 Pre-Study Suggestions

Review the following if needed:
1) Acetoacetic Ester Synthesis **ORG 9.4**
2) Similar Pair Options **SB A.2.7**
3) What information is needed from the passage?
4) Solve the problem.

Solution Discussion

The information from the passage is the Scheme 1. Please refer to it if needed.

The generalities and the specifics of the reaction were discussed in Q 137; please refer to it. The key to the structure shown is that the enolate carbon has two ethyl groups attached to it. This means there is double alkylation of the enol (enolate) **(ORG 7.1)**.

Option A is incorrect. The isobutyl iodide has the following structure:

$$CH_3CH_2CHICH_3$$

The general form of the product

formed from acetoacetate is:

$$CH_3COCH_2\text{-}R$$
(*see* the discussion in Scheme 1)

The product then would be:

$$CH_3$$
$$/$$
$$CH_3COCH_2\text{-}CH$$
$$\backslash$$
$$CH_2CH_3$$

Where the horizontal line is where the I was bonded.

Option B is incorrect. The structure of methyl iodide is CH_3I. When two alkylations result, two of these groups replace two of H's on the general form of the acetoacetate as found in option A. The product resulting would be:

$$CH_3$$
$$/$$
$$CH_3COCH$$
$$\backslash$$
$$CH_3$$

Option D is incorrect. The structure of isopropyl iodide is CH_3CHICH_3. The product formed by an alkylation is:

$$CH(CH_3)_2$$
$$/$$
$$CH_3COCH_2$$

It is not clear if the option wants to have a dialkylation; at any rate, the proper product is not formed either way.

Option C is correct. The structure of ethyl iodide is CH_3CH_2I. The product would be:

$$CH_2CH_3$$
$$/$$
$$CH_3COCH$$
$$\backslash$$
$$CH_2CH_3.$$

This is the product desired.

Biological Science Passage 4.BS.VII

Test Taking Skills Comment

This is a Similar Pair Options **(SB A.2.7)** question with options B and C being a similar pair. This is a reasonable guess.

Q140 Pre-Study Suggestions

Review the following if needed:
1) Inductive Effects **CHM 3.3**
2) Steric Strain **ORG 6.2.3**
3) Solubility of Organics **ORG 3.1.1, 6.1, 8.1, 9.4, 10.1, 11.1.2, 12.1.1**
4) Acid Strength **CHM 6.1 - 6.6**
5) Three or More Step Analysis **SB A.1.4**
6) Complex Sounding Option(s) **SB A.2.2**
7) Internally Inconsistent **SB A.2.5**
8) Similar Pair Options **SB A.2.7**
9) What information is needed from the passage?
10) Solve the problem.

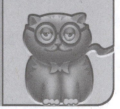

Solution Discussion

The key information is from the third paragraph:

"Acetoacetic ester may also ... butyllithium, respectively."

Option B is incorrect. This option is Internally Inconsistent **(SB A.2.5)**. First of all, the active hydrogen is less acidic. The addition of an alkyl group would decrease the acidity of the active hydrogen by increasing the electron density at the enolate carbon. This is the reverse of an inductive effect **(CHM 3.3)**. If the hydrogen was more acidic, a weaker base would be appropriate.

Option C is incorrect. This option is also Internally Inconsistent **(SB A.2.5)**. If the monoalkylated product increased steric strain **(ORG 6.2.3)**, then a smaller base would be more effective. Since the butyllithium is larger than the sodium hydride, this would not be the rea-

son for using the sequence described in the passage.

Option D is incorrect. This is also an Internally Inconsistent **(SB A.2.5)** option as a monoalkylated product should be less soluble in ethanol based on solubility of organics **(ORG 3.1.1, 6.1, 8.1, 9.4, 10.1, 11.1.2, 12.1.1)** (please refer to that discussion).

Option A is correct. When the first alkyl group is added, the active hydrogen remaining will be less acidic and will require a stronger base to remove it.

Test Taking Skills Comment

Each of the incorrect options has an element of Internal Inconsistency **(SB A.2.5)** as previously discussed. Options A and B constitute a reasonably Similar Pair Options **(SB A.2.7)** and would be a good guess.

Q141 Pre-Study Suggestions

Review the following if needed:
1) Respiratory System (Pulmonary) **BIO 12**
2) Mechanics of Breathing **BIO 12.4**
3) Membrane Transport **BIO 1.1**
4) Gas Exchange in Lungs **BIO 12.3**
4) Dichotomy of Options **SB A.2.3**
5) Solve the problem.

Solution Discussion

Option A is incorrect. The simple diffusion **(BIO 1.1.1)** of the gases is the mechanism of transport across the capillaries **(BIO 7.5.2)** and the linings of the lungs. *See* gas exchange in lungs **(BIO 12.3)**.

Option B is incorrect. There is no active transport **(BIO 1.1.2)** of gases in the lung. *See* gas exchange in lungs **(BIO 12.3)**.

Option C is incorrect. The deflation of the lungs, expiration (*see* mechanics of breathing; **BIO 12.4**) occurs under positive pressure.

Option D is correct. When the chest wall is expanded by muscular action, a vacuum is created in the pleural space. This creates a nega- tive pressure that inflates the lungs - *see* mechanics of breathing **(BIO 12.4)**.

Test Taking Skills Comment

This is a dichotomy of options **(SB A.2.3)**. Options A and B should be eliminated as they do not relate to mechanics of breathing **(BIO 12.4)** but relate to gas exchange in lungs **(BIO 12.3)** which are different but related functions of the respiratory system (pulmonary) **(BIO 12)**.

Q142   Pre-Study Suggestions

Review the following if needed:
1) Bacteria **BIO 2.2**
2) Virus **BIO 2.1**
3) Prokaryotic **BIO 2.2**
4) Eukaryotic **BIO 1**
5) Similar Pair Options **SB A.2.7**
6) Best Option **SB A.1.2**
7) Solve the problem.

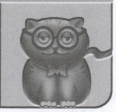

Solution Discussion

Option B is incorrect. This is generally true as most bacteria **(BIO 2.2)** have rigid cell walls and viruses **(BIO 2.1)** do not. There are some bacteria that do not have cell walls. This could be an answer unless there is a better one.

Option C is incorrect. Neither bacteria nor viruses have nuclear membranes. Bacteria **(BIO 2.2)** are prokaryotic **(BIO 2.2)**. Viruses have an outer protein covering/coat.

Option D is incorrect. Either bacteria or viruses could contain RNA and protein.

Option A is correct. Viruses do not reproduce by fission and bacteria may do so. This is the Best Option **(SB A.1.2)** although option A would reliably differentiate between a virus and bacterium if present.

Test Taking Skills Comment

This could be a Similar Pair Options **(SB A.2.7)** as options B and C both relate to membranes/coverings. But a guess is a guess and will be incorrect at times. On the average, the test taking techniques will help you guess correctly more often than not. This is a Best Option **(SB A.1.2)** question as previously discussed.

Q143   Pre-Study Suggestions

Review the following if needed:
1) Hormones **BIO 6.3**
2) Renal System **BIO 10.3**
3) Excretory System Homeostasis **BIO 10**
4) Aldosterone **BIO 6.3.2**
5) Internally Inconsistent **SB A.2.5**
6) Dichotomy of Options **SB A.2.3**
7) Three or More Step Analysis **SB A.1.4**
8) Solve the problem.

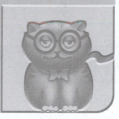

Solution Discussion

Option B is incorrect. Aldosterone **(BIO 6.3.2)** causes the kidney tubules **(BIO 10.2, 10.3)** to reabsorb sodium. With a load of sodium (as NaCl), this effect would not offset the extra load - in fact, it would make it a lot worse. This is Internally Inconsistent **(SB A.2.5)** based on your Study Knowledge **(SB A.2.2)**.

Option C is incorrect. This is also Internally Inconsistent **(SB A.2.5)**. If aldosterone **(BIO 6.3.2)** causes the excretion (secretion) of sodium, it would logically increase in the presence of excess sodium. This is how body systems work.

Option D is incorrect. Same as option B. Also, aldosterone does not cause secretion of sodium, so this is Internally Inconsistent **(SB A.2.5)** based on your Study Knowledge **(SB A.2.2)**.

Option A is correct. Aldosterone **(BIO 6.3.2)** is stimulated by low volume or low salt and is suppressed by the opposite states.

Test Taking Skills Comment

This is double Dichotomy of Options **(SB A.2.3)**. If you knew that aldosterone causes the reabsorption of sodium, then you eliminate options B and D. If you also knew that aldosterone was stimulated by low volumes or low sodium, then you would have eliminated options C and D. The only option left is A. The Internally Inconsistent **(SB A.2.5)** options are previously discussed. This is a Three or More Step Analysis **(SB A.1.4)** which makes it more difficult:

1) determine if 'yes' or 'no' is correct;
2) determine if the reason given is consistent with the yes/no;
3) determine if the option is True or False **(SB A.1.2)**; and,
4) determine if the option is Correct or Incorrect **(SB A.1.2)**.

Q144

Pre-Study Suggestions

Review the following if needed:
1) Virus **BIO 2.1**
2) DNA **BIO 1.2.2**
3) T Cells (T lymphocytes) **BIO 8**
4) Internally Inconsistent **SB A.2.5**
5) Similar Pair Options **SB A.2.7**
6) Complex Sounding Option(s) **SB A.2.2**
7) Solve the problem.

Solution Discussion

Option A is incorrect. This is a Complex Sounding Option(s) **(SB A.2.2)**. Even if there were enzymes present, which you do not have to know from Study Knowledge **(SB A.2.2)**, how would 'enzymes that destroy T cells' allow the virus to reproduce? There is no way to know this, and this is why this is complex sounding.

Option B is incorrect. This is Internally Inconsistent **(SB A.2.5)** as the Stem **(SB A.1.1)** states the virus is an RNA virus; where did the viral DNA come from? This option does not explain this fact.

Option C is incorrect. This is even more of a Complex Sounding Option(s) **(SB A.2.2)**. How are you to know that core proteins rather than DNA is present? You don't. Viruses **(BIO 2.1)** must contain RNA or DNA; this makes no sense and is Internally Inconsistent **(SB A.2.5)** because you are already told that this is an RNA virus and not a DNA virus.

Option D is correct. The reverse transcriptase is the enzyme found in retroviruses that converts their RNA into DNA to merge with the host DNA or use the host DNA machinery for making mRNA and proteins.

Test Taking Skills Comment

This question has Internally Inconsistent **(SB A.2.5)** and Complex Sounding Option(s) **(SB A.2.2)** answer choices as previously discussed. There is also a Similar Pair Options **(SB A.2.7)** in that options B and C both deal with 'DNA'. In this question, the technique does not work, but on the average, you will do better with the use of them.

Membrane Bound Organelles
(only in Eukaryotes)

- Nucleus: Cell's Architect = DNA

- Mitochondrion: Power House = ATP

- Lysosomes: Suicide Sacs = digestion

- Endoplasmic Reticulum: Synthesis Center = protein (rER)

- Golgi Apparatus: Export Department = protein to the PM

BIO 1.2.1

Q145 — Pre-Study Suggestions

Review the following if needed:

1) Menstrual Cycle **BIO 14.3**
2) Hypothalamus Hormones **BIO 6.1, 6.3.1**
3) Anterior Pituitary Hormones **BIO 6.3.1**
4) Adrenal Hormones **BIO 6.3.2**
5) Ovarian Hormones **BIO 14.3**
6) Thyroid Hormone **BIO 6.3.3**
7) Three Out of Four Type Question **SB A.2.8**
8) Similar Pair Options **SB A.2.7**
9) Solve the problem.

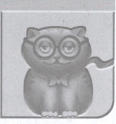

Solution Discussion

Option A is incorrect. The thyroid gland **(BIO 6.3.3)** is not involved in the menstrual cycle **(BIO 14.3)**.

Option C is incorrect. Same as option A.

Option D is incorrect. The adrenal hormones **(BIO 6.3.2)** are not involved in the menstrual cycle directly.

Option B is correct. The hypothalamus hormones **(BIO 6.1, 6.3.1)** (gonadotropic releasing hormones), the anterior pituitary hormones **(BIO 6.3.1)** (FSH and LH) and ovarian hormones **(BIO 14.3)** (estrogen and progesterone) are all related to the menstrual cycle.

Test Taking Skills Comment

This is a Three Out of Four Type Question **(SB A.2.8)** with B, C and D all having 'pituitary'. Option A is an outlier without pituitary - outliers are usually incorrect. A and B are an obvious Similar Pair Options **(SB A.2.7)**, but they are not part of the three out of four, and there is a second similar pair with options A and C (thyroid). Each of these observations makes the use of a similar part nonproductive.

Q146 — Pre-Study Suggestions

Review the following if needed:
1) Genetics **BIO 15**
2) Incompletely Dominant **BIO 15.1**
3) Gene Linkage **BIO 15.3**
4) Dihybrid Crosses **BIO 15.3**
5) Guess Question **SB A.2.4**
6) Solve the problem.

Solution Discussion

Assume the following:

R = red
W = white

where R and W are incompletely dominant **(BIO 15.1)**, and

L = long leaf
s = short leaf

where L is dominant to s.

The parents (P₁) were:

WWLL x RRss

The only gametes from these parents were:

WL xRs.

The F₁ must be WRLs.

Then the cross of F₁ would result in:

WRLs x WRLs.

The gametes of F₁ are:

WL, Ws, RL, Rs.

The Punnett Square will be:

	WL	Ws	RL	Rs
WL	WWLL	WWLs	WRLL	**WRLs**
Ws	WWLs	WWss	**WRLs**	WRss
RL	WRLL	**WRLs**	RRLL	RRLs
Rs	**WRLs**	**WRss**	RRLs	RRss

White long = WWLL, WWLs
White short = WWss
Red long = RRLL, RRLs
Red short = RRss
Pink long = WRLL, WRLs
Pink short = WRss.

This is very time consuming and would be the wrong way to do the problem unless you had a lot of time. You should be able to look at the gametes and determine the genotypes and phenotypes:

Gametes: WL, Ws, RL, Rs.

Since any gamete may combine with any other including itself, you can determine the possible combinations as shown beforehand. There would normally be four different phenotypes [for a dihybrid cross **(BIO 15.3)** with dominance and recessive relationship **(BIO 15.1, 15.3)** alleles]. But, the incompletely dominant **(BIO 15.1, 15.3)** alleles **(BIO 15.3)** increase this number by two.

Option D is correct. See the previous discussion.

Options A, B and C are incorrect. See previously.

Test Taking Skills Comment

This could be time consuming. You should eliminate options A and B because it should be clear you will have four or more phenotypes given the gametes for a dihybrid cross **(BIO 15.3)** with dominance and recessive relationships **(BIO 15.1, 15.3)** alleles **(BIO 15.3)**. This could be a Guess Question **(SB A.2.4)**.

Blood Types

"Type **O** is the universal d**O**n**O**r!"

Type A serum has anti-B antibodies (Abs); type B has anti-A; type O has both anti-A and anti-B; and type AB has neither Abs. Since there are no antigens on type O red blood cells, all blood types can receive a type O transfusion without having an Ab-Ag reaction (blood clumping, agglutination).

BIO 15.2